AF413048

The Elite Young Athlete

Medicine and Sport Science

Vol. 56

Series Editors

J. Borms Brussels
M. Hebbelinck Brussels
A.P. Hills Brisbane
T. Noakes Cape Town

The Elite Young Athlete

Volume Editors

N. Armstrong Exeter
A.M. McManus Hong Kong

19 figures and 22 tables, 2011

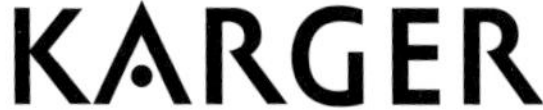

Basel · Freiburg · Paris · London · New York · Bangalore ·
Bangkok · Shanghai · Singapore · Tokyo · Sydney

Medicine and Sport Science

Founded 1968 by E. Jokl, Lexington, Ky.

Prof. Neil Armstrong
Northcote House
The Queen's Building
University of Exeter
Exeter EX4 4QJ (UK)

Dr. Alison M. McManus
Institute of Human Performance
University of Hong Kong
Hong Kong SAR (China)

This book was generously supported by **GATORADE**

Library of Congress Cataloging-in-Publication Data

The elite young athlete / volume editors, N. Armstrong, A.M. McManus.
    p. ; cm. -- (Medicine and sport science, ISSN 0254-5020 ; v. 56)
  Includes bibliographical references and indexes.
  ISBN 978-3-8055-9550-6 (hard cover : alk. paper) -- ISBN 978-3-8055-9551-3
(e-ISBN)
  1. Pediatric sports medicine. I. Armstrong, Neil. II. McManus, A. M.
(Alison M.) III. Series: Medicine and sport science ; v. 56. 0254-5020
  [DNLM: 1. Athletic Performance--physiology. 2. Adolescent. 3. Athletic
Injuries--prevention & control. 4. Child. 5. Nutritional Requirements. 6.
Risk Factors. W1 ME649Q v.56 2011 / QT 260]
  RC1218.C45E45 2011
  617.1'027--dc22
                                    2010041123

Contents

List of Contributors

Neil Armstrong
University of Exeter, UK

Alan R. Barker
University of Exeter, UK

Linda Cronin
Roehampton University, London, UK

Vincenzo Denaro
Campus Bio-Medico University, Rome, Italy

Bareket Falk
Brock University, St. Catharines, Ont., Canada

Raffy Dotan
Brock University, St. Catharines, Ont., Canada

Asker Jeukendrup
University of Birmingham, UK

Umile Guiseppe Longo
Campus Bio-Medico University, Rome, Italy

Nicola Maffulli
Barts and the London School of Medicine and Dentistry, UK

Nuno Matos
University of Exeter, UK

Alison M. McManus
University of Hong Kong, Hong Kong

Sébastien Ratel
Université Blaise Pascal, Clermont Ferrand, France

Thomas W. Rowland
Bay State Medical Centre, Springfield, Mass., USA

Filippo Spiezia
Campus Bio-Medico University, Rome, Italy

Richard J. Winsley
University of Exeter, UK

Craig A. Williams
University of Exeter, UK

Preface

Participation in sport is an important component of children's experience and sport provides a positive environment for the promotion of young people's health and well-being. Sport is by its nature competitive and even during youth it is performed at different levels with elite young athletes at the peak of the performance pyramid. Elite young athletes are those who have superior athletic talent, undergo specialised training, receive expert coaching and are exposed to early competition. Outstanding sport performances have been achieved by elite young athletes and many young people fulfil their potential, gain great pleasure from elite youth sport and are subsequently successful in sport during adulthood. Other similarly talented young people are denied access to elite youth sport through selection policies influenced by body size, stage of maturation or relative age. Others drop-out prematurely through early specialisation in a sport inappropriate for their late adolescent or adult physique. Elite young athletes undergoing intensive training programmes and high-frequency participation in sports competitions from an early age are associated with potential risk of abnormal development, injury or exceptionally sudden death.

Research in paediatric exercise science and medicine has increased dramatically over the last 25 years. Experimental techniques initially pioneered with adults and new non-invasive technologies have been successfully modified for use with children and adolescents. These developments have opened up new avenues of research into exercise performance during childhood and adolescence but data on elite young athletes are relatively sparse. Elite young athletes are therefore a special population worthy of further study.

This volume of *Medicine and Sport Science* is devoted to the elite young athlete and each comprehensively referenced chapter critically examines the extant literature and analyses what we know about factors underlying the performance of elite young athletes. Where data are not available on elite young athletes, the contributors extrapolate from research carried out with healthy young people or young adult athletes. All contributors are active researchers in the field covered by their chapter and, where appropriate, they draw upon their own research data to enrich the text and provide further insights into sport performance during youth.

In the opening two chapters Armstrong and McManus review the physiology of elite young male and female athletes and note that data on young female athletes are remarkably sparse compared with those on males. They use the extant literature and apply their own research to critically examine the hypothesis that in both sexes success in elite sport during childhood and adolescence is influenced by a range of age- and maturity- related physical and physiological variables. Jeukendrup and Cronin then discuss the essential role of nutrition in the health of young athletes and conclude that current sport nutrition knowledge is largely extrapolated from the adult population and that more specific research is needed to optimise nutrition practises with young athletes. They carefully compare and contrast paediatric and adult exercise metabolism and identify where elite young athletes might benefit from different nutritional advice to that given to elite adult athletes.

In order to enhance their performance elite young athletes, at different stages of maturation, either in teams or individually, engage in intensive training programmes which are often based on a limited scientific foundation. In the next chapter, Armstrong and Barker discuss data on the effects of endurance training on performance during childhood and adolescence. In the absence of secure data on elite young athletes, they analyse the outcomes of well-designed studies of healthy young people and present an evidence-based exercise training programme designed to enhance the aerobic fitness of young athletes. In the following chapter, Ratel focuses on high-intensity and high-resistance training during youth. He concludes that with expert guidance this training mode is a safe and effective means of developing muscle strength and power output and enhancing sport performance but he also highlights the potential risks of unsupervised training of this type. Next, Winsley and Matos review the phenomenon of overtraining, analyse the underlying traits and discuss the potential outcomes for overtrained young athletes. In the final chapter in this section, Barker and Armstrong emphasize the importance of monitoring the performance of elite young athletes. They critically examine field- and laboratory-based assessment of aerobic fitness and performance during maximal intensity exercise and discuss the issues underlying appropriate physiological support for elite young athletes.

Elite young athletes are currently required to compete in different environments and time zones but compared with the number involving adults well-designed studies relating to the preparation of young people for optimum performance are sparse. Falk and Dotan review the literature on thermoregulation and demonstrate that although adults and children employ different thermoregulatory strategies in dealing with heat stress young athletes are physiologically as capable as adults to handle these challenges. Williams addresses the potential effects of environmental stressors on the performance of young athletes and notes the paucity of research and the need for further experimental studies with this population. However, based on the extant data, he presents guidelines to aid young athletes' training and enhance their performance when challenged by unusual sleep patterns, jet lag, air pollution and altitude.

The final section of this volume addresses some of the risks associated with intensive training and performance during childhood and adolescence. Rowland reviews strategies for preventing sudden cardiac death during exercise and discusses the optimal content of pre-participation evaluations. He examines the aetiologies of sudden cardiac death in young athletes and debates the controversies surrounding the prevention of these tragedies. Engagement in several hours per week of strenuous exercise including competitive sport during growth and maturation inevitably increases the risk of injury. In the final chapter, Maffulli and his colleagues identify the aetiology of sport-specific injuries to the elite young athlete and overview the diagnosis and management of common sport injuries.

The editors acknowledge that within the space available herein it is not possible to address fully the science underpinning the performance of elite young athletes. The aim of this volume is therefore to reference what we know and do not know in key areas of the topic in order to inform and challenge sport scientists, coaches, medics and other professionals involved in supporting elite young athletes. If this volume of *Medicine and Sport Science* stimulates research programmes devoted to the promotion of both the performance and long-term health and well-being of elite young athletes, it will have served its purpose.

Neil Armstrong, Exeter
Alison M. McManus, Hong Kong

Chapter 1

Armstrong N, McManus AM (eds): The Elite Young Athlete.
Med Sport Sci. Basel, Karger, 2011, vol 56, pp 1–22

Physiology of Elite Young Male Athletes

Neil Armstrong[a] · Alison M. McManus[b]

[a]Children's Health and Exercise Research Centre, University of Exeter, Exeter, UK; [b]Institute of Human Performance,
University of Hong Kong, Hong Kong, SAR, China

Abstract

Performance in sport takes place within a matrix of bio-cultural characteristics but boys' success in elite youth sport is underpinned by a range of age- and maturity-related physical and physiological variables which act in a sport-specific manner to influence performance. Stature, body mass, and muscle mass increase with growth and maturation and earlier maturing boys are generally taller, heavier, and more muscular than boys of the same chronological age who mature later. Earlier maturing boys also benefit from changes in body shape which are advantageous in many sports. Marked increases in muscle strength and muscle power are expressed during adolescence. The muscle enzyme profile needed to promote the anaerobic generation of energy is enhanced as children move through adolescence into young adulthood. Aerobic fitness benefits from age and/or maturation-related increases in stroke volume, haemoglobin concentration, and muscle mass. These individual differences are most pronounced at 12–15 years when participation in elite youth sport is at its peak. Many boys fulfil their potential, gain great pleasure from elite youth sport and become elite adult sportsmen. Other equally talented boys are denied access to elite youth sport through selection policies which are influenced by stage of maturation or age relative to the beginning of the selection year. Others drop-out prematurely through early specialisation in a sport inappropriate for their late adolescent or adult physique. Boys are not mini-men and coaches and parents should focus on providing opportunities for all boys and on nurturing talent irrespective of the ticking of individual biological clocks.

Participation in organized, competitive sport often begins as early as 6–7 years of age. Indeed, a national newspaper recently reported that the English Premier League football clubs Newcastle United and Aston Villa had both signed 6 year-olds who, 'already had their sights on the national team'. By their teens some boys have experienced several years of intensive training and high-level competition. Over this period performance in sport progressively, but asynchronously, improves with age, growth, and maturation. This can be illustrated by perusing chronological age group world best athletic performances (fig. 1) and observing not only significant increases in performance with age but differing rates of improvement as boys move from childhood through adolescence into young adulthood.

Having the appropriate physical and physiological attributes is not, of course, the only significant factor in becoming an elite young athlete. Initial selection for, and retention in, elite sport takes place within a matrix of bio-cultural characteristics, which include health status, family size, parental support, socio-economic status, and psychological readiness. Well-designed exercise training and skills promotion programmes in relation to age, growth and maturation are vital ingredients of success in

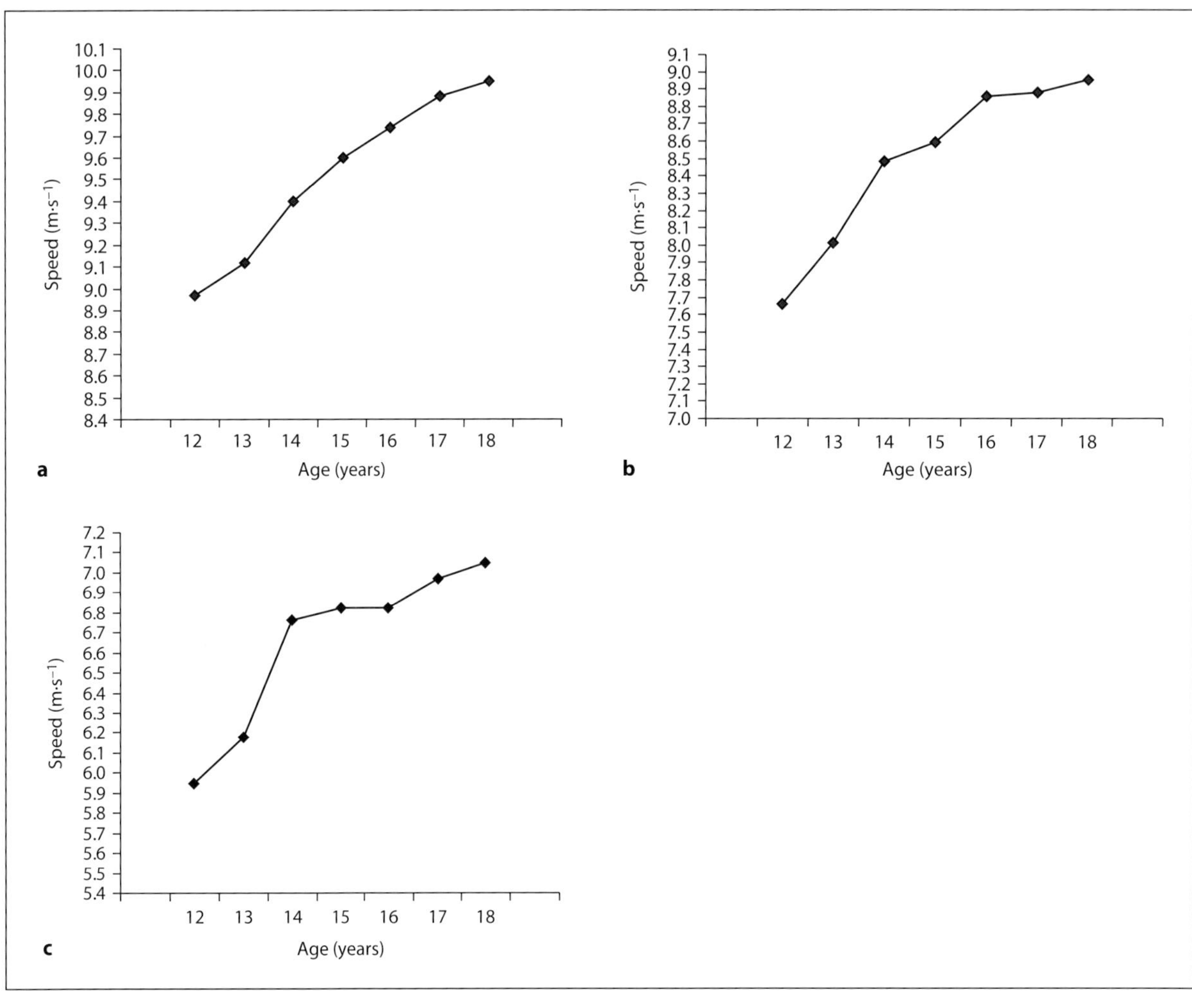

Fig. 1. Average speed of world best performances by age. **a** 100 m, **b** 400 m, **c** 1,500 m.

youth sport. However, successful performance in sport during childhood and adolescence is underpinned by a range of physical and physiological factors, such as body size, shape and composition, muscle strength, and aerobic and anaerobic exercise metabolism, which operate in a sport-specific manner. These variables will be the primary focus of this chapter.

Body Size, Shape and Composition

During the first 2 years of life body length increases by about 37–38 cm so that by age 2 years the child has attained approximately 50% of adult stature. Thereafter, all boys follow a similar pattern and, with the exception of the small mid-growth spurt between 6 and 8 years, there is a steady deceleration of growth to a rate of about 5–6 cm per year until the adolescent growth spurt. There are wide individual variations but, in developed countries, the onset of boys' adolescent growth spurt occurs between 10.3 and 12.1 years with peak height velocity (PHV) being reached between 13.4 and 14.4 years. During the growth spurt boys increase in stature by about 7 cm in the first year, 9 cm in the second year and 7 cm in the final year. The rate of growth decreases to 3 cm in the next year then to 2 cm per year until adult stature is attained at 18–20 years [1, 2].

Growth status (size attained at a given age) is monitored by making comparisons with reference percentiles where the 50th percentile represents the average size at any chronological age. Young male athletes in most sports (e.g. swimming, tennis, ice hockey, rowing) are generally taller than their non-athletic peers although in some sports there is variation by playing position (e.g. soccer, basketball). Gymnastics is the only youth sport that consistently presents a profile of stature below the 50th percentile but these data must be considered in the context of the selective criteria applied to this sport, including selection at an early age for small body size and physique characteristics associated with later maturation. There are no secure data to suggest that intensive training is a strong enough stimulus to influence attained stature or rate of growth in stature [3, 4].

Body mass triples during infancy and by the end of the second year it has quadrupled. From age 2 years, there is a slight but constantly accelerating rate of increase in mass prior to the adolescent growth spurt. The adolescent spurt in mass is similar to that of stature but normally occurs about 0.2–0.4 years later. The increase in boys' body mass is primarily due to gains in skeletal and muscle mass with a reduction in percentage body fat from about 16 to 12–14% of total body mass. Training, supplemented with calorie restriction in some sports such as wrestling, can influence relative fatness and young sportsmen tend to be thinner than their non-athletic peers. Body mass reflects a similar pattern to stature with young athletes in most sports being thinner but having body masses that equal or exceed the 50th percentile. Gymnasts and ballet dancers consistently present body masses below the 50th percentile but whereas gymnasts tend to have appropriate mass-for-stature ratios ballet dancers have low mass-for-stature ratios. Male swimmers, soccer players and tennis players were, in a longitudinal study, showed to be close to average for body mass until age 15 years with their body mass subsequently increasing to well above the 50th percentile between 15 and 19 years of age [4, 5].

Bone mineral density (BMD) progressively increases from birth through childhood and adolescence and into early adult life but adolescence is a very important period for the development of bone mass. Studies of boys have reported increases in BMD in the region of 5–70% of total adult value during adolescence although the magnitude of change varies according to skeletal site. Bone mass adapts to the mechanical strain placed upon it by skeletal loading by activating osteocytes which subsequently alter the delicate balance between bone resorption and bone formation. Changes in bone mass are localised to the induced strain and there may be net bone formation and net bone loss occurring simultaneously in different parts of the skeleton. Intermittent loading, high in magnitude and high in rate has been showed to produce a substantial osteogenic effect. Therefore, short bursts of explosive exercise are effective for bone development [6, 7].

The effect of intensive training and participation on BMD is sport-related. Racquet sport athletes and little league baseball players have been observed to have up to 20% higher BMD in their dominant arm than control subjects [8]. Swimming is not as beneficial to bone health as mass-supporting activities and BMD has consistently been reported to be higher in young gymnasts than in swimmers or control subjects [9, 10]. Soccer has been observed to promote bone health [11] and elite junior weight lifters have been reported to have 13–30% greater spine and femoral

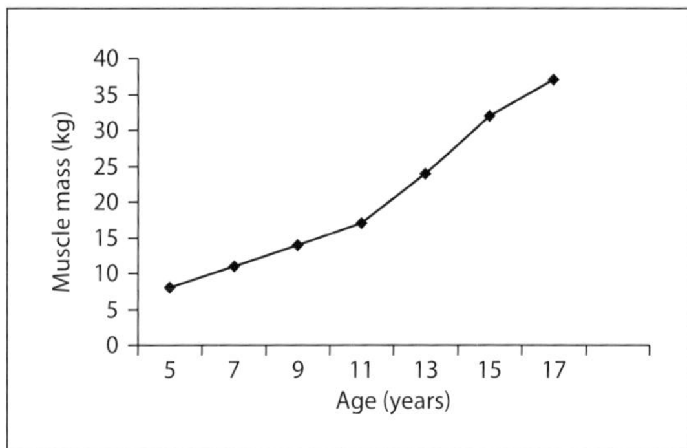

Fig. 2. Variation in muscle mass with age. Drawn from data in Malina et al. [5].

neck BMD than age-matched non-weightlifters [12]. It appears that the earlier a boy starts with appropriate exercise the more bone is accumulated. Increasing the amount of appropriate exercise during youth enhances bone accrual and promotes adult bone health through the achievement of a greater peak bone mass [6, 13].

Over the age range 7–17 years boys' percentage muscle mass has been estimated to increase from 42 to 54% of body mass with a marked spurt in muscle mass during adolescence [5], as illustrated in figure 2. Although growth hormone, somatomedins, insulin, and thyroid hormones are important regulators of muscle growth, the dramatic increase in testosterone during adolescence is the most crucial influence on muscle size [14]. The maximal force that can be generated by skeletal muscle is primarily a function of muscle size although during growth and maturation neurogenic factors, such as the ability to activate motor units, influence the relationship between muscle size and muscle strength. The expression of strength is also dependent upon lever ratios in the skeleton [15, 16]. Nevertheless, numerous longitudinal studies have demonstrated a significant relationship between muscle cross-sectional area and the development of strength [17, 18]. Peak muscle mass velocity (PMV) occurs several

months later than PHV and peak strength velocity lags behind PMV by 0.4 years such that marked sport-related advantages are not likely to become apparent until relatively late in adolescence [19, 20].

Physique is a significant contributor to success in several sports, particularly aesthetic activities such as gymnastics, diving, and figure skating where young competitors present similar somatotypes to elite adult performers. This suggests that boys may be selected for certain sports based on their physiques. There is less variation in somatotype among young sportsmen compared to the general population and in most youth sports mesomorphy is prominent, endomorphy is low and there is a large variation in ectomorphy. Exceptions are the higher weight categories in weight lifting and throwing events in track and field. Through increasing muscle mass and decreasing fat mass, it is conceivable that training may influence scores in mesomorphy and endomorphy but significant changes in somatotype through training remain to be proven [13, 21].

In summary, biological clocks run at different rates and earlier maturing boys enjoy changes in body size, body composition, and body shape that are advantageous in many sports. For example, at puberty boys experience an increase in limb length, a marked adolescent spurt in shoulder breadth, and an increase in muscle size which is reflected by a corresponding increase in strength. Even small differences in shoulder breadth can result in large differences in upper trunk muscle. When this is combined with the greater leverage of longer arms one of the reasons for earlier maturing boys' better performances than later maturing boys in throwing, rowing, and racquet sports becomes readily apparent. With few exceptions, elite male athletes in many youth sports are advanced in biological maturity status or at least average ('on time'). Other than gymnasts, few later maturing boys are successful in sport during early adolescence. However, later maturing boys are, if they retain interest in sport participation, often successful in some sports (e.g. track athletics) by the age of 16–18 years due to the reduced significance of maturity-associated variation in body size on performances at this time. There is no convincing evidence to suggest that the initiation of adolescence or the rate of boys' progress through adolescence is affected by intensive training or sport participation [3, 13].

Muscle Strength

Muscle strength is a complex construct which is recognised by Farpour-Lambert and Blimkie [22] as referring to the ability of muscles to exert force either for the purpose of resisting or moving external loads (including the body) or to propel objects (including one's own body) against gravity. Both alone and in combination with variables such as anaerobic and aerobic fitness, strength is an important determinant of success in sport, particularly during adolescence. Superior strength can act in a direct manner by providing the increased force necessary in many sports to differentiate the elite athlete from the less successful performer. It can also act permissively by providing increased joint stability and therefore minimizing the risk of musculoskeletal injuries and facilitating re-entry into sport after injury.

Muscle activation results in one of three types of muscle action namely, isometric, concentric, and eccentric. An isometric muscle action is where the intrinsic muscle tension matches the external resistance and although the muscle is in an active state there is no change in the external length of the muscle. Isometric muscle actions stabilize joints and are therefore important in sports such as gymnastics, wrestling, and golf. A concentric action is where the distance between the origin and insertion of muscle becomes shorter and the generated muscle tension is greater than the opposing resistance. Concentric muscle actions result in dynamic movement of parts of the body at constant (isokinetic) or variable velocity.

Concentric actions of variable velocity are more common in both sports and everyday life but the development of sophisticated dynamometers which can control velocity of action has increased interest in the measurement of isokinetic performance. Concentric actions such as knee extension during kicking a ball are fundamental to many sports. Eccentric muscle actions are where the intrinsic muscle tension is less than the external resistance, the muscle lengthens and the distance between limbs or the joint angular displacement increases. Eccentric muscle actions are common in sport and include running downhill and the dipping action at the knee in preparation for a jump shot in basketball [22].

Strength may be defined as, 'the maximal force, torque or moment developed by a muscle or muscle groups during one maximal voluntary or evoked action of unlimited duration, at a specified velocity of movement' [22, p. 38]. But, it should be noted that isometric, concentric and eccentric muscle actions provide measures of strength which reflect muscle activation under specific testing conditions of variable muscle length, joint position and/or movement velocity. Correlations between strength measures from different muscle actions and/or muscle groups may be low [23]. Nevertheless, regardless of muscle action and whether individual strength measurements or composite strength from several muscle groups are examined, data describing the development of strength during childhood and adolescence are consistent [16, 24].

In common with other performance measures, muscle strength is highly correlated with chronological age during childhood and adolescence. Strength increases in an almost linear manner from early childhood until about 13–14 years of age when there is a marked acceleration through the late teenage period. This is followed by a slower increase into the early or late 20s (fig. 3a). When related to the timing of the adolescent growth spurt, data are consistent and show that peak strength development occurs about 1.0–1.5

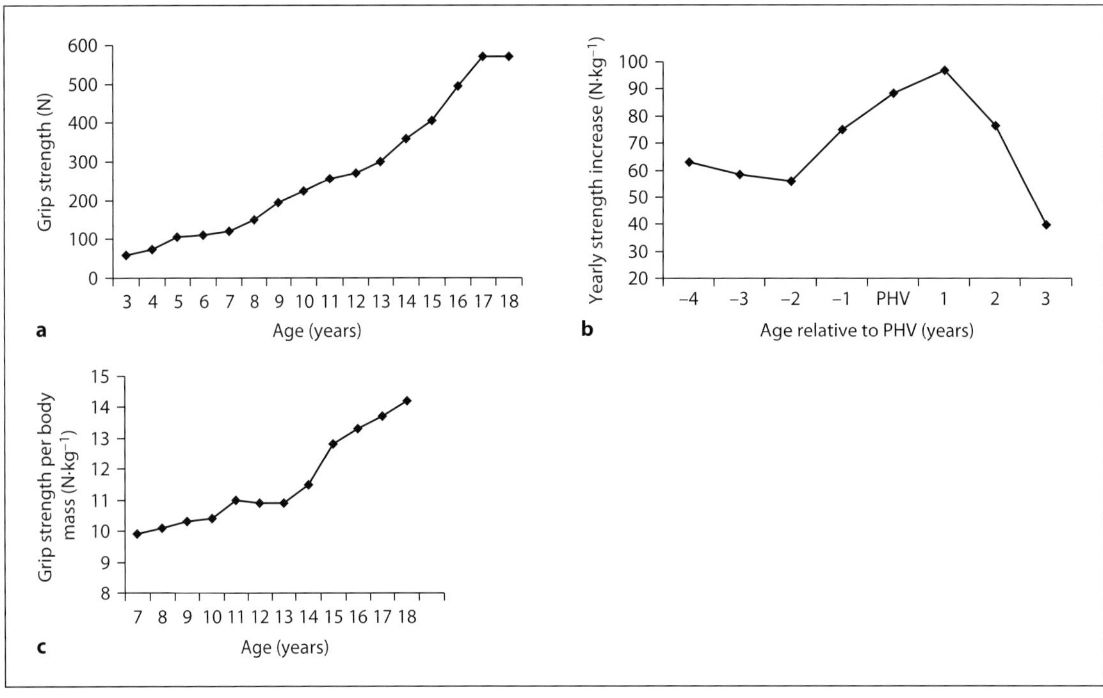

Fig. 3. Muscle strength in relation to age, peak height velocity, and age. **a** Grip strength in relation to age. Drawn from data in Blimkie [16]. **b** Upper body and lower body strength in relation to peak height velocity. Drawn from data in Carron and Bailey [25]. **c** Grip strength in relation to body mass. Drawn from data in Blimkie [16].

years after PHV (fig. 3b) and more in accord with PWV and PMV [24, 25].

Age-specific correlations between muscle strength and body mass tend to be low to moderate during childhood, then increase and peak during puberty before decreasing in the post-pubertal period. Correlations between strength and stature follow a similar pattern although they tend to be weaker than those observed between strength and body mass. The interpretation of physiological data in relation to body size is complex [26] but in the context of sport performance it is often informative to consider physiological variables in direct relationship with the body mass to be transported. Figure 3c illustrates how grip strength increases with age and demonstrates a marked pubertal spurt even when examined in relation to body mass. Similar results have been observed

for leg extension, elbow flexion, abdominal flexion and composite maximal voluntary strength in relation to body mass [16, 27].

The persistence of a pubertal spurt in muscle strength even after 'correcting' for body size indicates the importance of other variables in the development of strength. Perusal of figures 2 and 3a illustrates the similarity in the growth curves of muscle size and strength gain. Muscle cross-sectional area is strongly correlated with strength although there is still some debate about whether strength in relation to muscle cross-sectional area increases with age [20]. Changes in muscle pennation with increased muscle size during growth influences the expression of strength in relation to muscle cross-sectional area especially during adolescence but this has not been extensively addressed in young people [16, 20].

There is evidence that during isometric exercise 16-year-olds can voluntarily activate a greater percentage of knee extensor motor units than 11-year-olds [16]. Muscle fibres increase 4- to 5-fold in size from early childhood to adolescence, although the magnitude may vary between upper and lower limbs, reaching peak size during late adolescence or young adulthood [28]. Similarly, the percent distribution of type II fibres increases and attains adult values during late adolescence [29]. Although there are no data available on the relationship between muscle fibre type distribution, or fibre area and voluntary strength in children, type IIX and type IIA fibres in the quadriceps of adults have been showed to have respectively 10 and three times greater shortening velocity than type I fibres [30]. If this difference in magnitude of fibre type shortening speed is similar during adolescence it will enhance velocity-dependent strength performance of muscle composed of varying distributions of muscle fibre types and confer an advantage to more mature young people in sports demanding high speed strength and power activities (e.g. basketball, volleyball) [16].

In summary, earlier maturing boys have greater muscle mass and strength than their average and later maturing peers of the same chronological age, with the most marked differences occurring between 13 and 16 years of age. The advantages of greater muscle mass and strength are readily apparent in most youth sports.

Exercise Metabolism

Sport performances of varying intensities and durations are supported by different overlapping energy systems and the relative contribution of these systems is dependent on age and maturation. For example, a 100 m sprint is supported by the catabolism of phosphocreatine (PCr) and anaerobic glycolysis/glycogenolysis with only about 10% of the energy being provided by aerobic metabolism.

A 400-metre sprint is also predominantly dependent on the anaerobic energy systems but with 30–40% of energy being derived from aerobic sources. The 1,500 m is principally an aerobic event (>80% aerobic) although increases in pace (e.g. final sprint) have high anaerobic components. Understanding the development of exercise metabolism during childhood and adolescence can therefore provide valuable insights into potential sport performance.

At the onset of exercise, muscle contraction is supported by the energy released during the hydrolysis of adenosine triphosphate (ATP). The intramuscular stores of ATP are small and for maximal exercise to be sustained beyond 2 s ATP must be re-synthesized before total depletion. Anaerobic re-synthesis of ATP from PCr stores in the muscles occurs almost instantaneously once exercise commences but PCr is depleted rapidly during maximal exercise. PCr re-synthesis of ATP reaches its zenith within 2 s and declines thereafter so that during the last 10 s of a 30 s maximal sprint the contribution of PCr to ATP re-synthesis is only about 2% of that during the first 2 s. The anaerobic catabolism of glycogen/glucose to pyruvate is rapidly initiated and reaches its peak rate of ATP re-synthesis within 5 s. To sustain glycolysis, pyruvate is either reduced to lactate or oxidized in the tricarboxylic acid cycle to carbon dioxide and water. The rate of muscle lactate production during exercise is therefore dependent on the balance between anaerobic and aerobic metabolism of pyruvate. The greater the oxidation of pyruvate the less lactate produced. As relative exercise intensity increases muscle lactate production rises and some of the lactate diffuses out of the active muscle fibres and into the blood, where, in relation to exercise intensity, it provides a useful indicator of aerobic fitness.

The aerobic re-synthesis of ATP is relatively slow to adapt to the demands of exercise and, in children, the time constant of the response is about 20–25 s. The rate at which ATP can be re-synthesized aerobically in the mitochondria is much slower than that of anaerobic ATP re-synthesis but aerobic metabolism can use carbohydrates, lipids (i.e. free fatty acids, FFAs), and even amino acids as substrates, although protein catabolism contributes less than 5% of energy provision during exercise. Aerobic metabolism therefore has a much greater capacity for energy generation than anaerobic metabolism. Although it makes a relatively minor contribution during short-term, high intensity exercise the aerobic contribution to ATP re-synthesis progressively increases with time. In children, the aerobic contribution is dominant during exercise of longer than 1 min.

Substrate utilization during submaximal exercise is dependent on a number of factors including exercise duration, diet, level of training, and the relative intensity of the exercise. Muscle glycogen is the principal fuel during the early stages of sub-maximal exercise but as time progresses FFAs become the main energy source for exercise below the lactate threshold (T_{LAC}). If exercise intensity rises above the T_{LAC}, the contribution of FFAs falls and carbohydrates become the dominant energy source. The relative contribution to total energy derived from carbohydrates and lipids during sub-maximal, near steady-state exercise can be estimated from the respiratory exchange ratio (RER) measured at the mouth and computed using non-protein respiratory quotient values. Using this technique, studies have consistently reported significantly lower RER values (and therefore a higher FFA contribution to energy) in boys than men during exercise at both the same relative and absolute intensity [31]. More recent work using ^{13}C stable isotopes, as well as RER, has substantiated these findings [32]. According to Stephens et al. [33], the development of an adult fuel-utilization profile occurs sometime in the transition between mid-puberty and late-puberty and is complete on reaching full maturity. From an energy supply perspective, during sports involving long duration, low intensity exercise enhanced FFA consumption may compensate for reduced glycolytic capacity. Young people's lipid stores vary with maturation but it has been estimated that adults' lipid stores are sufficiently large to fuel 30 marathons.

Direct knowledge of boys' ATP, PCr and glycogen stores is limited to a series of muscle biopsy studies of 11- to 15-year-olds carried out in the 1970s by Eriksson and colleagues [34–37]. They reported resting ATP stores in the quadriceps femoris which were invariant with age at around 5 $mmol \cdot kg^{-1}$ wet weight of muscle and very similar to values others had recorded in adults. The concentration of ATP remained essentially unchanged following 6 min bouts of sub-maximal exercise but minor reductions were observed following maximal exercise. Eriksson and co-workers concluded that boys' PCr concentration at rest was similar to that of adults. However, closer scrutiny of the data reveals an age-dependency with reported PCr concentrations rising by 63% from 14.5 $mmol \cdot kg^{-1}$ wet weight of muscle at 11 years to near adult values of 23.6 $mmol \cdot kg^{-1}$ wet weight in the 15-year-olds. The PCr concentration gradually declined following exercise sessions of increasing intensity with values less than 5 $mmol \cdot kg^{-1}$ wet weight reported following maximal exercise. More recently, using the technique of magnetic resonance spectroscopy (MRS), Gariod et al. [38] corroborated the finding of Eriksson's group of invariant ATP concentration with age but in conflict reported strikingly similar PCr concentrations in children and adults.

Eriksson's group reported muscle glycogen concentrations at rest averaging 54 $mmol \cdot kg^{-1}$ wet weight of muscle at 11 years progressively increasing to 87 $mmol \cdot kg^{-1}$ wet weight at 15 years, which is comparable to values recorded in adults. Following exercise, a decrease was observed in all groups but the decrease was three times greater in the oldest compared to the youngest boys thus indicating enhanced glycogenolysis with age. The age-related increase in the glycolytic contribution to metabolism was reflected by reported muscle lactate concentrations of 8.8, 10.7, 11.3 and 15.5 $mmol \cdot kg^{-1}$ wet weight of muscle for boys aged 11.6, 12.6, 13.5 and 15.5 years, respectively [37].

Eriksson [35] reported levels of the enzymes succinate dehydrogenase (SDH) and phosphofructokinase (PFK) to be 20% higher and 50% lower, respectively, than the adult values his group had observed previously. This implies that children might have a low glycolytic and enhanced oxidative capacity during exercise. However, in a more recent investigation, Haralambie [39] observed no age-related change in PFK activity but reported a series of oxidative enzymes to be more active in adolescents than in adults. In a subsequent study, Berg and Keul [40] reported oxidative enzyme activity to be negatively correlated with age, thus substantiating Haralambie's observations. But, in accord with Eriksson they observed glycolytic enzymes to be positively correlated with age.

The work of Haralambie and Berg and Keul provides the opportunity to gain further insights into muscle metabolism through the exploration of ratios of specific glycolytic/oxidative enzyme activities. A re-calculation of Berg and Keul's data indicates pyruvate kinase/fumarase ratios of 3.585, 3.201 and 2.257 for adults, adolescents and children, respectively. In other words, the glycolytic/oxidative enzyme activity ratio was 59% higher in young adults than in children and 42% higher in adolescents than in children. Haralambie's data allow a comparison of the activity of the potential rate-limiting enzymes of glycolysis and the tricarboxylic acid cycle, namely, PFK and isocitrate dehydrogenase (ICDH). The ratio PFK/ICDH was 93% (and significantly) higher in adults than in adolescents at 1.633 and 0.844, respectively.

In summary, the weight of evidence suggests that children have lower glycolytic enzyme activity than adolescents but are able to oxidize pyruvate and FFAs at a higher rate than adolescents who have an enhanced aerobic capacity compared to adults. Boys therefore appear to be disadvantaged, compared to men and late adolescents, in sports involving short-duration, high intensity events fuelled by glycogenolysis/glycolysis. But, in terms of substrate utilization, they are well equipped for performance in long duration, low-to-moderate intensity sporting activities.

High Intensity Exercise

Short-Term Maximal Intensity Exercise

The ability to perform short-term maximal intensity exercise is fundamental to virtually all sports (e.g. football, rugby, hockey) but the difficulty of measuring physiological variables during non-steady state exercise and the ethical restrictions of involving children in investigations using invasive techniques has limited understanding of the mechanisms underpinning performance. Research has focused on tests which assess power output during maximal exercise and a plethora of tests involving jumping, running, and cycling have been developed. All performance tests have flaws but the data generated in relation to body size, age and maturation are generally consistent [41]. The '30 s all-out' Wingate anaerobic test (WAnT), which allows the determination of cycling peak power (CPP), usually over a 1-, 3- or 5-second period, and cycling mean power (CMP), over the 30-second test period, has emerged as the most popular test of young people's maximal intensity exercise. Data from variants of this test can be used to explore peak power output changes during growth and maturation.

The performance of maximal intensity exercise improves with age and, as illustrated in figure 4, there is a linear increase in CPP from age 7 until about 13 years when a second and steeper linear increase in CPP through to young adulthood is observed [42]. In a longitudinal study, Armstrong et al. [43] reported 12-year-olds to generate 45% of the CPP and 47% of the CMP they achieved at 17 years. Few data are available on maximal intensity exercise with the arms (e.g. as required in swimming) but they appear to follow the same

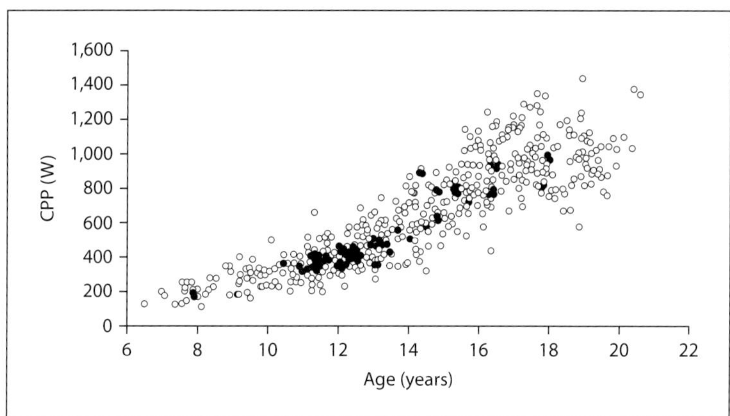

Fig. 4. Relationship between cycling peak power and age. From Van Praagh [42], by permission of *Human Kinetics*.

trend with the upper limbs generating 60–70% of the power of the legs [44].

A cross-sectional study of 12-year-olds reported earlier maturing boys to have greater CPP and CMP independent of differences in body mass [45]. When the same children were retested at ages 13 and 17 years a multi-level modelling analysis [26] revealed that the CPP and CMP increased by 121 and 113%, respectively, by age 17 years. However, once age, body mass and body composition had been controlled for maturation, as estimated from pubic hair development, did not exert an independent effect on either CPP or CMP [43]. Two other longitudinal studies by the same research group reported that even with age, body mass, and body composition statistically controlled for using multi-level modelling thigh muscle volume exerted an independent and positive effect on peak power output [46, 47].

The physiological mechanisms underlying the increase in CPP with age are complex. In addition to the biochemical issues underpinning the rapid re-synthesis of ATP and the variables outlined in earlier sections on muscle size, composition, contractile properties, and strength; factors such as the length-force, force-velocity, and power-velocity relationships of muscle must also be considered in the expression of power output [48].

Incremental Exercise to Exhaustion

Magnetic resonance spectroscopy (MRS) is a non-invasive technique that provides in real time and in vivo a window through which muscle can be interrogated during exercise. MRS studies are constrained by exercising within a small bore tube and the need to synchronize the acquisition of data with the rate of muscle contraction. This can be challenging with young participants but a recent study has demonstrated good test-re-test reliability with pre-pubertal children [49] and experiments using MRS are providing new insights into developmental muscle metabolism during incremental exercise to exhaustion [50].

The principal nucleus used in metabolic studies is the naturally occurring phosphorus nucleus, ^{31}P which enables the monitoring of the molecules that play a central role in exercise metabolism, namely, ATP, PCr, and inorganic phosphate (P_i). During an incremental exercise test to exhaustion, P_i increases with a corresponding decline in PCr. The expression of muscle P_i/PCr against power output provides an index of mitochondrial

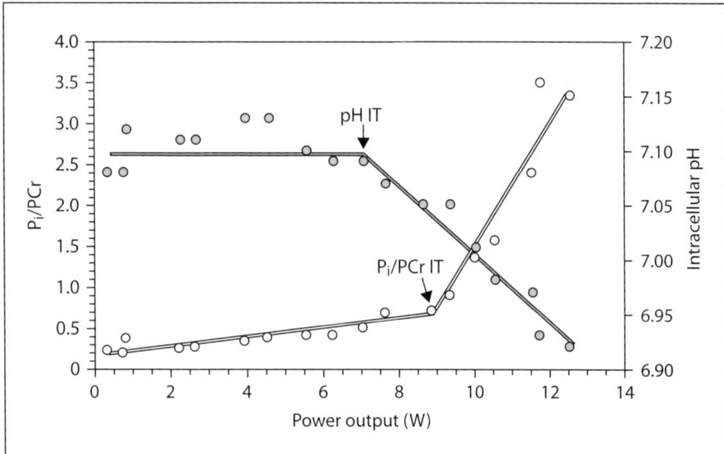

Fig. 5. P_i/PCr ratio and pH in relation to power output with intracellular thresholds indicated. From Armstrong and Fawkner [51], by permission of Oxford University Press.

function. That is, a muscle with a greater oxidative capacity will require a lower change in P_i/PCr for a given increment in power output. In addition, the chemical shift of the P_i spectral peak relative to the PCr peak reflects the acidification of the muscle and allows the determination of the intracellular pH. The change in pH during exercise provides an indication of muscle glycolytic activity but it is not a direct measure of glycolysis [50].

An incremental exercise test to exhaustion results in non-linear changes in the ratio P_i/PCr plotted against power output and in pH plotted against power output. As power output increases, an initial shallow slope is followed by a second steeper slope and the transition point is known as the intracellular threshold (fig. 5). The intracellular thresholds for muscle P_i/PCr ($IT_{Pi/PCr}$) and muscle pH (IT_{pH}) are valuable in vivo indicators of the oxidative capacity of muscle and have been showed to occur in children at relative power outputs similar to the T_{LAC} or ventilation threshold in whole body exercise [51].

Few ^{31}P-MRS studies have rigorously monitored children during incremental exercise but despite methodological differences the data are consistent [53–55]. During low to moderate intensity exercise (i.e. below $IT_{Pi/PCr}$ and IT_{pH}) no appreciable differences have been observed in the muscle phosphate and pH responses of boys compared to men. During quadriceps exercise, Barker et al. [55] normalized power output to quadriceps muscle mass and reported that the power output and energetic state at the intracellular thresholds were independent of age. However, during high intensity exercise (i.e. above $IT_{Pi/PCr}$ and IT_{pH}) age-related differences in the muscle phosphate and pH responses were apparent with men exhibiting a greater anaerobic contribution to exercise metabolism than boys. Taken collectively, these data indicate that the modulation of muscle metabolism during incremental exercise between boys and men is dependent on the intensity of the exercise. During low-to-moderate intensity exercise oxidative metabolism is not age-related but, during exercise above the $IT_{Pi/PCr}$, boys are characterized by a lower increase in P_i/PCr for a given increase in power output compared to men. The fall in pH for a given increase in power output following the IT_{pH} is lower in boys than in men. Maturational effects on incremental exercise metabolism have not been demonstrated in boys but earlier maturing girls have been showed to display pH dynamics that are akin to those of adult women [55].

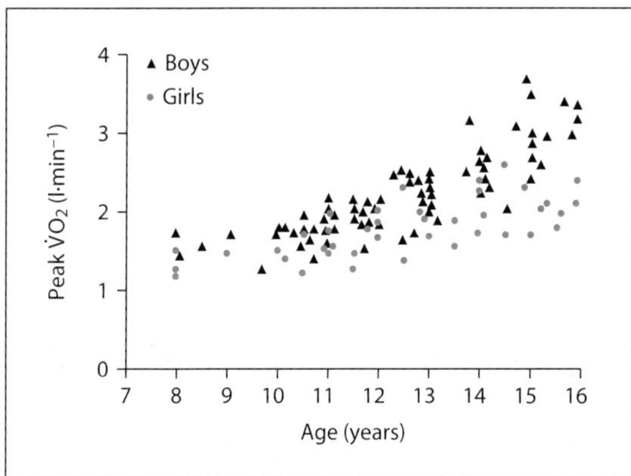

Fig. 6. Relationship between peak oxygen uptake and age. From Armstrong and Welsman [64], by permission of Williams & Wilkins.

In the only study to examine the muscle energetics of trained and untrained boys, Kuno et al. [54] noted no significant differences for muscle $PCr/(PCr+P_i)$ or pH at exhaustion between trained and untrained boys at 12, 13, 14 and 15 years of age.

In summary, the data underpinning performance in both short-tem maximal intensity exercise and high intensity incremental exercise to exhaustion support the view that exercise performance in these domains will improve with age, growth and maturation.

Aerobic Fitness

Aerobic fitness may be defined as the ability to deliver oxygen to the muscles and to utilize it to generate energy through aerobic metabolism to support muscle activity during exercise. Aerobic fitness therefore depends on the pulmonary, cardiovascular, and haematological components of oxygen delivery and the oxidative mechanisms of exercising muscle. Peak oxygen uptake (peak $\dot{V}O_2$), the highest rate at which a child or adolescent can consume oxygen during exercise, is recognized as the best single indicator of young people's aerobic fitness [56, 57].

Peak $\dot{V}O_2$ limits the rate of provision of aerobic energy during exercise and a high peak $\dot{V}O_2$ is a pre-requisite of elite performance in many sports (e.g. several events in athletics and swimming) but it does not describe fully all aspects of sport-related aerobic fitness. Peak $\dot{V}O_2$ is neither the best measure of a child's ability to sustain submaximal aerobic exercise nor the most sensitive means to detect improvements in aerobic fitness after a training programme. Despite its origins in anaerobic metabolism in the muscles, blood lactate accumulation is a valuable indicator of aerobic fitness and it can be used to monitor improvements in muscle oxidative capacity with exercise training in the absence of changes in peak $\dot{V}O_2$ [57, 58]. Furthermore, the requirements for success in sport depend as much on the ability to change rapidly the intensity of the exercise (e.g. soccer, rugby) as on the ability to achieve or maintain maximal aerobic performance for sustained periods. Under these circumstances it is the transient kinetics of $\dot{V}O_2$ which reflect the integrated response of the oxygen delivery system and the metabolic requirements of the exercising muscle [59].

Peak Oxygen Uptake

Cardiorespiratory components of young people's peak $\dot{V}O_2$ in relation to growth and maturation have been recently and comprehensively reviewed. The circulatory factors controlling and limiting responses to exercise are no different in child and adolescent athletes than in non-athletes and ventilation factors are not generally considered to limit exercise in young people despite recent concerns about exercise-induced arterial hypoxaemia [60–63].

The peak $\dot{V}O_2$ of children and adolescents has been extensively documented and figure 6 represents almost 5,000 treadmill-determined peak

$\dot{V}O_2$ scores of 8- to 16-year-olds. The figure must be interpreted cautiously, as the data points are reported means from studies with varying sample sizes, but it clearly illustrates an almost linear increase in boys' peak $\dot{V}O_2$ in relation to age. The regression equations generated by Armstrong and Welsman [64] indicate that boys' peak $\dot{V}O_2$ (litres $\bullet$ min^{-1}) increases by about 150% from 8 to 16 years.

The few longitudinal studies available reflect the cross-sectional data and indicate that the largest annual increases in peak $\dot{V}O_2$ occur between 13 and 15 years. It has been suggested that the greatest increase in peak $\dot{V}O_2$ accompanies the attainment of PHV but several studies have noted a consistent growth in peak $\dot{V}O_2$ from 3 years before to 2 years after PHV [60]. Comparative aerobic and anaerobic data are available in a single longitudinal study where the CPP, CMP, and peak $\dot{V}O_2$ of the same boys were determined at 12, 13 and 17 years [43]. CPP and CMP increased respectively by 121% and 113% whereas the corresponding increase in peak $\dot{V}O_2$ was somewhat less at 70% indicating a more marked increase in maximal anaerobic metabolism than aerobic metabolism as boys move from childhood into late adolescence. It is well-documented that elite young athletes in some sports (e.g. swimming, long and middle distance running) tend to have higher peak $\dot{V}O_2$ than athletes in other sports and non-athletes but whether this is due to selection or subsequent training is unknown [65, 66].

Peak $\dot{V}O_2$ is strongly correlated with body size and correlation coefficients describing its relationship with stature or body mass typically exceed 0.70. Conventionally, researchers have attempted to control for body mass by dividing peak $\dot{V}O_2$ by mass and expressing it as the simple ratio ml $\bullet$ kg^{-1} $\bullet$ min^{-1}. When peak $\dot{V}O_2$ is expressed in this manner a different picture emerges from that apparent when absolute values (litres $\bullet$ min^{-1}) are studied. Mass-related peak $\dot{V}O_2$ remains essentially unchanged (at about 48–50 ml $\bullet$ kg^{-1} $\bullet$ min^{-1}

in untrained boys) from 8 to 18 years. This interpretation is important in the context of sports in which body mass needs to be moved but it has clouded the physiological understanding of peak $\dot{V}O_2$ during growth and maturation.

Armstrong and Welsman [67] used multi-level modelling to analyze their longitudinal data set of 11- to 17-year-olds' peak $\dot{V}O_2$ and demonstrated a positive effect of age with body mass and stature controlled for. When stage of maturation (pubic hair development) was introduced to the model positive, incremental effects of stage of maturation on peak $\dot{V}O_2$ were demonstrated independent of age and body size. When skinfold thicknesses were introduced to the model, stage of maturation remained a significant covariate in all but stage 5 but the magnitudes of the effects were reduced, indicating the relationship between maturation and lean body mass. With body mass, skinfold thicknesses, and maturation accounted for peak $\dot{V}O_2$ was shown to still increase with age. In this analysis muscle mass was the predominant influence on the increase in peak $\dot{V}O_2$ through adolescence but both chronological age and stage of maturation were additional explanatory variables independent of body size and fatness. This conclusion is in accord with the observed differences in 11- and 17-year-olds' performance in sports dependent on aerobic fitness.

Blood Lactate

Lactate is continuously produced in skeletal muscle, even at rest but, with the onset of exercise, increases in glycolytic re-synthesis of ATP result in a correspondingly greater production of lactate in active muscle fibres. Lactate accumulates within the muscle and diffuses into the blood where, during sub-maximal exercise, it can be analyzed to provide an estimate of aerobic fitness. Lactate accumulation in blood is, however, a function of several dynamic processes including muscle production, muscle consumption, rate of diffusion

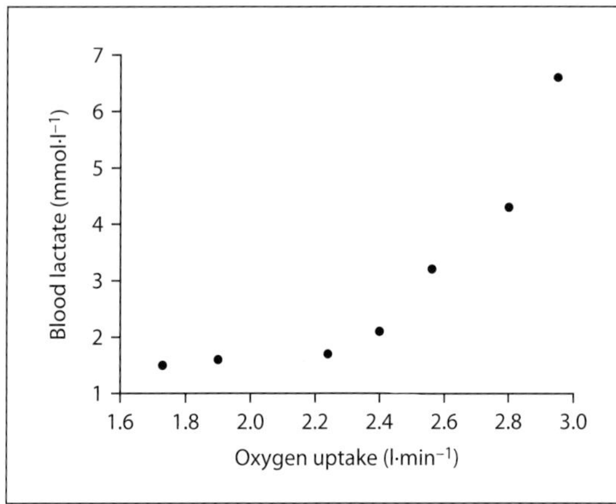

Fig. 7. Blood lactate response to exercise in relation to peak oxygen uptake.

into the blood and rate of removal from the blood. Lactate cannot be assumed to have a consistent or direct relationship with rates of either muscle lactate production or concentration.

Armstrong and Welsman [67] critically examined the analysis and assessment of young people's blood lactate accumulation during and following exercise. They demonstrated that measures of blood lactate concentration and the subsequent determination of lactate reference values, such as T_{LAC} (the first observable increase in lactate above resting levels during incremental exercise) and maximal lactate steady state (MLSS, the highest exercise intensity that can be sustained without incurring a progressive accumulation of blood lactate), must be interpreted with caution [57].

During a progressive, incremental exercise test lactate accumulates in the blood as illustrated in figure 7. In the early stages of the test there are typically minimal changes in lactate but as the test progresses a point is reached where lactate starts to accumulate rapidly with a steep rise to exhaustion. Following appropriate training, the curve is shifted to the right such that any given

exercise intensity is achieved with lower blood lactate.

Training-induced improvements in aerobic fitness result in lower blood lactate accumulation at all levels of sub-maximal exercise so any point on the lactate curve might be used to detect and monitor intra-individual improvements. However, in order to make comparisons among individuals or groups, reference values such as T_{LAC} are conventionally reported and monitored. Both T_{LAC} and MLSS can provide sensitive indicators of aerobic fitness and valuable markers of the transition from moderate to heavy and heavy to very heavy exercise respectively.

T_{LAC} in relation to peak $\dot{V}O_2$ is well-established as a measure of boys' aerobic fitness but MLSS has not been documented extensively with young people [57, 8]. Fixed reference values of lactate accumulation, such as 4 mmol•l⁻¹, have been proposed as reflecting MLSS and recommended for use with adults but they are not applicable to children where studies, using a plethora of methodologies, have reported mean values of MLSS ranging from 2.1 to 5.0 mmol•l⁻¹ [57]. T_{LAC} and MLSS are used routinely to monitor training programmes in sports such as swimming but to be effective tools they need to be individually determined and interpreted as there are wide inter-individual variations, particularly in young athletes.

Children accumulate less blood lactate than adults during both sub-maximal and maximal exercise and there is a negative correlation between T_{LAC} as a percentage of peak $\dot{V}O_2$ and age. Most studies have reported MLSS to occur at a lower concentration of blood lactate but at a higher percentage of peak $\dot{V}O_2$ in young people than in adults [57] but a recent study has suggested that the MLSS is independent of age [68]. Despite some indications that muscle [34] and blood [69] lactate responses are related to indices of maturation, the role of maturation in influencing blood lactate accumulation during exercise remains inconclusive [57].

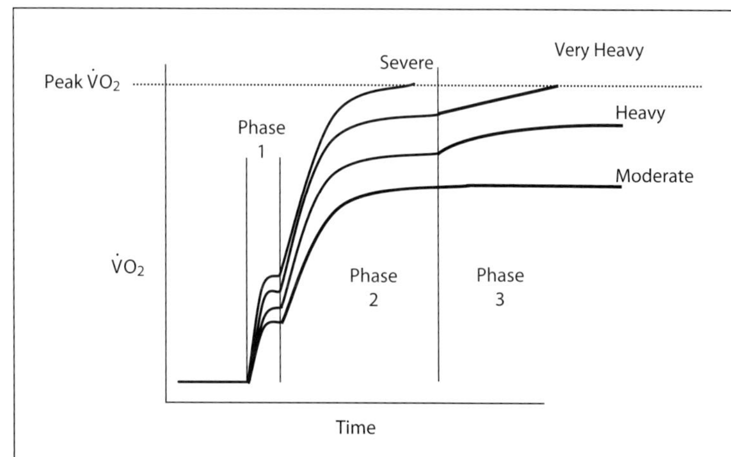

Fig. 8. Oxygen uptake kinetic response at the onset of constant intensity exercise with reference to exercise intensity domains. From Fawkner and Armstrong [71], by permission of Adis International.

Oxygen Uptake Kinetics

Oxygen uptake kinetics is important in all sports which require step changes in exercise intensity (e.g. changes of pace in soccer, rugby, tennis). In the laboratory $\dot{V}O_2$ kinetics is studied by the use of a step transition where a period of low intensity exercise, such as unloaded pedalling, is followed by a sudden increase in exercise intensity to a pre-determined level. The $\dot{V}O_2$ kinetics response to the step increase in exercise intensity is then interpreted in relation to four exercise domains, namely moderate, heavy, very heavy and severe intensity exercise. The upper threshold of moderate intensity exercise is the T_{LAC} which also acts as the lower threshold of the heavy exercise intensity domain. The MLSS or, more often in young people the critical power [70] serves as the upper marker of heavy exercise. Exercise above the MLSS or critical power but below peak $\dot{V}O_2$ falls into the very heavy exercise intensity domain. In the severe exercise intensity domain the projected $\dot{V}O_2$ is greater than peak $\dot{V}O_2$ and the $\dot{V}O_2$ kinetics response is terminated with the rapid achievement of peak $\dot{V}O_2$ (fig. 8). Rigorously determined data from children are only available for moderate and heavy intensity exercise [59, 71].

At the onset of a step transition in exercise there is an almost immediate increase in $\dot{V}O_2$ measured at the mouth. This cardiodynamic phase (phase 1), which lasts about 15 s in children, is closely associated with an increase in cardiac output which occurs prior to the arrival at the lungs of venous blood from the exercising muscles. Phase I is independent of muscle $\dot{V}O_2$ and is predominantly a result of the increase in pulmonary blood flow with exercise. Phase I is followed by an exponential increase in $\dot{V}O_2$ (phase II) that drives $\dot{V}O_2$ to the steady state value (phase III). Phase II (the primary component) arises with the arrival at the lungs of hypoxic and hypercapnic blood from the exercising muscles. Phase II kinetics are described by their time constant, which is the time taken to achieve 63% of the change in $\dot{V}O_2$, and they reflect, within about 10%, the kinetics of $\dot{V}O_2$ at the muscles. In phases I and II, ATP re-synthesis cannot be fully supported by oxidative phosphorylation and the additional energy requirements are met from oxygen stores, PCr, and glycolysis. The oxygen equivalent of these energy sources is known as the oxygen deficit and the faster the time constant the smaller the oxygen deficit.

During moderate intensity exercise, pulmonary $\dot{V}O_2$ reaches a steady state within about 2 min with an oxygen cost (gain) of about 10 ml $\cdot$ min^{-1} $\cdot$ W^{-1} above that found during unloaded pedalling. During heavy intensity exercise, the phase II gain is similar to that observed during moderate intensity exercise However, the oxygen cost increases over time as a slow component of $\dot{V}O_2$ is superimposed upon the primary component and the achievement of a steady state might be delayed by 10–15 min. The mechanisms underlying the slow component remain speculative but appear to be a function of muscle fibre distribution, motor unit recruitment and the matching of oxygen delivery to active muscle fibres [59, 71].

With step transitions to both moderate and heavy intensity exercise, children demonstrate a faster phase II time constant and a greater phase II oxygen gain than adults both of which indicate an enhanced capacity for oxidative phosphorylation in children [59, 72]. In addition, with a step transition to heavy intensity exercise Fawkner and Armstrong [73] observed, over 2 years, a slowing of the phase II time constant and a reduction in the phase II oxygen gain in boys who were prepubertal at the onset of the study. Furthermore, a slow component was observed on both test occasions, contributing about 10% of the final $\dot{V}O_2$ on the first occasion and about 15% of the final $\dot{V}O_2$ 2 years later. These findings, which have been replicated over an age range of 14–16 years by the same group [74], are consistent with the presence of an age-dependent influence on the muscles' potential for oxygen utilization although the independent effects of maturation on $\dot{V}O_2$ kinetic responses to moderate and heavy intensity exercise remain to be explored.

In adults, it has been demonstrated that with the implementation of appropriate modelling techniques, the phase II pulmonary $\dot{V}O_2$ response has a close relationship with PCr kinetics at the onset of exercise during knee extensor exercise in a MR scanner [75]. Children display a lower $\dot{V}O_2$ signal amplitude than adults, which makes a simultaneous assessment of $\dot{V}O_2$ and PCr kinetics in a MR scanner infeasible. However, it has been demonstrated that children's PCr kinetics during prone quadriceps exercise and $\dot{V}O_2$ kinetics during upright cycle ergometry are similar, at least during moderate intensity exercise [51].

To date, only two ^{31}P-MRS studies, from the same research group, have examined age-related differences in quadriceps muscle PCr kinetics during exercise and similar responses in boys and men have been reported for both moderate intensity [76] and heavy intensity [77] exercise. These results suggest that skeletal muscle metabolism is not related to age. However, it is worth noting that during heavy exercise 24–30% differences in the PCr time constants were reported between the boys and men which while not statistically different infer possible biological significance. Maturational differences in muscle metabolism during constant intensity exercise have not been investigated using ^{31}P-MRS.

In summary, age, growth and maturation each exert a positive and independent effect on aerobic fitness as reflected by peak $\dot{V}O_2$. Peak $\dot{V}O_2$ expressed in ratio with body mass (ml $\cdot$ kg^{-1} $\cdot$ min^{-1}) is remarkably consistent from 8 to 18 years of age, in this context younger boys might not be penalized in sports which involve the movement of body mass (but see the following section for comments on running economy in relation to age). Blood lactate accumulation during sub-maximal exercise increases with age and T_{LAC} occurs at a higher percentage of peak $\dot{V}O_2$ in boys than in men suggesting that boys are well-equipped for sports involving sustained sub-maximal exercise. Boys' faster $\dot{V}O_2$ kinetics during a step change to either moderate or heavy intensity exercise results in a lower oxygen deficit and indicates an enhanced potential for muscle oxygen utilization in young people.

Fatigue and Recovery from Exercise

There are no metabolic factors that limit the ability of children to perform low to moderate intensity ($<T_{LAC}$), continuous exercise for prolonged

periods of time and they can run at a slow speed for long periods [78]. However, the time an individual can maintain a given running speed above 80% of his maximal aerobic speed is correlated with age [79]. Children's performance in long duration sporting events which require intensities of exercise $>T_{LAC}$ therefore improves with age.

Children are less economical than adolescents and adults during walking and running. This reflects several age-related differences and Bar-Or and Rowland [80] have suggested that the most important are excessive co-contraction of antagonist muscle groups, a high stride frequency, and, in young children, an inconsistent stride-to-stride walking pattern reflecting their immature neuromotor control. In non-weight-bearing activities, such as swimming and cycling, there is evidence to suggest that children and adults have similar cardiovascular responses at the same relative exercise intensity [81, 82]. Nevertheless, children have a lower metabolic reserve than adolescents and Astrand [83] noted that an 8-year-old boy could increase his basal metabolic rate only 9.4 times during maximal running whereas a 17-year-old boy could attain 13.5 times his basal metabolic rate. Therefore, at the same absolute exercise intensity (or running or cycling speed) the child will be operating at a higher percentage of his maximal aerobic power and will fatigue earlier than adolescents and adults.

In an earlier section we showed that maximal intensity exercise performance improves with age but boys have consistently been found to fatigue less than men during successive bouts of high intensity exercise. Physiologic functions that return to resting values faster in boys than men include heart rate, $\dot{V}O_2$, carbon dioxide output, ventilation, plasma volume, blood lactate accumulation, and blood pH [80].

Ratel et al. [84, 85] carried out a series of studies of high intensity, intermittent exercise in which they demonstrated that short-term power output and/or running velocity is dependent on age, mode of exercise, and time allowed for recovery. During 10 maximal 10-second cycling sprints 10-year-old boys were able to sustain their CPP with 30 s recovery intervals whereas 15-year-old boys and 20-year-old men required a 5 min recovery period. When 11-year-old boys and 22-year-old men performed 10 consecutive maximal sprints with 15-second recovery intervals on both a cycle ergometer and a non-motorised treadmill, the men exhibited a significantly greater decrement in power output compared to the boys on both ergometers. In all exercise models the men experienced a greater increase in blood lactate accumulation and perceived exertion than the boys. Ratel et al. [86] concluded that the greater fatigue resistance in boys might be explained by lower neuromuscular activation, a higher percentage of type I muscle fibres, lower work rate in relation to lean leg volume during the earlier sprints, lower accumulation of blood lactate, and less depletion and faster re-synthesis of PCr via higher muscle oxidative activity.

The ability to recover faster from exercise is clearly of interest to those involved in elite youth sport, however, further research, using a range of exercise-recovery models and modes of exercise, is required to clearly map out the physiological mechanisms underlying recovery from intermittent high intensity exercise during growth and maturation. Recent work using ^{31}P-MRS has provided evidence of fatigue resistance through faster PCr re-synthesis, and therefore greater mitochondrial oxidative capacity, following maximal exercise in boys than in young men [87, 88].

Selection into Sports

Small body size can be advantageous in sports such as gymnastics and diving whereas a large body size is an asset in sports such as basketball, rugby, and swimming. Successful young athletes tend to reflect the morphological attributes of adults in the same sport but as morphologies are more dependent on genetic make-up than training [89], it appears that body size and physique play an important role in the initial selection into youth sport. As described in this chapter, body size, physique, and enhanced physiological endowments are strongly related to chronological age and biological maturation. Earlier maturing boys are generally large for their chronological age and benefit from enhanced physiological development therefore biological maturity can play an important role in the selection of youth sportsmen [90].

In addition to advanced biological maturity, chronological age relative to the selection year clearly influences the chances of being selected for elite age-grouped sports. Birth-date discrimination, a product of the time of year cut-off used by either the school system or sport leagues for class or competition grouping, is referred to as the 'relative age effect' and creates a marked advantage for those boys who are the oldest in their age group [91]. In the UK, the 1st September is the start of the school year and discrimination in selection by birth-date has been demonstrated in soccer, rugby and hockey with the older, Autumn-born boys over-represented in school teams compared to the younger Summer-born children [92]. This bias occurs regardless of the cut-off date for the season. For example, in the UK, Baxter-Jones and Helms [93] reported half of their sample of elite young tennis players and swimmers to be born in the first 3 months of a selection year beginning on 1st January. Similarly, in Canadian ice hockey 78% of the boys selected for elite junior squads were born in the first half of a selection year beginning in January [94].

Selection by chronological age relative to the selection year persists into adult elite sport and, perhaps, the most striking example can be found in football. Over a period of 6 years, 16–17 14-year-old boys were selected every year for the Football Association's School of Excellence. The birth distribution of the 103 boys selected revealed that 67% were born in the first quarter of the selection year, 89% in the first half of the year, and less than 2% in the last 3 months. The unequal distribution of birthdates persists into the senior game, in which almost 40% of English premier league footballers were born in the first quarter of the youth selection year. Similarly, those born in the early part of the selection year are over-represented in national teams (fig. 9). The residual birth-date bias seen in elite senior teams is likely to be the result of selection at a younger age. As successful youth players, those later picked for elite adult teams will have devoted more time to training, had a higher level of specialised coaching than their rejected peers, and will have become known to selectors of representative teams and professional clubs. Many talented boys are overlooked and subsequently drop-out of elite football simply because they are born late in the selection year.

Conclusions

Successful performance in sport during childhood and adolescence is dependent on a range of physical and physiological variables which are age-and maturation-related. Boys who mature earlier are generally taller, heavier and have higher mass-to-stature ratios than those who mature at a later age. The differences are most pronounced at 12–15 years when participation in elite youth sport is at its peak. In addition to greater body size, early maturing boys benefit from changes in body composition and shape that are advantageous in most popular youth sports. Marked increases in muscle strength and power are seen during adolescence. The muscle enzyme profile needed to optimally generate energy anaerobically to support high intensity exercise improves as children move through adolescence. Aerobic fitness (peak $\dot{V}O_2$) benefits from increases in muscle mass, stroke volume, and haemoglobin concentration. The greater strength, power, anaerobic and aerobic fitness

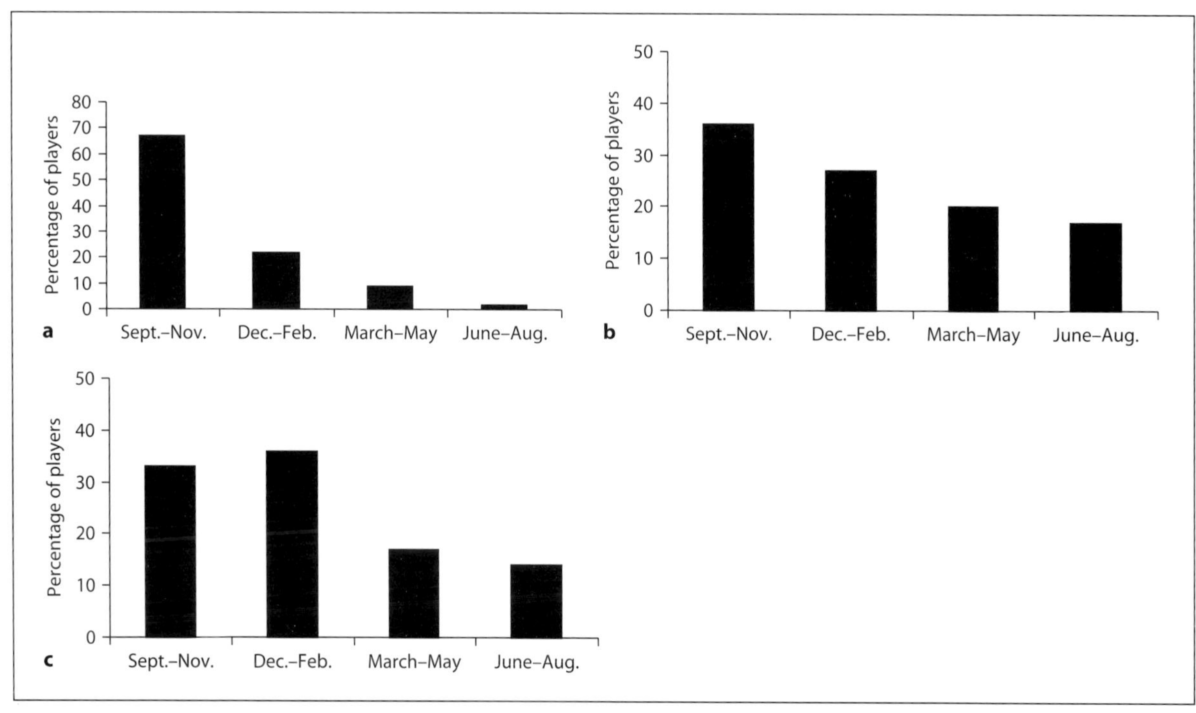

Fig. 9. Birth-date bias in English football. **a** Birth-date distribution of boys selected for the FA School of Excellence. **b** Birth-date distribution of English Premier League footballers. **c** Birth-date distribution of England World Cup squads.

of earlier maturing boys at the same chronological age as later maturing boys further enhances sport performance.

The limitations of using chronological age for grouping boys in sport has been recognized for over 100 years but although matching participants by body size/weight and/or biological maturity as well as by chronological age has been proposed implementation is confounded by methodological and ethical considerations [95].

Many young boys enjoy success and gain great pleasure from elite competitive sport, but other equally talented boys are denied access through selection policies which are influenced by stage of maturation and/or relative age effect. Others drop out of elite age-grouped sport prematurely through ill-advised early specialisation in sports which turn out to be inappropriate for their late-adolescent physiology, body size, composition or physique. Coaches and other adults who work with children should be aware of and alert to the effects of age, growth and maturation on sports performance and should focus on providing opportunities to foster participation for all boys and on nurturing talent irrespective of the ticking of individual biological clocks.

References

1 Baxter-Jones ADG: Growth and maturation; in Armstrong N, Van Mechelen W (eds): Paediatric Exercise Science and Medicine, ed 2. Oxford, Oxford University Press, 2008, pp 157–168.
2 Armstrong N, Welsman JR: Young People and Physical Activity. Oxford, Oxford University Press, 1997.
3 Malina RM: Physical growth and biological maturation of young athletes. Exerc Sport Sci Rev 1994;22:389–433.
4 Baxter-Jones ADG, Helms P, Maffulli N, Baines-Preece J, Preece M: Growth and development of male gymnasts, swimmers, soccer and tennis players: a longitudinal study. Ann Hum Biol 1995;22:381–394.
5 Malina RM, Bouchard C, Bar-Or O (eds): Growth, Maturation and Physical Activity, Champaign, Human Kinetics, 2004, pp 623–641.
6 Kemper HCG: Physical activity, physical fitness and bone health; in Armstrong N, Van Mechelen W (eds): Paediatric Exercise Science and Medicine, ed 2. Oxford, Oxford University Press, 2008, pp 365–374.
7 Kemper HCG: Skeletal development during childhood and adolescence and the effects of physical activity. Pediatr Exerc Sci 2000;12:198–216.
8 Watson R: Bone growth and physical activity in young males; in Mazess R (ed): International Conference on Bone Mineral Measurements. Washington, US Government Printing Office, 1974, pp 380–385.
9 Nichols JF, Spindler AA, La Fave KL, Sartoris DJ: A comparison of bone mineral density and hormone status of preadolescent gymnasts, swimmers and controls. Med Exerc Nutr Health 1995;4:101–106.
10 Grimston SK, Morrison K, Harder J, Hanley G: Mechanical loading regime and its relationship to bone mineral density in children. Med Sci Sports Exerc 1993;25:1203–1210.
11 McCulloch RG, Bailey DA, Whalen RL, Houston CS, Faulkner RA, Craven BR: Bone density and bone mineral content of adolescent soccer players, athletes and competitive swimmers. Pediatr Exerc Sci 1992;4:319–330.
12 Conroy BP, Kraemer WJ, Maresh CM, Fleck SJ, Stone MH, Frey AC: Bone mineral density in elite junior Olympic weightlifters. Med Sci Sports Exerc 1993;25:1103–1109.
13 Baxter-Jones ADG, Mundt CA : The young athlete; in Armstrong N (ed): Paediatric Exercise Physiology. 2006, pp 299–324.
14 Florini JR: Hormonal control of muscle growth. Muscle Nerve 1987;10:577–598.
15 Jones DA, Round JM: Muscle development during childhood and adolescence; in Hebestreit H, Bar-Or O (eds): The Young Athlete. Oxford, Blackwell, 2008, pp 18–26.
16 Blimkie CJR: Age- and sex-associated variation in strength during childhood: Anthropometric, morphologic, neurologic, biomechanical, endocrinologic, genetic, and physical activity correlates; in Gisolfi CV, Lamb DR (eds): Youth, Exercise, and Sport. Carmel, Benchmark Press, 1989, pp 99–161.
17 De Ste Croix MBA, Armstrong N, Welsman JR, Sharp P: Longitudinal changes in isokinetic leg strength in 10–14 year olds. Ann Hum Biol 2002;29:50–62.
18 Wood LE, Dixon S, Grant C, Armstrong N: Elbow flexion and extension strength relative to body size or muscle size in children. Med Sci Sports Exerc 2004;36:1977–1984.
19 Rasmussen B, Kaulsen K, Jespersen B, Jensen K: A longitudinal study of development in growth and maturation of 10- to 15-year old boys and girls; in Osied S, Carlsen HK (eds): Children and Exercise. Part XIII. Champaign, Human Kinetics, 1990, pp 103–111.
20 De Ste Croix MBA: Muscle strength; in Armstrong N, Van Mechelen W (eds): Paediatric Exercise Science and Medicine, ed 2. Oxford, Oxford University Press, 2008, pp 199–214.
21 Malina RM: Growth and maturation: do regular physical activity and training for sport have a significant influence? in Armstrong N, Van Mechelen W (eds): Paediatric Exercise Science and Medicine. Oxford, Oxford University Press, 2000, pp 95–106.
22 Farpour-Lambert NJ, Blimkie CJR: Muscle strength; in Armstrong N, Van Mechelen W (eds): Paediatric Exercise Science and Medicine, ed 2. Oxford, Oxford University Press, 2008, pp 37–53.
23 Asmussen E: Growth in muscular strength and power; in Rarick GL (ed): Physical Activity, Human Growth and Development. New York, Academic Press, 1973, pp 60–79.
24 Froberg K, Lammert O: Development of muscle strength during childhood; in Bar-Or O (ed): The Child and Adolescent Athlete. London, Blackwell, 1996, pp 25–41.
25 Carron AV, Bailey DA: Strength development in boys from 10 through 16 years. Monogr Soc Res Child Dev 1974;39:1–37.
26 Welsman JR, Armstrong N: Interpreting exercise performance data in relation to body size; in Armstrong N, Van Mechelen W (eds): Paediatric Exercise Science and Medicine, ed 2. Oxford, Oxford University Press, 2008, pp 13–22.
27 Blimkie CJR, Sale DG: Strength development and trainability during childhood; in Van Praagh E (ed): Pediatric Anaerobic Performance. Champaign, Human Kinetics, 1998, pp 193–224.
28 Oertel G: Morphometric analysis of normal skeletal muscles in infancy, childhood and adolescence: an autopsy study. J Neurol Sci 1988;88:303–313.
29 Jansson E: Age-related fiber type changes in human skeletal muscle; in Maughan RJ, Shirreffs S (eds): Biochemistry of Exercise. Part XI. Champaign, Human Kinetics, 1996, pp 297–307.
30 Larssson L, Moss RL: Maximum velocity of shortening in relation to myosin isoform composition in single fibres from human skeletal muscles. J Physiol 1993;472:595–614.
31 Boisseau N, Delamarche P: Metabolic and hormonal responses to exercise in children and adolescents. Sports Med 2000;30:405–422.
32 Timmons BW, Bar-Or O, Riddell MC: Oxidation rate of exogenous carbohydrate during exercise is higher in boys than men. J Appl Physiol 2003;94:278–284.

33 Stephens BR, Cole AS, Mahon AD: The influence of biological maturation on fat and carbohydrate metabolism during exercise in males. Int J Sports Med 2006;16:166–179.

34 Erikksson BO, Karlsson J, Saltin B: Muscle metabolism during exercise in pubertal boys. Acta Paediatr Scand 1971;217:154–157.

35 Eriksson BO: Physical training, oxygen supply and muscle metabolism in 11–13 year-old boys. Acta Physiol Scand 1972;384(suppl):1–48.

36 Eriksson BO, Saltin B: Muscle metabolism during exercise in boys aged 11 to 16 years compared to adults. Acta Paediatr Belg 1974;28:257–265.

37 Eriksson BO: Muscle metabolism in children: a review. Acta Physiol Scand 1980;283:20–28.

38 Gariod L, Binzoni T, Ferretti G, Le Bas JF, Reutenauer H, Cerretelli P: Standardisation of 31 phosphorus nuclear magnetic resonance spectroscopy determinations of high energy phosphates in humans. Eur J Appl Physiol 1994;68:107–110.

39 Haralambie G: Enzyme activities in skeletal muscle of 13–15 year old adolescents. Bull Eur Phsiopath Resp 1982;18:65–74.

40 Berg A, Keul J: Biochemical changes during exercise in children; in Malina RM (ed): Young Athletes. Champaign, Human Kinetics, 1988, pp 61–78.

41 Armstrong N, Welsman JR, Williams CA: Maximal intensity exercise; in Armstrong N, Van Mechelen W (eds): Paediatric Exercise Science and Medicine, ed 2. Oxford, Oxford University Press, 2008, pp 55–66.

42 Van Praagh E: Development of anaerobic function during childhood and adolescence. Pediatr Exerc Sci 2000;12:150–173.

43 Armstrong N, Welsman JR, Chia MYH: Short term power output in relation to growth and maturation. Br J Sports Med 2001;35:118–124.

44 Williams CA: Maximal intensity exercise; in Armstrong N, Van Mechelen W (eds): Paediatric Exercise Science and Medicine, ed 2. Oxford, Oxford University Press, 2008, pp 227–241.

45 Armstrong N, Welsman JR, Kirby BJ: Performance on the Wingate anaerobic test and maturation. Pediatr Exerc Sci 1997;12:112–127.

46 De Ste Croix MBA, Armstrong N, Welsman JR, Sharp P: Longitudinal changes in isokinetic leg strength in 10–14-year-olds. Ann Hum Biol 2002;29:50–62.

47 Santos AMC, Armstrong N, De Ste Croix MBA, Sharp P, Welsman JR: Optimal peak power in relation to age, body size, gender and thigh muscle volume. Pediatr Exerc Sci 2003;15:406–418.

48 Sargeant AJ: Anaerobic performance; in Armstrong N, Van Mechelen W (eds): Paediatric Exercise Science and Medicine. Oxford, Oxford University Press, 2000, pp 143–151.

49 Barker AR, Welsman JR, Welford D, Fulford J, Williams CA, Armstrong N: Reliability of ^{31}P-magnetic resonance spectroscopy during an exhaustive incremental exercise in children. Eur J Appl Physiol 2006;98:556–565.

50 Barker AR, Armstrong N: Insights into developmental muscle metabolism through the use of ^{31}P-magnetic resonance spectroscopy: a review. Pediatr Exerc Sci 2010;22:350–368.

51 Armstrong N, Fawkner SG: Exercise metabolism; in Armstrong N, Van Mechelen W (eds): Paediatric Exercise Science and Medicine, ed 2. Oxford, Oxford University Press, 2008, pp 213–226.

52 Barker AR, Welsman JR, Fulford J, Welford D, Williams CA, Armstrong N: Muscle phosphocreatine and pulmonary oxygen uptake kinetics in children at the onset and offset of moderate intensity exercise. Eur J Appl Physiol 2008;102:727–738.

53 Zancanato S, Buchtal S, Barstow TJ, Cooper DM: ^{31}P-magnetic resonance spectroscopy of leg muscle metabolism during exercise in children and adults. J Appl Physiol 1993;74:2214–2221.

54 Kuno S, Takahashi H, Fujimoto K, Akima H, Miyamuru M, Nemoto I, Itai Y, Katsuta S: Muscle metabolism during exercise using phosphorus 31 nuclear magnetic resonance spectroscopy in adolescents. Eur J Appl Phsyiol 1995;70:301–304.

55 Barker AR, Welsman JR, Fulford J, Welford D, Armstrong N: Quadriceps muscle energetics during incremental exercise in children and adults. Med Sci Sports Exerc 2010;42:1303–1313.

56 Armstrong N, Welsman JR, Winsley RJ: Is peak $\dot{V}O_2$ a maximal index of children's aerobic fitness? Int J Sports Med 1996;17:356–359.

57 Armstrong N, Welsman JR: Aerobic fitness; in: Armstrong N, Van Mechelen W (eds): Paediatric Exercise Science and Medicine, ed 2. Oxford, Oxford University Press, 2008, pp 97–108.

58 Pfitzinger P, Freedson P: Blood lactate responses to exercise in children. 2. Lactate threshold. Pediatr Exerc Sci 1997;9:299–307.

59 Armstrong N, Barker AR: Oxygen uptake kinetics in children and adolescents: a review, Pediatr Exerc Sci 2009;21:130–147.

60 Armstrong N, McManus AM, Welsman JR: Aerobic fitness; in: Armstrong N, Van Mechelen W (eds): Paediatric Exercise Science and Medicine, ed 2. Oxford, Oxford University Press, 2008, pp 269–282.

61 Fawkner SG: Pulmonary function; in Armstrong N, Van Mechelen W (eds): Paediatric Exercise Science and Medicine, ed 2. Oxford, Oxford University Press, 2008, pp 244–253.

62 Rowland TW: Cardiovascular function; in Armstrong N, Van Mechelen W (eds): Paediatric Exercise Science and Medicine, ed 2. Oxford, Oxford University Press, 2008, pp 255–267.

63 Rowland TW: Cardiorespiratory responses during endurance exercise: Maturation and growth; in Hebestreit H, Bar-Or O (eds): The Young Athlete. Oxford, Blackwell, 2008, pp 39–49.

64 Armstrong N, Welsman JR: Assessment and interpretation of aerobic fitness in children and adolescents. Exerc Sports Sci Rev 1994;22:435–476.

65 Baxter-Jones A, Goldstein H, Helms P: The development of aerobic power in young athletes. J Appl Physiol 1993;75:1160–1167.

66 Armstrong N, Davies B: An ergometric analysis of age group swimmers. Br J Sports Med 1981;15:20–26.

67 Armstrong N, Welsman JR: Peak oxygen uptake in relation to growth and maturation in 11–17 year old humans. Eur J Appl Physiol 2001;85:546–551.

68 Behnke R, Heck H, Hebestreit H, Leithauser RM: Predicting maximal lactate steady state in children and adults. Pediatr Exerc Sci 2009;21:493–505.

69 Williams JR, Armstrong N: The influence of age and sexual maturation on children's blood lactate responses to exercise. Pediatr Exerc Sci 1991;3:111–120.

70 Fawkner SG, Armstrong N: Assessment of critical power in children. Pediatr Exerc Sci 2002;14:259–268.

71 Fawkner SG, Armstrong N: Oxygen uptake kinetic response to exercise in children. Sports Med 2003;33:651–669.

72 Barstow TJ, Schuermann B: $\dot{V}O_2$ kinetics effects of maturation and aging; in Jones AM, Poole DC (eds): Oxygen Uptake Kinetics in Sport, Exercise and Medicine. London, Routledge, 2004, pp 331–352.

73 Fawkner SG, Armstrong N: Longitudinal changes in the kinetic response to heavy intensity exercise. J Appl Physiol 2004;97:460–466.

74 Breese BC, Williams CA, Barker AR, Welsman JR, Fawkner SG, Armstrong N: Longitudinal changes in the oxygen uptake response to heavy intensity exercise in 14–16 year old boys. Pediatr Exerc Sci 2010;22:314–325.

75 Rossiter HB, Ward SA, Doyle VL, Howe FA, Griffiths JR, Whipp BJ: Inferences from pulmonary oxygen uptake with respect to intramuscular (phosphocreatine) kinetics during moderate exercise in humans. J Physiol (London) 1999;518:921–932.

76 Barker AR, Welsman JR, Fulford J, Welford D, Armstrong N: Muscle phosphocreatine kinetics in children and adults at the onset and offset of moderate-intensity exercise. J Appl Physiol 2008;105:446–456.

77 Willcocks RJ, Williams CA, Barker AR, Fulford J, Armstrong N: Age- and sex- related differences in muscle phosphocreatine and oxygenation kinetics during high-intensity exercise in adolescents and adults. NMR Biomed 2010;23:569–577.

78 Roberts WO: Can children and adolescents run marathons? Sports Med 2007;37:299–301.

79 Leger L: Aerobic performance; in Docherty D (ed). Measurement in Pediatric Exercise Science. Champaign, Human Kinetics, 1996, pp 183–223.

80 Bar-Or O, Rowland TW (eds): Pediatric Exercise Medicine. Champaign, Human Kinetics, 2004, pp 3–70.

81 Kjendlie PL, Ingjer F, Madsen O, Stallman RK, Stray-Gundersen J: Differences in the energy cost between children and adults during front crawl swimming. Eur J Appl Physiol 2004;91:473–480.

82 Rowland TW, Staab JS, Unnithan VB, Rambusch JM, Siconlfi SF: Mechanical efficiency during cycling in boys and men. Med Sci Sports Exerc 1990;40:282–287.

83 Astrand PO: Experimental Studies of Physical Working Capacity in Relation to Sex and Age. Copenhagen, Munksgaard. 1952.

84 Ratel S, Williams CA, Oliver J, Armstrong N: Effects of age and mode of exercise on power output profiles during repeated sprints. Eur J Appl Physiol 2004;92:204–210.

85 Ratel S, Williams CA, Oliver J, Armstrong N: Effects of age and recovery duration on performance during multiple treadmill sprints. Int J Sports Med 2006;27:1–8.

86 Ratel S, Duche P, Williams CA: Muscle fatigue during high intensity exercise in children. Sports Med 2006;36:1031–1065.

87 Taylor DJ, Kemp GJ, Thompson CH, Radda GK: Ageing: effects on oxidative function of skeletal muscle in vivo. Mol Cell Bio 1997;174:321–324.

88 Ratel S, Tonson A, Le Fur Y, Cozzone PJ, Bendahan D: Comparative analysis of skeletal muscle oxidative capacity in children and adults: a ^{31}P-MRS study. Appl Physiol Nutr Metab 2008;33:720–727.

89 Rankinen T, Bray M, Hagberg J, Peruse L, Roth S, Wolfarth B, Bouchard C: The human gene map for performance and health-related fitness phenotypes: the 2005 update. Med Sci Sports Exerc 2006;38:1863–1888.

90 Ericsson KA: Deliberate practice and the modifiability of body and mind: toward a science of the structure and acquisition of expert and elite performance. J Sport Psych 2007;38:4–34.

91 Musch J, Grondin S: Unequal competition as an impediment to personal development: A review of the relative age effect in sport. Dev Rev 2001;21:147–167.

92 Wilson G: The birth date effect in school sports teams. Eur J Phys Educ 1999;4:139–145.

93 Baxter-Jones ADG, Helms P: Born too late to win. Nature 1994;370:186.

94 Sherar L, Baxter-Jones ADG, Faulkner R, Russell K: Do physical maturity and birth date predict talent in male youth ice hockey players? J Sports Sci 2007;25:879–886.

95 Beunen G, Malina RM: Growth and biological maturation: relevance to athletic performance; in Hebestreit H, Bar-Or O (eds): The Young Athlete. Oxford, Blackwell, 2008, pp 3–17.

Prof. Neil Armstrong
Executive Suite, Northcote House, The Queen's Building, University of Exeter
Exeter EX4 4QJ (UK)
Tel. +44 1392 263006, Fax +44 1392 263008, E-Mail N. Armstrong@exeter.ac.uk

Chapter 2

Armstrong N, McManus AM (eds): The Elite Young Athlete.
Med Sport Sci. Basel, Karger, 2011, vol 56, pp 23–46

Physiology of Elite Young Female Athletes

Alison M. McManus[a] · Neil Armstrong[b]

[a]Institute of Human Performance, University of Hong Kong, Hong Kong, SAR, China; [b]Children's Health and Exercise Research Centre,
University of Exeter, Exeter, UK

Abstract

The participation of girls in elite sport has increased exponentially over the past 30 years. Despite these increases a
tradition for recruiting boys for exercise studies persists
and our knowledge of the physiologic response to exercise in girls remains limited. Girls' physiology varies with
age and maturation and is underpinned by a divergent hormonal milieu which begins early in foetal life. Sexual dimorphism underlies much of the physiologic response to exercise, and becomes most acute during adolescence when
boys become taller, heavier, less fat and are more muscular
than girls. Young girl athletes are not simply smaller, less
muscular boys. The widening sex disparity in responses to
exercise during puberty cannot always be accounted for
by size. The woeful number of studies on girls and our prior
inability to non-invasively study the complexity of the cellular metabolic response to exercise means an integrative
understanding of girls' physiological responses to exercise remains elusive. Success in elite sport requires intense
training, which for a long time was thought to cause disruption to normal growth and maturation. It would appear
that exercise training, without other predisposing factors,
is unlikely to cause aberrations to either growth or maturation. Nevertheless, there is clear evidence of a boundary
between healthy and unhealthy levels of exertion when
coupled with caloric limitation. Sports in which intense
training is combined with the need for leanness may predispose girls to increased risk of skeletal and reproductive
health problems, and ensuring risk is minimised should be
a priority.   Copyright © 2011 S. Karger AG, Basel

The young female athlete is unique. She stands
out from her peers, who show declining levels of
physical activity from early puberty [1]. In comparison to boys, she remains under-represented
in competitive sport [2]. This persists to Olympic
level competition with 1,704 fewer women competing at the 2008 Beijing Olympics than men [3].
Moreover, there are fewer scientific data on physiologic issues associated with exercise in girls than
in boys. Traditionally, boys have been recruited
for exercise studies and a search of key databases
shows that this persists with comparatively fewer
articles investigating physiologic responses to exercise in girls. This preference for recruiting boys reflects social constraints which can be traced back to
Victorian values surrounding women, exercise and
health [4]. Central to the issue of women's involvement in sport was biology, bolstered by the idea
that a woman's structural and functional ability
was unable to tolerate strenuous exercise, presenting considerable risk to her reproductive health.
Indeed, whether or not chronic training causes less
than optimal structural and functional alterations
in girls remains the topic of lively debate [5–8].

Sexual dimorphism does indeed underlie
much of the physiological response to acute and
chronic exercise, and although a myriad of factors have been shown to influence the development of sport performance [9], structural and
functional capacity represent a significant contribution to the gender differences notable. Figure 1

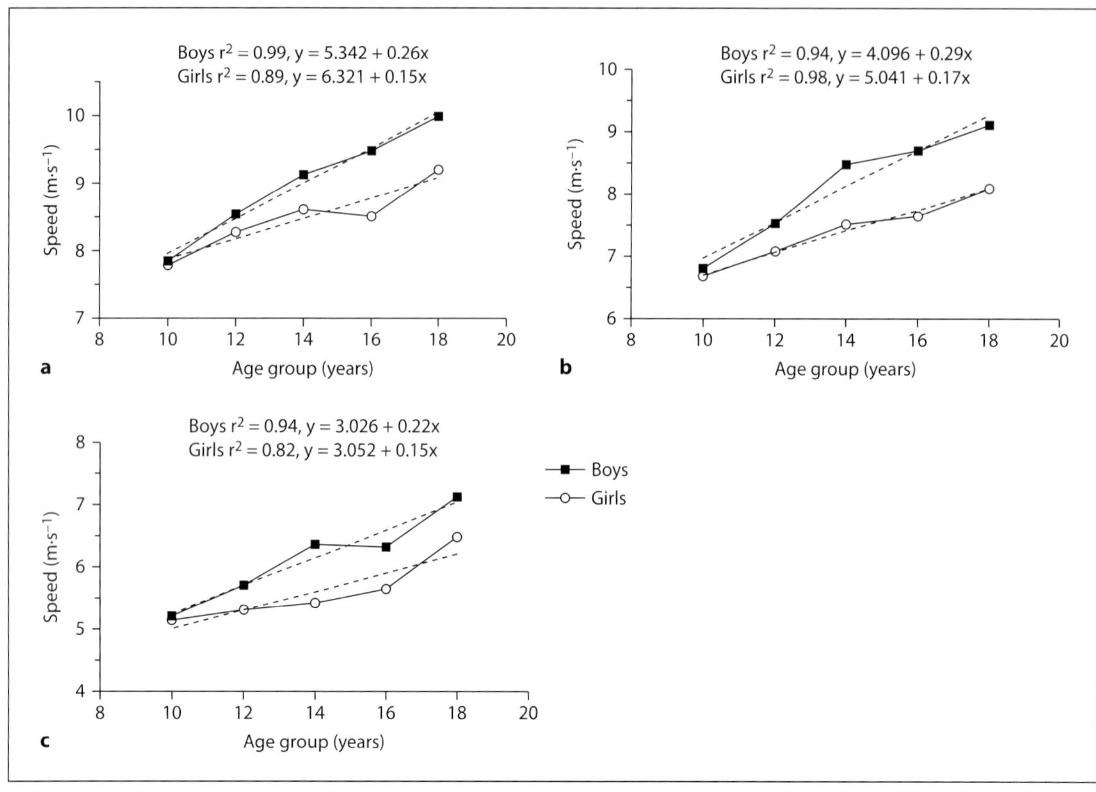

Fig. 1. Average running speed from North American age-group track and field records and world junior records over 100m (**a**), 400m (**b**) and 1,500m (**c**) for girls and boys.

illustrates the average running speed over 100, 400 and 1,500 m for girls and boys competing in age-group track and field championships in North America and world junior records [10, 11]. Analyses of these data show that regardless of distance, average running speed increases with age in both girls and boys (r^2 >0.82 for all distances). Prior to 11 years of age differences in average speed are minimal, thereafter disparity becomes more pronounced with boys 8–15% faster than girls from 13 years of age onwards. This is consistent with the 9–15% advantage in speed adult men have over women across a wide range of distances from 100 m to 200 km [12]. When the slopes of the regression lines were compared between the sexes by age, these were significantly different for 100 and 400 m with the rate of improvement greater in the boys than the girls (see fig. 1). The rate of improvement in running speed over 1,500 m was similar between boys and girls with a pooled slope of 0.19. That an interaction between distance, speed developmental trajectories and sex exists suggests intriguing physiological mechanisms.

A key question to be addressed is whether the superior performances of boys relate to qualitative discrepancies in functional capacity or alternatively, they are simply a function of the increased body size and disparate body composition that accompanies adolescent growth and maturation. Appropriate adjustment for differences in body size and composition dampen many apparent

McManus · Armstrong

physiological differences [13, 14]; however, young girl athletes are not simply smaller, less muscular boys. Girls' physiology varies with age and is underpinned by a divergent hormonal milieu which begins early in foetal life. There is evidence that in the two-cell stage of embryonic development, long before visual gonadal differentiation, the sex-determining region of the Y chromosome has already been transcribed [15]. Testosterone secretion commences at about 3 months in the male foetus, the absence of which in the female foetus allows maturation of the female reproductive organs, and by birth subtle differences in cardiac function and body composition already exist [16, 17]. The accentuated hormonal adjustments which occur during adolescence result in differential development and a widening sex disparity in many physiological responses to exercise, some of which cannot be accounted for by size.

The primary focus of this chapter is on physiologic issues that are associated with exercise in girls; but to illustrate sexual dimorphism, comparisons will be made with boys where relevant. The chapter begins with a brief overview of growth and maturation in girls, including a discussion of issues related to body composition and size. This is followed by a focus on the acute responses to sustained aerobic exercise, as well as short-duration high-intensity exercise in girls. The possible physiological mechanisms that underlie these responses, such as sex differences in pulmonary, cardiac, and peripheral function, as well as cellular metabolism are discussed. The chapter concludes with consideration of the contention that intensive training poses a substantial threat to the development and health of young girls.

Growth and Maturation

Growth hormone (GH), insulin-like growth factor I (IGF-I), the sex steroids and insulin are all potent anabolic hormones. Their complex interactions enable linear growth, bone mineralization, increases in muscle and metabolic adaptations during childhood and adolescence and much of this hormonal mélange is sex dependent [18]. For example, the physiological effects of the sex steroids testosterone and oestrogen differ markedly, with evidence that combined testosterone and GH administration causes increases in IGF-I concentrations, resulting in enhanced anabolism, greater increases in fat free mass and higher whole body protein synthesis in boys [19]. Oestrogen administration, on the other hand, has been shown to have no effect on whole body protein synthesis in girls [19]. Sex dimorphic growth and development is most pronounced during adolescence, which forms the primary focus of the following sections.

Stature and body mass follow a double-sigmoid growth pattern in girls and boys, with rapid gains in infancy, slower yearly gains of about 5–6 cm in stature and 2.25–2.75 kg in body mass through childhood, and a second rapid gain in adolescence [20]. Girls usually begin adolescent growth before boys and progress at a faster rate than boys [21, 22]. At the peak of the adolescent growth spurt, girls gain approximately 8–9 cm in a year in stature. Boys only gain about 3 cm more in stature during the adolescent growth spurt, but are about 11–13 cm taller by adulthood because of their extra pre-adolescent growth [23]. From onset to completion, adolescent growth in stature lasts about 4–4.5 years in girls, until rising levels of oestrogen induce epiphyseal fusion marking an end to the growth in stature, usually around a skeletal age of 15 years [18, 21]. Peak body mass velocity is in lag by some 4–6 months with peak height velocity and total body mass gains of 16 kg are usual during the adolescent growth spurt in girls [24].

Other body proportions such as sitting height, leg length, biacromial and bicristal breadths follow a similar growth pattern to stature. Leg length and sitting height differ little between girls and boys during childhood [23]. At the onset of adolescence rapid growth in leg length precedes trunk growth. Boys surpass girls in leg length by about 12 years of age and in sitting height around

14 years of age. Yet, the ratio of sitting height to stature is higher in girls than boys through adolescence indicating relatively shorter legs in girls for the same stature. Girls have a marginally wider bicristal breadth than boys from late childhood to late adolescence, when boys catch-up [23]. In contrast, boys experience much more dramatic increases in biacromial breadth compared to girls [23]. When bicristal breadth is expressed as a ratio of biacromial breadth (hip-to-shoulder ratio), in comparison to boys values are higher in girls from early childhood, with bicristal breadth approximately 72–73% of biacromial breath, remaining quite stable through adolescence. In boys a decline in this ratio is noted from about 70% at 11 years of age, to 65% by 16 years of age, which is an outcome of the disproportionately faster growth of biacromial breadth [23]. Interestingly, although stature as well as mass-to-stature ratio differ between girls involved in different competitive sports, minimal differences in other proportions such as arm span and seated height have been reported [25, 26]. Greater mass-to-stature ratios can confer performance benefit in some sports such as throwing events; however, the combined effect of broader hips and shorter legs that usually accompany a greater mass-for-stature and characterize early maturation in girls, is generally disadvantageous. Although data are sparse, young female athletes in running events or gymnastics are generally more likely to be characterized by longer legs, lower hip-to-shoulder ratios and lower mass-for-stature.

Assessment of maturity stage is vital but poses considerable challenge. Skeletal age is the biological marker of choice, but is hindered by ethical constraints related to ionizing radiation exposure. The timing and tempo of sexual maturation in girls has most commonly been described using the visual descriptive stages of secondary sexual characteristics. These were first documented by Reynolds and Wines [27], and then further refined by J.M. Tanner and are better known as Tanner stages [28]. There is a large normal variation in the timing and tempo of sexual maturation in girls, as well as clearly documented sex differences. Like linear growth, girls normally begin sexual maturation before boys and progress toward full maturity at a faster tempo than boys [22].

A recent large-scale longitudinal study of Caucasian and African-American children suggests that the average girl begins breast development at 9.8 years, whilst the average boy begins genital development at about 10.3 years [21]. Pubic hair growth usually occurs around 10.2 years in girls and around 11.3 years in boys. The onset of the initial stages of sexual maturity in these American girls is somewhat earlier than previously published data for European girls, for whom breast budding was reported to occur at about 10.5 years and Tanner Stage two for pubic hair at 10.8 years [28, 29]. This discrepancy probably reflects the different racial mix of the groups, in addition to a possible secular trend for a declining age of onset of maturation [30].

Asynchronous maturation of secondary sex characteristics in girls is common and has been defined as a difference of at least 4 months between breast and pubic hair development. About 51–66% of girls follow an asynchronous maturation pattern [21, 31]. Most (about 70%) follow a thelarchal pathway, with breast development beginning prior to pubic hair growth (adrenarche). Asynchrony usually persists into Tanner stage 3, the onset of which is on average 11.3 years for breast development, with pubic hair stage three occurring some 2 months later [31]. As the latter stages of sexual maturity are attained, development becomes more synchronous. A minority of girls (approximately 30%) follow an adrenarchal asynchronous pathway, in which pubic hair development precedes breast development. Thelarchal asynchrony is believed to result from initial advanced stimulation of gonadotropin and oestrogen, thereby enabling earlier breast development. The converse is true of adrenarchal asynchrony, where the advanced production of testosterone and adrenal hormones promotes earlier pubic hair growth. Age of onset of menses usually occurs during Tanner stage three for breast development. For those girls following the thelarchal pathway, menses occurs at an earlier age, around 12.6 years. Those following the adrenarchal pathway usually begin menses around 13.1 years [21, 31]. Lower oestrogen levels are noted in girls following an adrenarchal maturation pathway which persists throughout adolescence. This affords a body composition advantage, characterized by a lower sum of skinfolds, percent body fat and waist-to-hip ratio [31]. Girls involved in intensive training are generally characterized by lower percent body fat, but there is little evidence to suggest that they preferentially follow an asynchronous adrenarchal pathway [32].

The presence of asynchronous sexual maturation has implications when comparing young athletes with non-athletes, as well as making comparisons between girls and boys. Whether alignment is on the basis of a single marker (e.g. pubic hair development), the creation of a composite score for both pubic hair and breast development, or on differing secondary sex characteristics (such as genitalia and breast development), the assumption is that the timing of the appearance of a particular characteristic, as well as the tempo, is homogeneous. This is clearly not always the case, and it has been suggested that alignment of sexual maturation to other biological or somatic markers of maturation (e.g. age at menarche or peak height velocity) is more appropriate [33]. Menarchal age is convenient if retrospective, otherwise, like peak height velocity, a prospective research design is necessary. Assessment of maturational stage continues to present a real methodological challenge to paediatric exercise physiologists.

Body Composition and Size

Fat

Small sex differences in fat mass and percent body fat are evident from mid-childhood, with levels rising substantially in girls during adolescence. Body fat gains by the end of puberty usually result in 26–31% body fat in the average adolescent girl [34, 35]. Young athletes are generally leaner than the average non-athletic girl, but this is dependent on the chosen sport. Values as low as 14.3% have been reported for 15-year-old rhythmic gymnasts, with gymnasts generally showing lower body fat than other athletes [34]. Body fat values from 21 to 25% have been reported for dancers, distance runners and cross-country skiers from the ages of 10–17 years [36–39]. Higher values have been reported for 13- to 17-year-old high-school athletes competing in lacrosse, soccer, softball, swimming, track and field and volleyball (mean 27.4 ± 0.7%) [40].

Sex steroids are major determinants of body fat distribution, with the increases in body fat generally subcutaneous and in the gluteal and femoral regions in girls. Fat mass, combined with a smaller leg length-to-stature ratio, lowers the centre of gravity in girls, thereby affording better balance. However, fat mass is also negatively related to heat dissipation, which may prove disadvantageous in girls during endurance events in hot environmental conditions [41].

Fat tissue has relatively uniform properties throughout life, with negligible water content and a tissue density of 0.9007 kg$\cdot$l^{-1} [42]. Recent reference data from Wells et al. [42] have shown that in comparison lean tissue shows sex-specific chemical maturation, with decreases in water content and increases in density with increasing age. These new data have implications for the assessment of body fat since previous reference data extrapolated rather than directly assessed age specific tissue densities and hydration. Wells et al.'s [42] work provides the first comprehensive empirical data set for lean tissue properties for 4- to 23-year-old boys and girls, with lean tissue density values in girls of 1.0905 kg$\cdot$l^{-1} at 8–9 years, rising to 1.1021 kg$\cdot$l^{-1} at 16–17 years. Lean tissue hydration values declined with age from 75.2% at 8–9 years to 73.7% at 16–17 years in girls. Importantly, this study has shown that these new values differ from previously simulated values. The lean tissue density values of Wells et al. [42] were consistently higher, whilst the hydration data were consistently lower than those reported by Lohman [43]. Comparisons of % fat calculated from densitometry with the Lohman [43] formula led to a between-study error of –1 to 2.5% fat in the average girl. Wells et al. [42] provide important new reference values for the assessment of body fat by both hydrometry (total body water, bioelectrical impedance) and densitometry which should ensure greater clarity in future analyses.

Muscle

At birth, boys tend to have a greater lean mass than girls. This difference remains small but detectable throughout childhood with about a 10% greater lean mass in boys than girls prior to puberty [17]. The sharp increase in muscle mass disparity between the sexes during puberty indicates a primary role of the gonadal steroidal hormones. Muscle mass in girls increases from about 25 kg at 10 years of age to about 45 kg by 18 years of age [42]. Reported values for 15- to 17-year-old female athletes are not dissimilar, ranging from 42 to 53 kg [23]. These gains in muscle tissue represent an increase of about 5% in muscle mass. The relative contribution of muscle mass to total body mass usually declines once consideration is given to the relative contribution of fat mass. In comparison, the androgen-mediated growth of muscle in boys results in muscle mass reaching about 55% of total body mass at maturity [44]. The greater overall skeletal muscle mass in adolescent boys creates a potential cascade of functional differences apparent in adults such as differing muscle fibre size, activities of metabolic enzymes, lipid content and oxidation, relative expression of myosin isoforms, and fatigability [45–50]. Maturation of these features remains poorly understood.

The use of ultrasonography and magnetic resonance imaging (MRI) are providing insight into changes in muscle architecture with growth. A recent study using ultrasonography demonstrated that muscle thickness (a marker of physiological cross-sectional area) and pennation angle were correlated with age from 4 to 10 years in both sexes [51]. Findings from MRI studies have shown similarly that muscle cross-sectional area increases with age from childhood through adolescence, and more so in boys than girls [52]. Pennation angle on the other hand has not been found to differ between the sexes [51]. Whilst muscle cross-sectional area and pennation angle are related to age, this has not been shown in muscle fibre length [51]. Muscle fibre length has been found to have high inter- and intra-individual variation, which may reflect a greater malleability in response to external stimuli such as the extent and intensity of exercise [51].

Morphological change in the muscle impacts upon function. Maximal strength, for example, is dependent on the specific joint angle (force-length relationship), contraction type, muscle cross-sectional area and velocity. The length of the muscle fibre is proportional to the absolute maximum contraction velocity, whilst the pennation angle dictates the proportion of force transmitted to the tendon. Muscle strength, expressed as torque, increases with age in children, but gains are greater in boys. This has been presumed to be an outcome of the greater muscle cross-sectional area [53]. Alternatively, there may be intrinsic sex differences in the fibre composition and fatigue characteristics of skeletal muscle that materialize during adolescence that also influence the ability to increase torque.

In adults, several studies have reported higher glycolytic enzyme activity and lower oxidative enzyme activity in men compared to women, supporting the contention that men have a lower proportion of type I fibres [50, 54]. Data on muscle fibre typing in children are limited because of the invasive nature of the biopsy methodology, but there is evidence to show that differentiation of fibre type occurs during the first few years of life. About 10% of skeletal muscle fibres remain undifferentiated up until puberty, with no sex difference notable in the percentage of type I fibres (slow-twitch oxidative fibres) during childhood [55]. By adolescence females have a lower % of type I muscle fibres than males [45, 56] and the type II muscle fibres of young men are bigger than their type I fibres, something not evident in young women [56, 58].

Although boys gain more in strength than girls during adolescence, elite girl athletes are stronger than their less athletic peers. For example, average quadriceps and biceps isometric strength was reported to be 22% greater in elite gymnasts and swimmers and 18% greater in tennis players compared to less athletic school children [59]. Interestingly this study found no differences in strength between sports in the girls, even when co-varied for body mass. The relationship between strength and body mass, or strength-to-mass ratio, has been seen as an important predictor of sport performance particularly in gymnastics, middle- and long-distance running. Indeed, elite adult women runners such as Yvonne Murray and Greta Waitz were 17–18% below the average body mass for their stature at the peak of their running careers, which suggests relative strength was high. The work of Bencke et al. [60] has shown that 11-year-old girl gymnasts were the smallest, lightest and possessed the highest explosive strength compared to other athletes, suggesting high relative strength confers advantage in some sports in girls.

Bone

Bone characteristics differ little between boys and girls prior to puberty, but then follow two sex-divergent growth paths. During the adolescent growth spurt boys experience increases predominantly in bone diameter and cortical thickness due to periosteal apposition [17]. Girls on the other hand experience increases in cortical thickness, a decrease in medullary diameter, and little increase in periosteal diameter as a result of oestrogen inhibition of periosteal apposition [17, 61]. It should be noted that bone accretion and endocortical features appear to be site specific with data showing endocortical resorption at the mid-femur and proximal tibia in girls through puberty, but no endocortical resorption at the radial diaphysis [62, 63].

During puberty, bone mineral content (BMC) accrual rate is in lag with muscle accrual rate, suggesting that muscle enlargement, and concomitant increases in muscle force, are important for bone development [64]. Indeed, the 'functional muscle-bone unit' hypothesis suggests muscle force is a primary determinant of bone mass, structure and strength [65]. Young female runners and gymnasts have been shown to have elevated bone mass and enlarged bone size at specific sites such as the radius and lumbar spine in gymnasts [66] and the femur in runners [67], reflecting the specific mechanical-loading patterns these sports require. This has led some to conclude that muscular force alone explains the impact loading effect on bone [68–70]. On the contrary, recent research has shown that bone mass, size and strength increases in the upper extremity in gymnasts are independent of maturation, stature and muscle cross-sectional area and substantiates the hypothesis that other non-muscular loading factors may also account for skeletal adaptations [71, 72].

Puberty is the most favourable period for augmented bone mineralization, with about one quarter of adult bone being laid down. Bone mineral accrual is sex and maturity dependent and appears to be enhanced by oestrogen. It is clear that the early pubertal and pre-menarchal years are particularly important for young girls in terms of optimizing their bone mineralization and weight-bearing exercise plays a key complementary role in this process [73].

By the time the adolescent growth spurt is complete the body size, shape and composition of boys and girls is different. Boys have become taller, have longer legs, broader shoulders, are heavier, and have less fat and more muscle than girls. The effect of these discrepancies on performance is substantial, and it is important in understanding girls' physiologic responses to exercise that we are able to effectively partition the impact of size from function. Traditionally in exercise physiology this has been achieved by expressing the physiological measure of interest (y) as a ratio of an appropriate marker of body size (x) to give the ratio y/x. Tanner suggested in 1949 that the use of such ratio standards to scale physiological measurements to size was 'theoretically fallacious and unless in exceptional circumstances, misleading' [74]. Yet this has largely been ignored with much of the comparison between men and women, or boys and girls based on ratio standards [75, 76]. An implicit assumption with the ratio standard is that the relationship is linear and the y intercept is zero. Additionally, ratio standards should only be used when the coefficient of variation (V) for body size (x), divided by the coefficient of variation (V) for the physiological variable (y), equals the Pearson product moment correlation coefficient (r) for the two variables, expressed by the equation $V_x/V_y = r_{x,y}$. These assumptions are rarely met and the outcome is scaling distortion, which may have obscured our understanding of the physiologic responses of girls [77].

Theoretically, morphological and physiological variables are scaled according to the general allometric equation $y = ax^b$, where y is the morphological or physiological variable of interest, x is the chosen size denominator, b is the scaling exponent and a is the constant [78]. When this equation is solved the resultant power function ratio (y/x^b) is derived. Various studies have shown that with careful consideration of the denominator, alternative approaches, such as the allometric power function ratio or more complex multilevel modelling of longitudinal data, are more appropriate than ratio scaling when comparisons of various physiological outcomes between individuals of differing body size are sought [79, 80]. These alternatives should, wherever possible, be utilised.

Acute Responses to Aerobic Exercise

Peak oxygen uptake (peak $\dot{V}O_2$), the highest $\dot{V}O_2$ elicited during an exercise test to exhaustion in children, is well-established as the best single measure of aerobic fitness [81]. In comparison to boys, girls are characterised with a smaller absolute peak $\dot{V}O_2$. Predicted values range from 1.5 to 2.2 litres $\bullet$ min^{-1} in 10- to 16-year-old girls and are lower than boys by 11, 19, 23 and 27% at ages 10, 12, 14 and 16 years of age, respectively [82]. Peak $\dot{V}O_2$ is strongly correlated with body size and composition and thus, much of the divergence in values reflects this. When expressed as a ratio standard with body mass (ml $\bullet$ kg^{-1} $\bullet$ min^{-1}), peak $\dot{V}O_2$ shows a progressive decline in girls from 13 years of age, with values dropping from approximately 45 to 35 ml $\bullet$ kg^{-1} $\bullet$ min^{-1} [83]. In contrast, mass-related peak $\dot{V}O_2$ in young female runners has been found to be relatively constant with values of 56.3, 57.1, 56.9 and 54.3 ml $\bullet$ kg^{-1}·min^{-1} at ages 10, 12, 14 and 16 years, respectively [84]. Likewise, peak $\dot{V}O_2$ has been shown to be fairly stable between 11 and 16 years of age in elite girl swimmers and tennis players [85], with values of 51–52 ml $\bullet$ kg^{-1} $\bullet$ min^{-1} and 47–49 ml $\bullet$ kg^{-1} $\bullet$ min^{-1}, respectively. When multilevel modelling was used to account for mass, stature and biological age, the elite girl swimmers and tennis players showed increases in peak $\dot{V}O_2$ until late puberty when increases became non-significant [85]. Similarly, in the less athletic population when more appropriate allometric adjustment is used to partition size effects in body mass and stature, peak $\dot{V}O_2$ has been found to increase significantly from 11 to 13 years in girls, and then remain constant with no decline into adulthood evident [81].

Dramatic pubertal changes in muscle, fat and mass contribute to the widening of the sex difference in peak $\dot{V}O_2$. When a marker of body fat was included in a multilevel regression model which incorporated body mass, stature and age, the sex difference in peak $\dot{V}O_2$ was reduced, but the greater increase in boys' peak $\dot{V}O_2$ with growth compared to girls was still not fully explained [83]. Equally, longitudinal data have shown that even when differences in body mass and fat mass are controlled for allometrically, girls utilise less oxygen than boys during submaximal exercise, and this becomes more pronounced with age [86]. Understanding the physiologic mechanisms that underlie these size-independent sex differences in peak and submaximal $\dot{V}O_2$ requires consideration of the coordinated systems response, which includes pulmonary, cardiac and peripheral adjustments to the demands in muscular energy. A discussion of key features of each follows.

Pulmonary

It was generally assumed that because exercise training exerts little influence on lung structure or function that the lungs exert minimal influence on oxygen transport. However, there is evidence that lung function adaptation does occur as a consequence of exercise training in girls [87]. Moreover recent investigation of sex differences in pulmonary structure and function in adults has shown considerable effects on gas exchange and the integrated ventilatory response during exercise, in particular exercise-induced arterial hypoxia [88]. There are well-documented sex differences in anatomical aspects of the pulmonary system which occur during lung growth [89]. The consequence of sex dependent pubertal thoracic growth is a larger thoracic width in boys. When coupled with a greater muscle mass for generating lower lung function, boys have approximately 25% greater lung volumes than girls who are matched for stature [89]. By adult life, in addition to the smaller lung volumes, stature and age independent lower resting diffusion capacity (corrected for haemoglobin), lower maximal expiratory flow rates [90], and a greater occurrence of exercise-induced hypoxia has been shown in women [91]. Equally, there is also evidence that when matched for size and aerobic power women do not have reduced diffusion capacity or impaired ventilation perfusion during exercise [92].

In children, like adults, exercise pulmonary gas exchange depends on pulmonary ventilation ($\dot{V}_E$) and at maximal work rates high rates of ventilation are usual. Maximal values of 49–95 litres $\bullet$ min^{-1} have been recorded for girls between the ages of 9 and 16 years [93] and there is a consistent sex difference with values somewhat higher in boys (58–105 litres $\bullet$ min^{-1}) for the same age span. It should be noted that cross-study comparisons are difficult given the dependence of ventilation on the protocol and data such as these need to be interpreted cautiously. Maximum ventilation remains higher in boys, whether controlled for body size using a ratio standard or allometric adjustment with either stature and/or body mass [94, 95]. Thus, the higher peak $\dot{V}O_2$ in boys is indeed supported by a higher $\dot{V}_E$.

During exercise, an expiratory flow limitation is apparent in adult women but not men, resulting in a greater oxygen cost of breathing and the onset of arterial desaturation [88, 96]. Recent evidence has provided a comparison between pre-pubertal boys and girls and found no difference in the occurrence or severity of expiratory flow limitation between girls and boys and no changes in arterial saturation during exercise to maximum [97]. Others have found little evidence of exercise induced arterial hypoxaemia in pre-pubertal girls, or lower ventilatory efficiency at maximum [98, 99]. When Armstrong et al. [94] compared ventilatory parameters during submaximal exercise at the same absolute intensities they noted that girls demonstrated higher ventilatory equivalents for oxygen and carbon dioxide, i.e. poorer ventilatory efficiency in comparison to boys. However, when they compared submaximal ventilatory efficiency during the same relative exercise intensities, values were remarkably similar between the sexes. This suggests that differences apparent at absolute submaximal exercise intensities simply reflect the higher relative percentage of maximum that girls are working at and do not denote true inefficiency.

There is little evidence that prior to puberty pulmonary structure or function limits oxygen uptake, however, considerable evidence has shown pulmonary function influences gas exchange in adult women, suggesting that maturational adjustments occur. At present however, there is little evidence to substantiate this.

Blood Volume and Haemoglobin

Assessment of blood volume in children and adolescents is complex and the variability in techniques means there are considerable discrepancies between studies. There are conflicting results regarding changes in blood volume with age. Some have shown that blood volume per unit body mass increases with age [100], others have found no change [101], whilst others report decreasing blood volume with age [102]. Likewise, data on sex differences in blood volume between girls and boys are mixed. When normalised using a ratio standard with body mass, differences between girls and boys were apparent from about 6 years of age, with values lower in the girls [103]. In contrast, when normalised using a ratio standard for lean body mass, sex differences are no longer apparent for pre-pubertal children, or at any maturational stage [103].

In boys, haemoglobin rises through adolescence to about 152 g•l^{-1} by 16 years of age [104]. Girls, on the other hand, usually demonstrate a plateau in haemoglobin concentration with values of about 137 g•l^{-1} by 16 years of age [104]. Highly trained adolescent female athletes also show lower haemoglobin concentration values compared to trained boys, with about a 7% difference [105]. Fully saturated, 1 g of haemoglobin carries 1.34 ml of oxygen, and one would presume that the smaller increase in haemoglobin in girls would result in a reduced oxygen carrying capacity in comparison to boys. However, it has been shown that haemoglobin concentration is not a significant predictor of peak $\dot{V}O_2$ in 11- to 17-year-olds once body size and composition and maturation have been controlled for [83].

Cardiac and Vascular Considerations

There are clear differences in cardiac function at rest and during exercise between girls and boys, with differences apparent even prior to puberty. The electrical conduction system is influenced by sex steroid hormones, with girls normally having higher resting heart rates than boys – somewhere in the magnitude of 90 beats per minute at around 10–12 years of age [106]. This is thought to relate to intrinsic differences in the sinus node pacemaker [107], a difference notable at birth with newborn boys displaying lower baseline heart rates than girls [16]. The higher resting heart rate in girls is often explained as an artefact of differences in cardiac dimensions, and indeed the ratio of heart mass to body mass has been found to be higher in boys than girls at birth, remaining so through adolescence [106]. Heart volume has also been found to be greater in boys with values of 342 and 403 ml for pre-pubertal girls and boys, respectively, and of 466 and 561 ml for pubertal girls and boys, respectively [108]. When adjusted for body mass these differences were found to persist through puberty (female 10.0 ml•kg^{-1}; male 10.8 ml•kg^{-1}). Inconsistencies in the findings, however, are present and others have found no differences in either left ventricular mass [109] or heart volume [110].

Echocardiographic studies that have shown greater left ventricular mass in boys compared

Table 1. Oxygen uptake, stroke index, cardiac index and arteriovenous oxygen difference at maximal cycle ergometer exercise

Reference	Sex	n	Age (years)	SI ($ml \cdot m^{-2}$)	HR (bpm)	CI ($litres \cdot min^{-1} \cdot m^{-2}$)	a-v O_2 difference ($ml \cdot 100\ ml^{-1}$)	Peak $\dot{V}O_2$ ($litres \cdot min^{-1} \cdot kg^{-1}$)	Peak $\dot{V}O_2$ ($litres \cdot min^{-1}$)
Cumming [111]	F	29	11.8±3.1	46±3[†]	174±11	8.61±8.1[†]	–	–	–
	M	31	12.6±3.5	56±13	170±17	10.1± 1.8	–	–	–
Rowland et al. [112]	F	24	11.7±0.5	55±9[†]	198±9	10.9±1.7[†]	12.3±1.9	40.4±5.8[†]	1.84±31
	M	25	12.0±0.4	62±9	199±11	12.3±2.2	12.2±1.7	47.1±6.1	1.98±28
Obert et al. [113] Pre-training experimental group	F	7	10.66±0.3	47±7[†]	204±5	9.4±1.4[†]	13.2±1.6	40.9±8.9[†]	–
	M	9	10.66±0.5	52±8	199±9	10.5±1.8	13.0±2.1	44.1±6.1	–
Pre-training control group	F	10	10.41±0.3	46±6[†]	202±7	9.4±1.2[†]	13.1±2.8[†]	42.4±5.6[†]	–
	M	9	10.5±0.3	49±5	202±7	9.7±0.8	15.6±1.5	51.5±6.3	–
Winsley et al. [114]	F	9	10.2±0.3	45±6	192±11	8.7±1.1	12.6±1.6[†]	–	1.23±.08[†]
	M	9	10.1±0.5	47±8	195±11	8.9±1.4	14.8±2.1	–	1.41±.18

SI = Stroke index; HR = heart rate; CI = cardiac index; a-v O_2 difference = arterio-venous oxygen difference; $\dot{V}O_2$ = oxygen uptake. [†] Significant differences noted.

to girls have suggested that the reduced cardiac mass in girls may be associated with reduced contractility, reduced pre-load or increased afterload [106]. All of these could result in a reduced stroke index (SI) and therefore reduced cardiac index (CI). Cardiac index has generally been found to be higher in boys than girls at maximal exercise (table 1) and in the absence of sex differences in maximal heart rate, it would appear that SI most likely accounts for this difference. Absolute maximal SI index has been reported to be between 7 and 13% less in girls than boys. When corrected for body fat, this difference was reduced to 5.2% [112], but remained nonetheless. Interestingly, the lower maximal SI index apparent in girls has not always been found to relate to left ventricular dimensions, which suggests sex differences may instead relate to other factors such as the peripheral pump, systemic vascular resistance or differing adrenergic responses [113, 115].

Evidence of cardiac re-modelling following training has provided some insight into the role systemic vascular resistance may play in SI differences between boys and girls [113]. Following 13 weeks of training, both pre-pubertal boys and girls increased LV end-diastolic diameter and left ventricular mass. However, only LV end-diastolic diameter was related to percent increase in SI. Percent increase in SI was also inversely related to systemic vascular resistance, suggestive of vascular adaptations in response to high-intensity training. Of note, the decrease in systemic vascular resistance was greater in the boys than the girls, which may account for the greater increase in maximal SI in the boys.

The vasoregulatory capacity of the arterial and arteriolar vessels manipulates peripheral resistance. When blood is effectively distributed to the working muscle, peripheral resistance is reduced, which unloads the heart improving the capacity of the heart to increase SI. This is achieved by improving the flow of blood to and through the muscle and both the vasculature and skeletal muscle pump are involved. Interestingly, no sex differences in arterial compliance have been noted in pre- and early-pubertal children [116], although the beneficial role of oestrogen in vasodilation is well established and female advantage in arterial compliance is apparent in adults [117].

The skeletal muscle pump utilises the rhythmic muscle contractions to empty the venous vessels, aiding blood muscle hyperaemia and venous return. There is scant information on the skeletal muscle pump in children, but evidence in boys suggests, like adults, the skeletal muscle pump is associated with improved CI [118, 119]. In Rowland et al.'s [119] study, arterio-venous oxygen (a-v O_2) difference, a composite index of the haematological components of oxygen delivery, remained constant during unloaded exercise suggesting the increases in muscle oxygen supply were met by the increasing blood volume. Conversely, as exercise intensity increased with loading, a-v O_2 difference increased indicating decreased effectiveness of the muscle pump in satisfying the metabolic demands of the working muscle.

Whilst some studies have found no differences in estimated a-v O_2 difference at maximal or submaximal intensities between pre-pubertal girls and boys [112, 120], there are conflicting findings. Data recently published from a thoracic impedance measure of peak CI and MRI markers of cardiac size [114] demonstrated that pre-pubertal boys had a 16.7% higher a-v O_2 difference than girls. This was the only distinguishing factor to explain the significantly higher peak $\dot{V}O_2$ in the boys compared to the girls and unlike other studies no difference in either CI or SI were apparent at maximal exercise. It is interesting to note that a-v O_2 difference was 16% lower in the girls of the control group (table 1) in the study of Obert et al. [113]. These findings are intriguing, but confirmatory studies are needed to help understand the inconsistencies in the extant data.

Muscle Cellular Metabolism during Moderate Intensity Exercise

Characterizing muscle metabolism during exercise is extremely challenging and for a long time hampered by the need for invasive measurement of enzymatic activity. ^{31}P magnetic resonance spectroscopy (MRS) has enabled the study of high energy phosphates non-invasively in human skeletal muscle. This technique can provide an estimation of skeletal muscle metabolic activity via examination of creatine phosphate (PCr), inorganic phosphate (P_i) and intracellular pH, and has been validated in both adults and children [121, 122]. There remain methodological challenges in the paediatric population, which have been outlined by Armstrong and Fawkner [123], but the data available are providing fascinating insight into cellular metabolic processes.

Children, like adults show high correspondence between MRS determined muscle phosphocreatine (PCr) activity and the pulmonary oxygen uptake (p$\dot{V}O_2$) kinetic response [124, 125]. This implies that p$\dot{V}O_2$ kinetics also provide a marker of energy utilization at the muscular level, one which may prove very useful in understanding the interplay between cardiopulmonary and metabolic processes during exercise. More comprehensive descriptions of oxygen uptake kinetic assessments have been provided elsewhere [126] and only the salient issues related to girls' responses are summarized here. The p$\dot{V}O_2$ kinetic response is tri-phasic, but only phases II and III pertain to muscle oxygen uptake kinetics. During moderate intensity exercise, the phase II p$\dot{V}O_2$ kinetic response involves an exponential increase in oxygen uptake toward steady state, which signifies increases in muscle $\dot{V}O_2$. The primary response is described by a time constant (τ), representing the time taken (s) to achieve 63% of the change in $p\dot{V}O_2$. The attainment of a steady state denotes phase III. At higher workloads, i.e. those above the maximal lactate steady state, the $p\dot{V}O_2$ kinetic response alters, with phase III showing a delayed increase, eventually resulting in a $p\dot{V}O_2$ value higher than predicted on the basis of exercise intensity. This 'slow component' represents an increasing inefficiency in energy turnover and negatively correlates with increases in $\dot{V}O_2$ per unit increases in work, suggesting fatigue. To ensure confidence in the kinetic parameters estimated, the level of measurement rigour needed is high [126]. Few of the available oxygen uptake kinetics studies with children provide this and as such information on girls is very limited.

There is little evidence of a sex difference in $p\dot{V}O_2$ kinetic responses during moderate intensity exercise in children [127]. Neither have sex differences been found in boys and girls for MRS determined pH, P_i to PCr ratio (P_i/PCr) or PCr kinetic time constant at either the onset or offset of moderate intensity exercise [128]. In contrast, a study of the kinetic responses to high-intensity exercise found sex differences [129]. Results showed phase II $p\dot{V}O_2$ kinetics were approximately 20% slower in pre-pubertal girls compared to boys and the relative contribution of the $p\dot{V}O_2$ slow component to the end exercise $p\dot{V}O_2$ in the girls was about 30% greater. This is suggestive of a lower tolerance of fatigue in the girls, but the mechanisms underlying this response are not yet understood. One hypothesis suggests that these differences reflect a difference between boys and girls in the energetic profiles of the recruited muscles.

Barker et al. [130] have explored high-intensity exercise responses of the quadriceps muscle using MRS in children, but showed in accord with the $p\dot{V}O_2$ kinetic work, that girls responded with a greater anaerobic metabolic contribution than

boys. These findings were partly attributed to the inequalities in maturity status, with relatively immature boys compared to the girls. Maturation of the cellular anaerobic response was noted in the girls in this study, who progressed from a response that was attenuated prior to puberty, but adult-like with ensuing maturation. This was not apparent in the boys, most likely an artefact of the narrow age range of the boys (9–12 years). Generally, high-intensity work requires the recruitment of fast twitch muscle fibres that are faster and larger, with a greater glycolytic and lower oxidative capacity. As discussed earlier, there is evidence of sex differences in muscle fibre type and size which vary with age and maturation, and clearly comparison of cellular metabolism during high-intensity exercise in girls and boys who are more closely aligned in terms of maturation is something which deserves further enquiry.

To summarise, there are differences between boys and girls in the aerobic responses to exercise which cannot be accounted for solely by size. Ventilatory parameters do not appear to influence peak $\dot{V}O_2$ in pre-pubertal children, however, there is scant information on the maturation of ventilatory responses in girls. It has been suggested that peripheral factors may be more important in defining aerobic fitness than cardiac function [131], but these are poorly understood in children and in particular in girls.

Acute Responses to High-Intensity Exercise

Most sports require short-duration bursts of high-intensity effort, which are supported by high muscle energy turnover. The direct examination of muscular energetics during short-duration high-intensity exercise is complex and instead investigations have largely concentrated on mechanical output markers of short duration exercise performance. The most commonly employed tests are the Wingate cycle ergometer test (WAnT) and cycle ergometer force-velocity tests, both eliciting markers of leg power. Wingate test values for leg peak power in girls aged 11–16 years have ranged from 260 to 542 W [132–136], whilst comparable values between 250 and 555 W have been recorded using force-velocity tests in similarly aged girls [137–140]. Mean power values from the Wingate test have ranged from 228 to 341 W in 11- to 16-year-old girls [132, 136]. It is interesting to note that neither peak nor mean power appear to be unusually high in young girls who are engaged in elite tennis, swimming or gymnastics training [141]. Higher values have been recorded for elite handball players and elite sprinters [133, 141], which could not be fully explained by age and body composition; however, when comparison was made with published values for less athletic girls, peak and mean power for these elite girl athletes were not substantially different.

Longitudinal data have shown that leg peak power increases with age in both boys and girls, but the increases in boys are greater than in girls. In a study of 7- to 18-year-olds, peak power was shown to increase by 273% in girls from 7 to 16 years of age, and then to plateau [142]. In comparison, boys showed increases of 375% over this period with no plateau at 16 years. Armstrong et al. [132] examined changes in leg peak power from 12 to 17 years of age and noted increases of 66% in girls, whilst boys increased peak power by 120% over the same period. The increases noted by Armstrong et al. [132] are similar in magnitude to those of Martin et al. [142] when the same age range is considered. Similar age-related increases in mean power have been noted, again with increases in boys almost double those of girls between the ages of 12 and 17 years [132]. Sex differences in peak leg power do not appear to emerge until about 14 years of age [141], whilst mean power is greater in boys than girls from about 13 years of age [132]. Clearly age is an important predictor of short-term power in young people. The influence of stature and mass as predictors of peak and mean power have also been established [132, 143], highlighting the need to consider both body mass and composition when assessing short-term power. De Ste Croix and colleagues [143] have shown that in addition to the effects of body mass, sum of skinfolds and age, MRI determined thigh muscle volume exerts considerable influence on young people's short-term power output. Furthermore, De Ste Croix and colleagues [143] have shown using multi-level modelling that in addition to the effects of body mass, sum of skinfolds and age, MRI-determined thigh muscle volume has a significant impact on young people's short-term power output during cycling.

There are very few data on skeletal muscle metabolism during short-duration high-intensity exercise in girls. A MRS study of pH and P_i/PCr ratio during supramaximal plantar flexion exercise in pre-pubertal and pubertal girls found that the maturational differences in pH and P_i/PCr values were not statistically significant [144]. The authors concluded that glycolytic metabolism was not maturity dependent; rather, it was dependent on muscle cross-sectional area. A more recent study of the PCr kinetics and intracellular pH response during high-intensity exercise also showed a non significant sex difference in pH. It is worthy of note that in both studies [144, 145] there was considerable variability within small samples which may be masking biological significance. Wilcox et al. [145] did demonstrate that the PCr cost per watt was higher in the girls compared to the boys [145]. These findings suggest lower efficiency in the girls compared to the boys, which may be an outcome of differences in muscle fibre type, muscle activation patterns or leg vasodilatory response. However, this study failed to demonstrate that the differences in the slow component of the PCr response between children and adults were statistically significant, raising doubt that age-related change in muscle fibre recruitment substantially influences skeletal muscle metabolism during high-intensity exercise.

Does Intensive Training Pose a Threat to the Development and Health of Young Girls?

Growth

Many young athletes begin formal training before 10 years of age, with young elite gymnasts, swimmers and tennis players entering their respective sport between the ages of 6 and 7.5 years [146]. In a number of countries young girls are recruited into specialised sport schools as young as 5 years of age [147]. These elite young athletes train intensively all year round, for many hours, with weekly training volumes of 24 h not being unusual [148]. Whether intensive training such as this distorts normal growth and maturation remains a topic of much debate [7, 149].

Evidence of reduced or delayed growth in some young athletes, such as gymnasts, has been suggested to be a direct outcome of the intensive training these youngsters have endured [5, 50, 151]. Counter-argument contends that growth reductions or delay in young athletes simply reflect their late maturation [136, 152–154]. The Training of Young Athletes (TOYA) study found that elite young female swimmers and tennis players were generally taller than the general population throughout the growth period (close to the 75th percentile for stature), whilst gymnasts were generally smaller (below the 50th percentile for stature) from 10 to 17 years of age [146]. What was noteworthy was that by 18 years of age, the gymnasts were above the 50th percentile for stature and when aligned by biological age (years from attainment of menarche), gymnasts, swimmers and tennis players showed no significant differences in height. The catch-up growth noted in the gymnasts was indicative of late maturation and apparent in girls who are not involved in competitive training, but who mature late. Both the fathers and mothers of gymnasts have been found to be significantly shorter than the parents of other athletes and genetic predisposition for stature has been not only been shown to be preserved, but often

exceeded [146, 155]. Combined, this evidence indicates that the tendency for short stature in gymnasts is not, as argued by some [151], evidence of a training-induced alteration in growth, but more likely a reflection of a genetic predisposition for later development and short stature.

Reproductive Health

Menstrual dysfunction in young athletes has also been interpreted as evidence that intensive training in young girls is harmful to reproductive health [156]. Menstrual dysfunction includes delayed menarche (onset after 16 years), luteal phase defects, oligomenorrhea and amenorrhea (table 2). Several studies have concluded that female gymnasts, swimmers and ballet dancers have delayed menarche. De Ridder et al. [29] observed that, in comparison to a control group of girls matched for maturation and fatness, girls involved in competitive gymnastics exhibited delayed menarche. An early hypothesis suggested that because these young girls had low levels of body fat they did not attain a critical level of body fat (22%) necessary for menstruation. The wide variability noted in body fat at menarche [35] has provided proof that a threshold of 22% body fat is incorrect. Additionally, there is sufficient experimental evidence in women to show that it is not body fat but caloric deprivation that affects reproductive health [157].

Genetic predisposition for late menarche in athletes has also been explored. When age of menarche in a group of elite gymnasts was correlated with maternal menarchal age, it was, on average, in lag by 0.81 years [158]. This lag was double that noted for elite swimmers and triple that for elite tennis players. These data suggest that despite a genetic predisposition for delayed menarche, this does not fully explain the extent of the delay, signalling that training may indeed delay menarche in gymnasts. However, Baxter-Jones et al. [158] went on to show that when the time period between menarchal age and retirement from the sport were

Table 2. Components of the female athlete triad, diagnosis and prevention

Component of the triad	Diagnosis	Warning signs	Prevention
Energy availability [160]	Energy availability is defined as energy intake minus exercise energy expenditure, with a threshold of 30 kcal·kg^{-1} LBM·day^{-1}.	Low body mass (>85% of ideal body mass for stature). Fatigue.	Monitor dietary intake. Monitor training volume. Focus on healthy eating and caloric balance. Educate youngsters about nutritional fads. Reinforce message that body mass is only one aspect of good performance. Educational information on nutrition and energy expenditure, e.g. http://kidshealth.org/teen/food/sports/triad.html
Eating disorders [173]	*Anorexia nervosa* Refusal to maintain body mass over a minimally normal mass for age and stature. Intense fear of gaining mass or becoming fat. Disturbed body image. Secondary amenorrhea. *Bulimia nervosa* Recurrent episodes of binge eating (eating a large amount of food in a discrete period of time and lacking control over eating during the episode). Recurrent inappropriate compensatory behaviour such as self-induced vomiting, laxatives or excessive exercise. The binge-eating and purging behaviours occur at least twice a week for 3 months.	*Anorexia* Dramatic loss in body mass. Preoccupation with food, calories and body mass. Wears baggy clothes. Fine, downy facial hair. Mood swings. Avoidance of food-related social activities. *Bulimia* Noticeable loss in body mass. Excessive worry over weight. Bathroom visits after eating. Depression. Strict dieting followed by binging. Dental erosion.	Promote healthy body image. Removal of body mass/fat monitoring by coaches. Provide opportunities for developing self-coping strategies. Deemphasize body mass and thinness. Provide opportunities for nutritional counselling.
Menstrual dysfunction [174]	Oligomenorrhea – irregular menses (length between cycles >35 days). Primary amenorrhea – absence of menstruation by 15 years in girls with secondary sexual characteristics. Secondary amenorrhea- absence of menstrual cycles for 3 cycles after onset of menses.	Irregular or absent menstrual cycle.	Ask athletes to keep a training diary and include monitoring of menstrual cycle. Help girls understand that secondary amenorrhea is not normal. Provide education on reproductive health and the link between menstruation and bone health. Provide dietary education and help girls understand the link between diet and reproductive health.

Component of the triad	Diagnosis	Warning signs	Prevention
	Luteal phase dysfunction – shortened secretory phase of the menstrual cycle, typically less than 10 days.		
Low bone mineral density [175]	If comparison with age, gender, stature and race specific Z-scores yields values ≤2.0 this is classified as a low bone mineral density for chronological age. Osteoporosis is diagnosed if low BMD for chronological age is accompanied by one or more of the following fracture histories: long bone fracture of the lower extremities; vertebral compression fracture and two or more long–bone fractures of the upper extremities.	Secondary amenorrhea. Stress fracture. History of fractures.	Provide educational information on osteoporosis. Provide information on nutrition for bone health, particularly focusing on calcium-rich foods. Monitor diet and provide opportunities for nutritional counselling.

considered, 92% of the girls began menarche prior to retiring. The authors concluded that training was therefore unlikely to cause the delay in menarche noted in the gymnasts, instead there was simply a chronological age difference in the timing of events. It would appear that exercise training, without other predisposing factors, is unlikely to be the cause of menstrual dysfunction.

The Female Athlete Triad

The female athlete triad was established in the early 1990s as a syndrome of three separate, but inter-related conditions, namely menstrual dysfunction, disordered eating and premature osteoporosis [159]. An updated position statement from the American College of Sports Medicine (ACSM) has revised the definition of the triad as the presence of one or more of (1) low energy availability (with or without eating disorders), (2) amenorrhea, and (3) osteoporosis (table 2) [160]. Prevalence estimates of components of the female triad are very dependent on the athletic group studied, with higher rates in sports where low body mass is the norm. For instance, 25% of young women in endurance, weight class or aesthetic sports had clinical eating disorders, compared to 9% of the general population [161]. Secondary amenorrhea has been reported to be as high as 69% in dancers and less than 1% in the general population [162, 163]. Osteoporosis has been found in about 13% of female athletes, although this is not too different from the normal population [164] and in pre-menopausal women low bone mineral density for age is a more appropriate marker than osteoporosis.

Much of the available data on the female triad is on college-age or young adult athletes, with few reports targeting adolescents. Two key studies of high school athletes have shown a considerable number of girls present with components of the female triad. In a study of 170 13- to 18-year-olds, 18% had disordered eating, 24% had oligomenorrhea or amenorrhea and 22% had low bone mass for their age based on WHO diagnostic criteria [165]. A higher rate of occurrence of low energy availability (55%) was noted in a study of 80 similarly aged young athletes, with 16% diagnosed with amenorrhea and using the same WHO diagnostic criteria, 16% presented with low bone mineral density [166]. The existence of the female athlete triad in these young girls is particularly worrying given this is a time when substantial amounts of bone should be accrued.

Energy deficiency appears to be particularly harmful when combined with excessive exercise, and leads to reduced oestrogen levels, athletic amenorrhea and bone demineralisation Loucks et al. [167] have shown that there is an energy availability threshold of 20–25 $kcal \cdot kg^{-1}\ LBM \cdot day^{-1}$, below which skeletal and reproductive health is compromised. This group conducted a number of studies in which women underwent energy availability manipulations, decreasing energy availability from 45 to 20 $kcal \cdot kg^{-1}\ LBM \cdot day^{-1}$ or from 45 to 10 $kcal \cdot kg^{-1}\ LBM \cdot day^{-1}$. These reductions caused blunting of LH pulsatility [168] and a de-linking of bone resorption and formation [169]. The existence of an energy availability threshold may help to explain why not all athletes develop athletic amenorrhea even when following the same training programme and provides a useful marker for nutritional health.

Recent conjecture that the triad is a 'myth' [8] has caused intense debate [164, 170, 171]. This contention stems from a number of criticisms, including flaws in the epidemiological evidence, assumptions that low energy availability implies disordered eating and a lack of experimental evidence in athletes. Much of the epidemiological evidence of the prevalence of the female triad is for individual components of the triad, rather than for the synchronous appearance of all three which, it has been argued, over-inflates the extent of the problems. When occurrence of all three components is examined, prevalence falls dramatically [172]. On the other hand, the definition of the female athlete triad states explicitly that presence of one component is sufficient for diagnosis and the revised guidelines provided by the ACSM, have removed disordered eating and replaced it with energy availability, accepting that low energy availability does not equate to a pathological eating disorder [160].

Definitive conclusions on whether elite participation causes aberrations to skeletal and reproductive health are not possible. Nevertheless, there is clear evidence of a boundary between healthy and unhealthy levels of exertion when coupled with caloric limitation. Exposure to excessive training and caloric limitation causes abnormality in skeletal and reproductive function and regardless of the magnitude of the problem, young girl athletes deserve protection. Protection likely entails athlete education, coach recognition of the triad and the monitoring of both training volume and nutritional health in young elite girls. Table 2 provides an overview of the components of the triad, with possible prevention strategies for young athletes, coaches and parents.

Conclusions

Girls have differential growth and development in comparison to boys, resulting in substantial differences in body size and composition. Whilst stronger and leaner than many of her non-athletic peers, the smaller stature, shorter legs, lower muscularity and greater relative fatness of the elite girl athlete means she is not as strong, nor as fast as her male counterpart. Some discordant responses to exercise are not solely explained by body size and/or composition and there is evidence of underlying qualitative differences which require further clarification.

A young girl's involvement in elite sport predisposes her to increased risk of skeletal and reproductive health problems, particularly in sports where intense training is coupled with the need for leanness. Ensuring girls involved in elite training are in an environment which optimises their athletic potential while minimising risk is a priority. This entails sufficient knowledge of the physiologic responses to exercise in girls, as well as thorough understanding of the female triad disorder, its aetiology and prevention. Despite the burgeoning literature in the field of paediatric exercise physiology, an integrative understanding of girls' physiological responses to exercise remains elusive. Traditional technologies have proved inadequate in providing a detailed understanding of the complexity of the cellular metabolic response to exercise and this is compounded by the need to separate qualitative changes from changes which are an artefact of a growing, maturing body. More recent application of non-invasive imaging techniques and breath-by-breath gas analysis is facilitating a more integrated understanding of the responses to exercise, but the number of studies to date with girls is woefully small. In addition, more needs to be learnt about the female triad and its antecedents in younger girls. The dearth of information on girls and emergence and availability of new technologies provides plenty of scope for future studies in paediatric exercise physiology.

References

1 Armstrong N, Welsman JR, Kirby BJ: Longitudinal changes in 11–13-year-olds' physical activity. Acta Paediatr 2000;89:775–780.

2 Women's Sport and Fitness Foundation: Participation. Factsheet November 2009:http://www.wsff.org.uk/documents/Participation_factsheet_November_09.pdf

3 Women's Sport and Fitness Foundation: WSSF viewpoint – women and the Olympics. Factsheet July 2009:http://www.wsff.org.uk/documents/Women_and_the_Olympics.pdf

4 Vertinsky P: The Eternally Wounded Woman: Women, Doctors and Exercise in the Late Nineteenth Century. Chicago, University of Illinois Press, 1994.

5 Theintz G, Howald H, Weiss U, Sizonenko P: Evidence for a reduction of growth potential in adolescent female gymnasts. J Pediatr 1993;122:306–313.

6 Damsgaard R, Bencke J, Matthiesen G, Petersen J, Müller J: Is prepubertal growth adversely affected by sport? Med Sci Sports Exerc 2000;32:1698–1703.

7 Baxter-Jones ADG, Maffulli N, Mirwald RL: Does elite competition inhibit growth and delay maturation in some gymnasts? Probably not. Pediatr Exerc Sci 2003;15:373–382.

8 DiPietro L, Stachenfeld NS: The myth of the female athlete triad. Br J Sports Med 2006;40:490–493.

9 McManus AM, Armstrong N: The elite child athlete; in Armstrong N, van Mechelen W (eds): Paediatric Exercise Science and Medicine, ed 2. Oxford, Oxford University Press, 2008, pp 489–502.

10 USA Track and Field Age Group Records. http://www.dyestat.com/rivals/227840.html#GIRLS

11 World Junior Records http://www.iaaf.org/statistics/index.html

12 Coast JR, Blevins JS, Wilson BA: Do gender differences in running performance disappear with distance? Can J Appl Physiol 2004;29:139–145.

13 George K, Sharma S, Batterham A, Whyte G, McKenna W: Allometric analysis of the association between cardiac dimensions and body size variables in 464 junior athletes. Clin Sci 2001;100:47–54.

14 Nevill AM, Holder RL: Scaling, normalizing, and per ratio standards: an allometric modeling approach. J Appl Physiol 1995;79:1027–1031.

15 Ao A, Erickson RP, Winston RML, Handysiade A: Transcription of paternal Y-linked genes in the human zygote as early as the pro-nucleate stage. Zygote 1994;2:281–287.

16 Turgeon JL, Carr MC, Maki PM, Mendelsohn ME, Wise PM: Complex actions of sex steroids in adipose tissue, the cardiovascular system and brain: insights from basic science and clinical studies. Endocr Rev 2006;27:575–605.

17 Wells JCK: Sexual dimorphism of body composition. Best Pract Res Clin Endocrinol Metab 2007;21:415–430.

18 Rogol A, Clark P, Roemmich J: Growth and pubertal development in children and adolescents: effects of diet and physical activity. Am J Clin Nutr 2000;72:S521–S528.

19 Mauras N: Growth hormone and testosterone: effects on whole body metabolism and skeletal muscle in adolescence. Horm Res 2006;66:42–48.

20 Baxter-Jones ADG: Growth and maturation; in Armstrong N, van Mechelen W (eds): Paediatric Exercise Science and Medicine, ed 2. Oxford, Oxford University Press, 2008, pp 157–168.

21 Susman EJ, Houts RM, Steinberg L, Belsky J, Cauffman E, Dehart G, Friedman SL, Roisman GI, Halpern-Felsher BL, Eunice Kennedy Shriver NICHD Early Child Care Research Network: Longitudinal development of secondary sexual characteristics in girls and boys between ages 9 1/2 and 15 1/2 years. Arch Pediatr Adolesc Med 2010; 164:166–173.

22 Sherar LB, Baxter-Jones AD, Mirwald RL: Limitations to the use of secondary sex characteristics for gender comparisons. Ann Hum Biol 2004;31:586–593.

23 Malina RM, Bouchard C, Bar-Or O (eds): Growth, Maturation and Physical Activity. Champaign, Human Kinetics, 2004, pp 39–81.

24 Sinclair D, Dangerfield P: Human Growth after Birth, ed 6. Oxford, Oxford University Press, 1988.

25 Claessons AL, Veer FM, Stijnen V, Lefevre J, Maes H, Steens G, Beunen G: Anthropometric characteristics of outstanding male and female gymnasts. J Sports Sci 1991;9:53–74.

26 Damsgaard R, Bencke J, Matthiesen G, Petersen J, Müller J: Body proportions, body composition and pubertal development of children in competitive sports. Scand J Med Sci Sports 2001;11:54–60.

27 Reynolds EL, Wines JV: Individual differences in physical changes associated with adolescence in girls. Am J Dis Child 1948;75:329–350.

28 Tanner JM: Growth at Adolescence, ed 2. Oxford, Blackwell Scientific Publications, 1962.

29 de Ridder C, Thijssen J, Bruning P, Van den Brande J, Zonderland M, Erich W: Body fat mass, body fat distribution, and pubertal development: a longitudinal study of physical and hormonal sexual maturation of girls. J Clin Endocrinol Metab 1992;75:442–446.

30 Kaplowitz P: Pubertal development in girls: secular trends. Curr Opin Obstet Gynecol 2006;18:487–491.

31 Biro FM, Lucky AW, Simbartl LA, Barton BA, Daniels SR, Striegel-Moore R, Kronsberg SS, Morrison JA: Pubertal maturation in girls and the relationship to anthropometric changes: pathways through puberty. J Pediatr 2003;142: 643–646.

32 Malina R: Physical growth and biological maturation of young athletes. Exerc Sport Sci Rev 1994;22:389–434.

33 Baxter-Jones ADG, Eisenmann JC, Sherar LB: Controlling for maturation in pediatric exercise science. Pediatr Exerc Sci 2005;17:18–30.

34 Klentrou P, Plyley M: Onset of puberty, menstrual frequency, and body fat in elite rhythmic gymnasts compared with normal controls. Br J Sports Med 2003; 37:490–494.

35 Sherar LB, Baxter-Jones AD, Mirwald RL: The relationship between body composition and onset of menarche. Ann Hum Biol 2007;34:673–677.

36 Matthews BL, Bennell KL, McKay HA, Khan KM, Baxter-Jones AD, Mirwald RL, Wark JD: The influence of dance training on growth and maturation of young females: a mixed longitudinal study. Ann Hum Biol 2006;33:342–356.

37 Barrack MT, Rauh MJ, Nichols JF: Cross-sectional evidence of suppressed bone mineral accrual among female adolescent runners. J Bone Min Res 2010;25:1850–1857.

38 Rusko H, Rahkila P, Karvinen E: Anaerobic threshold, skeletal muscle enzymes and fibre composition in young female cross-country skiers. Act Physiol Scand 1980;108:263–268.

39 Thorland WG, Johnson GO, Fagot TG, Tharp GD, Hammer RW: Body composition and somatotype characteristics of Junior Olympic athletes. Med Sci Sports Exerc 1981;13:332–338.

40 Malina RM: Regional body composition: age, sex and ethnic variation; in Roche AF, Heysnfield SB, Lohman TG (eds): Human Body Composition. Champaign, Human Kinetics, 1996, pp 217–255.

41 Falk B, Dotan R: Temperature regulation and elite young athletes; in Armstrong N, McManus AM (eds): The Elite Young Athlete. Med Sports Sci. Basel, Karger, 2011, vol 56, pp 126–149.

42 Wells JCK, Williams JE, Chomtho S, Darch T, Grijalva-Eternod C, Kennedy K, Haroun D, Wilson C, Cole TJ, Fewtrll MS: Pediatric reference data for lean tissue properties: density and hydration from age 5 to 20 y. Am J Clin Nutr 2010;91:610–618.

43 Lohman TG: Assessment of body composition in children. Pediatr Exerc Sci 1989;1:19–30.

44 Rogol AD: Growth at puberty: interaction of androgens and growth hormone. Med Sci Sports Exerc 1994;26:767–770.

45 Simoneau JA, Bouchard C: Human variation in skeletal muscle fibre-type proportion and enzyme activities. Am J Physiol 1989;257:E567–E572.

46 Staron RS, Hagerman FC, Hilida RS, Murray TF, Hostler DP, Crill MT, Ragg KE, Toma K: Fiber type composition of the vastus lateralis muscle of young men and women. J Histochem Cytochem 2002;48:623–629.

47 Schrauwen-Hinderling VB, Hesslink MKC, Schrauwen P, Kooi ME: Intramyocellular lipid content in human skeletal muscle. Obesity 2006;14:357–367.

48 Roepstorff C, Steffenson CH, Madsen M, Stallknecht B, Kanstrup L, Richter RA, Riens B: Gender differences in substrate utilization during submaximal exercise in endurance-trained subjects. Am J Physiol Endocrinol Metab 2002;282: E435–E447.

49 Hunter SK, Enoka RM: Sex differences in the fatigability of arm muscles depends on absolute force during isometric contractions. J Appl Physiol 2001;91:2686–2694.

50 Jaworowski Å, Porter MM, Holmbäck AM, Downham D, Lexell J: Enzyme activities in the tibialis anterior muscle of young moderately active men and women: relationship with body composition, muscle cross-sectional area and fibre type composition. Acta Physiol Scand 2002;176:215–225.

51 Legerlotz K, Smith HK, Hing WA: Variation and reliability of ultrasonographic quantification of the architecture of the medial gastrocnemius muscle in young children. Clin Physiol Funct Imaging 2010;30:198–205.

52 De Ste Croix MBA, Armstrong N, Welsman JR, Sharp P: Longitudinal changes in isokinetic leg strength in 10–14 year olds. Ann Hum Biol 2002;29:50–62.

53 O'Brien TD, Reeves ND, Baltzopoulos V, Jones DA, Maganaris CN: In vivo measurements of muscle specific tension in adults and children. Exp Physiol 2009;95:202–210.

54 Nygaard E: Skeletal muscle fibre characteristics in young women. Acta Physiol Scand 1981;112:299–304.

55 Vogler C, Bove KE: Morphology of skeletal muscle in children. Arch Path Lab Med 1985;109:238–242.

56 Glenmark B, Hedberg G, Jansson E: Changes in muscle fibre type from adolescence to adulthood in women and men. Acta Physiol Scand 1992;146:251–259.

57 Glenmark B, Hedberg G, Kaijster L, Jansson E: Muscle strength from adolescence to adulthood: relationship to muscle fibre types. Eur J Appl Physiol Occup Physiol 1994;68:9–19.

58 Lexell J: Human aging, muscle mass, and fibre type composition. J Gerontol 1995;50:11–16.

59 Maffulli N, King JB, Helms P: Training in elite young athletes (the training of young athletes (TOYA study): injuries, flexibility and isometric strength. Br J Sport Med 1994;28:123–136.

60 Bencke J, Damsgaard R, Saekmose A, Jørgensen P, Jørgensen K, Klausen K: Anaerobic power and muscle strength characteristics of 11 years old elite and non-elite boys and girls from gymnastics, team handball, tennis and swimming. Scand J Med Sci Sports 2002;12: 171–178.

61 Schoenau E: Bone mass increase in puberty: what makes it happen? Horm Res 2006;65(Suppl 2):2–10.

62 Kontulainen SA, Macdonald HM, McKay HA: Change in cortical bone density and its distribution differs between boys and girls during puberty. J Clin Endocrinol Metab 2006;91:2555–2561.

63 Högler W, Blimkie CJ, Cowell CT, Kemp AF, Briody J, Wiebe P, Farpour-Lambert N, Duncan CS, Woodhead HJ: A comparison of bone geometry and cortical density at the mid-femur between prepuberty and young adulthood using magnetic resonance imaging. Bone 2003;33:771–778.

64 Schoenau E, Neu MC, Manz F: Muscle mass during childhood: relationship to skeletal development. J Musculoskelet Neuronal Interact 2004;4:105–108.

65 Schoenau E: From mechanostat theory to development of the 'Functional Muscle-Bone-Unit'. J Musculoskelet Neuronal Interact 2005;5:232–238.

66 Ward KA, Roberts SA, Adams JE, Mughal MZ: Bone geometry and density in the skeleton of pre-pubertal gymnasts and school children. Bone 2005;36: 1012–1018.

67 Duncan CS, Blimkie CJR, Cowell CT, Burke ST, Briody JN, Howman-Giles R: Bone mineral density in adolescent female athletes: relationship to exercise type and muscle strength. Med Sci Sports Exerc 2002;34:286–294.

68 Haapasalo H, Kontulainen S, Sievanen H, Kannus P, Jarvinene M, Vuori I: Exercise-induced bone gain is due to enlargement in bone size without a change in volumetric bone density: a peripheral quantitative computed tomography study of the upper arms of male tennis players. Bone 2000;27:351–357.

69 Duncan CS, Blimkie CJR, Kemp A, Higgs W, Cowell CT, Woodhead H, Briody JN, Howman-Giles R: Mid-femur geometry and biomechanical properties in 15- to 18-yr-old female athletes. Med Sci Sports Exerc 2002;34:673–681.

70 Högler W, Blimkie CJR, Cowell CT, Inglis, Rauch F, Kemp AF, Wiebe P, Duncan CS, Farpour-Lambert N, Woodhead HJ: Sex-specific developmental changes in muscle size and bone geometry at the femoral shaft. Bone 2008;42:982–989.

71 Dowthwaite JN, Kanaley JA, Spadaro JA, Hickman RM, Scerpella TA: Muscle indices do not fully account for enhanced upper extremity bone mass and strength in gymnasts. J Musculoskelet Neuronal Interact 2009;9:2–14.

72 Daly RM, Saxon L, Turner CH, Robling AG, Bass SL: The relationship between muscle size and bone geometry during growth and in response to exercise. Bone 2004;34:281–287.

73 Bailey DA, Martin AD: Physical activity and skeletal health in adolescents. Pediatr Exerc Sci 1996;6:330–347.

74 Tanner JM: Fallacy of per-weight and per-surface area standards and their relation to spurious correlation. J Appl Physiol 1949;2:1–15.

75 Guenette A, Sheel AW: Exercise-induced arterial hypoxaemia in active young women. Appl Physiol Nutr 2007;32: 1263–1273.

76 Mota J, Guerra S, Leandro C, Pinto A, Ribeiro JC, Duarte JA: Association of maturation, sex, and body fat in cardiorespiratory fitness. Am J Human Biol 2002;14:707–712.

77 Armstrong N, Welsman JR: Aerobic fitness; in Armstrong N, van Mechelen W (eds): Paediatric Exercise Science and Medicine, ed 2. Oxford, Oxford University Press, 2008, pp 97–108.

78 Nevill AM, Bate S, Holder RL: Modeling physiological and anthropometric variables known to vary with body size and other confounding variables. Year Book Phys Anthropol 2005;48:141–153.

79 Tolfrey K, Barker A, Thom JM, Morse CI, Narici MV, Batterham AM: Scaling of maximal oxygen uptake by lower leg muscle volume in boys and men. J Appl Physiol 2006;100:1851–1856.

80 Rowland T, Goff D, Martel L, Ferrone L, Kline G: Normalization of maximal cardiovascular variables for body size in premenarchal girls. Pediatr Cardiol 2000;21:429–432.

81 Armstrong N, McManus AM, Welsman JR: Aerobic fitness; in Armstrong N, van Mechelen W (eds): Paediatric Exercise Science and Medicine, ed 2. Oxford, Oxford University Press, 2008, pp 269–282.

82 Armstrong N, Welsman JR: Young People and Physical Activity. Oxford, Oxford University Press, 1997.

83 Armstrong N, Welsman JR: Peak oxygen uptake in relation to growth and maturation in 11- to 17-year-old humans. Eur J Appl Physiol 2001;85:546–551.

84 Eisenmann JC, Pivarnik JM, Malina RM: Scaling peak $\dot{V}O_2$ to body mass in young male and female distance runners. J Appl Physiol 2001;90:2172–2180.

85 Baxter-Jones A, Goldstein H, Helms P: The development of aerobic power in young athletes. J Appl Physiol 1993;75: 1160–1167.

86 Welsman JR, Armstrong N: Longitudinal changes in submaximal oxygen uptake in 11- to 13-year-olds. J Sports Sci 2000; 18:183–189.

87 Courteix D, Obert P, Lecoq AM, Guenon P, Kock G: Effect of intensive swimming training on lung volumes, airway resistances and on the maximal expiratory flow-volume relationship in prepubertal girls. Eur J Appl Physiol 1997;76:264–269.

88 Sheel AW, Richards JC, Foster GE, Guenette JA: Sex differences in respiratory exercise physiology. Sports Med 2004;34:567–579.

89 Boezen HM, Jansen DF, Postma DS: Sex and gender differences in lung development and their clinical significance. Clin Chest Med 2004;25:237–245.

90 Harms CA: Does gender affect pulmonary function and exercise capacity? Respir Physiol Neurobiol 2006;151:124–131.

91 Guenette A, Sheel AW: Exercise-induced arterial hypoxaemia in active young women. Appl Physiol Nutr 2007;32: 1263–1273.

92 Olfert IM, Balouch J, Kleinsasser A, Knapp A, Wagner H, Wagner PD, Hopkins SR: Does gender affect human pulmonary gas exchange during exercise? J Physiol 2004;557:529–541.

93 Fawkner SG, Armstrong N: Pulmonary function; in Armstrong N, van Mechelen W (eds): Paediatric Exercise Science and Medicine, ed 2. Oxford, Oxford University Press, 2008, pp 243–254.

94 Armstrong N, Kirby BJ, McManus AM, Welsman JR: Prepubsecents' ventilatory responses to exercise with reference to sex and body size. Chest 1997;112:1554–1560.

95 Rowland TW, Cunningham LN: Development of ventilatory responses to exercise in normal white children. Chest 1997;111:327–332.

96 Hopkins SR, Harms CA: Gender and pulmonary gas exchange during exercise. Exerc Sport Sci Rev 2004;32:50–56.

97 Swain KE, Rosenkranz SK, Beckman B, Harms CA: Expiratory flow limitation during exercise in prepubescent boys and girls: prevalence and implications. J Appl Physiol 2010;108:1267–1274.

98 Laursen PB, Tsang GCK, Smith GJ, van Velzen MV, Ignatova BB, Sprules EB, Chu KS, Coutts KD, McKenzie DC: Incidence of exercise-induced arterial hypoxemia in prepubescent females. Pediatr Pulmonol 2002;34:37–41.

99 Guerro L, Naranjo J, Carranza MD: Influence of gender on ventilatory efficiency during exercise in young children. J Sports Sci 2008;26:1455–1457.

100 Karlberg P, Lind J: Studies of the total amount of hemoglobin and the blood volume in children. 1 Determination of total hemoglobin and blood volume in normal children. Acta Paediatr Scand 1955;44:17–34.

101 Sukarochana K, Parenzan L, Thakurdas N, Kiesewetter WB: Red cell mass determinations in infancy and childhood, with the use of radioactive chromium. J Pediatr 1961;59:903–908.

102 Linderkamp O, Versmold HT, Riegel KP, Betke K: Estimation and prediction of blood volume in infants and children. Eur J Pediatr 1977;125:227–234.

103 Raes A, Van Aken S, Craen M, Donckerwolcke R, Walle JV: A reference frame for blood volume in children and adolescents. BMC Pediatrics 2006;6:3.

104 Dallman PR, Siimes MA: Percentile curves for hemoglobin and red cell volume in infancy and childhood. Pediatrics 1979;94:26–31.

105 Boyadjiev N, Taralov Z: Red blood cell variables in highly trained pubescent athletes: a comparative analysis. Br J Sports Med 2000;34:200–204.

106 Rowland TW: Developmental Exercise Physiology. Champaign, Human Kinetics, 1996, pp 117–140.

107 Larsen JA, Kadish AH: Effects of gender on cardiac arrhythmias. J Cardiovasc Electrophysiol 1998;9:655–664.

108 Wirth A, Trager E, Scheele K, Mayer D, Diehm K, Reischle K, Weicker H: Cardiopulmonary adjustment and metabolic response to maximal and submaximal physical exercise of boys and girls at different stages of maturity. Eur J Appl Physiol 1978;39:29–39.

109 Telford RD, McDonal IG, Ellis LB, Chennells MH, Sandstrom ER, Fuller PJ: Echocardiographic dimensions in trained and untrained 12-year-old-boys and girls. J Sports Sci 1988,6.49–57.

110 Thoren CAR, Asano K: Functional capacity and cardiac function in 10-year-old-boys and girls with high and low running performance; in Ilmarinen J, Valimaki I (eds): Children and Sport: Pediatric Work Physiology. Berlin, Springer, 1984 pp 182–188.

111 Cumming GR: Hemodynamics of supine bicycle exercise in 'normal' children. Am Heart J 1977;93:617–622.

112 Rowland TW, Goff D, Martel L, Ferrone L: Influence of cardiac functional capacity on gender differences in maximal oxygen uptake in children. Chest 2000; 117:629–635.

113 Obert P, Mandigout S, Nottin S, Vinet A, N'Guyen L, Lecoq A: Cardiovascular responses to endurance training in children: effect of gender. Eur J Clin Invest 2003;33:199–208.

114 Winsley RJ, Fulfold J, Roberts AC, Welsman JR, Armstrong N: Sex differences in peak oxygen uptake in prepubertal children. J Sci Med Sport 2009;12: 647–651.

115 Gutin B, Owens S, Trieber F, Mensah G: Exercise hemodynamics and left ventricular parameters in children; in Armstrong N, Kirby B, Welsman J (eds): Children and Exercise. Part XIX. London, E & FN Spon, 1997, pp 460–464.

116 Osika W, Dangardt F, Montgomery SM, Volkmann R, Li MG, Friberg P: Sex differences in peripheral artery intima, media and intima media thickness in children and adolescents. Atherosclerosis 2009;203:172–177.

117 Gavin KM, Seals DR, Silver AE, Moreau KL: Vascular endothelial estrogen receptor alpha is modulated by estrogen status and related to endothelial function and endothelial nitric oxide synthase in healthy women. J Clin Endocrinol Metab 2009;94:3513–3520.

118 Nadland IH, Walloc L, Toska K: Effect of the leg muscle pump on the rise in muscle perfusion during muscle work in humans. Eur J Appl Physiol 2009;105: 829–841.

119 Rowland T, Lisowski R: Hemodynamic responses to increasing cycle cadence in 11-year old boys: role of the skeletal muscle pump. Int J Sports Med 2001;22: 405–409.

120 Armstrong N, Welsman JR: Cardiovascular responses to submaximal treadmill running in 11 to 13 year olds. Acta Paediatr 2002;91:125–131.

121 Constantin-Theodosiu D, Greenhaff PL, McIntyre DB, Round JM, Jones DA: Anaerobic energy production in human skeletal muscle in intense contraction: a comparison of ^{31}P magnetic resonance spectroscopy and biochemical techniques. Exp Physiol 1997;82:592–601.

122 Barker A, Welsman J, Welford D, Fulford J, Williams C, Armstrong N: Reliability of ^{31}P magnetic resonance spectroscopy during an exhaustive exercise test in children. Eur J Appl Physiol 2006;98: 556–565.

123 Armstrong N, Fawkner SG: Exercise metabolism; in Armstrong N, van Mechelen W (eds): Paediatric Exercise Science and Medicine, ed 2. Oxford, Oxford University Press, 2008, pp 213–226.

124 Jones AM, Poole DC: Oxygen uptake dynamics: from muscle to mouth-an introduction to the symposium. Med Sci Sports Exerc 2005;37:1542–1550.

125 Barker AR, Welsman JR, Fulford J, Welford D, Williams CA, Armstrong N: Muscle phosphocreatine and pulmonary oxygen uptake kinetics in children at the onset and offset of moderate intensity exercise. Eur J Appl Physiol 2008;102: 727–738.

126 Fawkner SG, Armstrong N: Oxygen uptake kinetic response to exercise in children. Sports Med 2003;33:651–669.

127 Fawkner SG, Armstrong N, Potter CR, Welsman JR: Oxygen uptake kinetics in children and adults after the onset of moderate-intensity exercise. J Sports Sci 2002;20:319–326.

128 Barker AR, Welsman JR, Fulford J, Welford D, Armstrong N: Muscle phosphocreatine kinetics in children and adults at the onset and offset of moderate-intensity exercise. J Appl Physiol 2008;105:446–456.

129 Fawkner SG, Armstrong N: Longitudinal changes in the kinetic response to heavy intensity exercise. J Appl Physiol 2004; 97:460–466.

130 Barker AR, Welsman JR, Fulford J, Welford D, Armstrong N: Quadriceps muscle energetic during incremental exercise in children and adults. Med Sci Sports Exerc 2011;42:1303–1313.

131 Rowland TW: Circulatory responses to exercise: are we misleading Fick? Chest 2005;127:1023–1030.

132 Armstrong N, Welsman JR, Williams CA, Kirby BJ: Longitudinal changes in young people's short-term power output. Med Sci Sports Exerc 2000;32:1140–1145.

133 Thorland WG, Johnson GO, Cisar CJ, Housh TJ, Tharp GD: Strength and anaerobic responses of elite young female sprint and distance runners. Med Sci Sports Exerc 1987;19:56–61.

134 Blimkie CJ, Roche P, Bar-Or O: The anaerobic power ratio in adolescent boys and girls; in Rutenfranz J, Mocellin R, Klimt F (eds): Children and Exercise XII. International Series on Sport Science. Champaign, Human Kinetics, 1986, pp 31–37.

135 Palgi Y, Gutin B, Young J, Alejandro D: Physiological and anthropometric factors underlying endurance performance in children. Int J Sports Med 1984;5:67–73.

136 Bar-Or O: Pediatric Sports Medicine for the Practitioner (Comprehensive Manual in Pediatrics). New York, Springer, 1983.

137 Doré E, Bedu M, França NM, Van Praagh E: Anaerobic cycling performance characteristics in prepubescent, adolescent and young adult females. Eur J Appl Physiol 2001;84:476–481.

138 Aucouturier J, Lazaar N, Doré E, Meyer M, Ratel S, Duché P: Cycling peak power in obese and lean 6–8 year-old girls and boys. Appl Physiol Nutr Metab 2007;32: 367–371.

139 Van Praagh E: Development of anaerobic function during childhood and adolescence. Pediatr Exerc Sci 1990;2:336–348.

140 Williams CA, Armstrong N: Optimised peak power output of adolescent children during maximal sprint pedalling; in Ring FJ (ed): Children in Sport. Proc 1st Bath Sports Medicine Conference. Bath, University of Bath, 1995, pp 40–44.

141 Bencke J, Damsgaard R, Saekmose A, Jørgensen P, Jørgensen K, Klausen K: Anaerobic power and muscle strength characteristics of 11 years old elite and non-elite boys and girls from gymnastics, team handball, tennis and swimming. Scand J Med Sci Sports 2002;12: 171–178.

142 Martin RJF, Doré E, Twisk J, Van Praagh E, Hautier CA, Bedu M: Longitudinal changes of maximal short-term peak power in girls and boys during growth. Med Sci Sports Exerc 2004;36:498–503.

143 De Ste Croix MBA, Armstrong N, Chia MYH, Welsman JR, Parsons G, Sharpe P: Changes in short-term power output in 10- to 12-year-olds. J Sport Sci 2001;19: 141–148.

144 Peterson SR, Gaul CA, Stanton MM, Hanstock CC: Skeletal muscle metabolism during short-term, high-intensity exercise in prepubertal and pubertal girls. J Appl Physiol 1999;87:2151–2156.

145 Wilcocks RJ, Williams CA, Barker AR, Fulford J, Armstrong N: Age- and sex-related differences in muscle phosphocreatine and oxygenation kinetics during high-intensity exercise in adolescents and adults. NMR Biomed 2010; 3:569–577.

146 Erlandson MC, Sherar LB, Mirwald RL, Maffulli N, Baxter-Jones AD: Growth and maturation of adolescent female gymnasts, swimmers, and tennis players. Med Sci Sports Exerc 2008;40:34–42.

147 Hong F: Innocence lost: child athletes in China. Sport Society 2004;7:338–354.

148 Lang M: Surveillance and conformity in competitive youth swimming. Sport Educ Society 2010;15:19–37.

149 Caine D, Bass S, Daly R: Does elite competition inhibit growth and delay maturation in some gymnasts? Quite possibly. Pediatr Exerc Sci 2003;15:360–372.

150 Klentrou P, Plyley M: Onset of puberty, menstrual frequency, and body fat in elite rhythmic gymnasts compared with normal controls. Br J Sports Med 2003;37:490–494.

151 Bass S, Bradney G, Pearce E, Hendrich E, Inge K, Stuckey S, Lo SK, Seeman E: Short stature and delayed puberty in gymnasts: influence of selection bias on leg length and the duration of training on trunk length. J Pediatr 2000;1136: 149–155.

152 Georgopoulos N, Markou K, Theodoropoulou A, Paraskevopoulou P, Varaki L, Kazantzi Z, Leglise M, Vagenakis AG: Growth and pubertal development in elite female rhythmic gymnasts. J Clin Endocrinol Metab 1999;84:4525–4530.

153 Georgopoulos NA, Markou KB, Theodoropoulou A, Vagenakis GA, Benardot D, Leglise M, Dikmopoulos JCA, Vagenakis AP: Height velocity and skeletal maturation in elite female rhythmic gymnasts. J Clin Endocrinol Metab 2001;86:5159–5164.

154 Theodoropoulou A, Markou KB, Vagenakis GA, Benardot D, Leglise M, Kourounis G, Vagenakis AP, Georgopoulos NA: Delayed but normally progressed puberty is more pronounced in artistic compared with rhythmic elite gymnasts due to the intensity of training. J Clin Endocrinol Metab 2005; 90:6022–6027.

155 Baxter-Jones ADG, Helms PJ: Effects of training at a young age: a review of the Training of Young Athletes (TOYA) Study. Pediatr Exerc Sci 1996;8:310–327.

156 Constantini NW, Warren MP: Menstrual dysfunction in swimmers: a distinct entity. J Clin Endocrinol Metab 1995;80: 2740–2744.

157 Loucks AB: Energy availability, not body fatness, regulates reproductive function in women. Exerc Sport Sci Rev 2003;31: 144–148.

158 Baxter-Jones ADG, Helms P, Baines-Preece J, Preece M: Menarche in intensively training gymnasts, swimmers and tennis players. Ann Hum Biol 1994;21: 407–415.

159 Otis CL, Drinkwater B, Johnson M, Loucks A, Wilmore J: American College of Sports Medicine position stand: the female athlete triad. Med Sci Sports Exerc 1997;29:i–ix.

160 Nattiv A, Loucks AB, Manore MM, Sanborn CF, Sundgot-Borgen J, Warren MP, American College of Sports Medicine: American College of Sports Medicine position stand: the female athlete triad. Med Sci Sports Exerc 2007;39: 1867–1882.

161 Sundgot-Borgen J, Torstveit MK: Prevalence of eating disorders in elite athletes is higher than in the general population. Clin J Sport Med 2004;14: 25–32.

162 Abraham SF, Beumont PJ, Fraser IS, Llewellyn-Jones D: Body weight, exercise and menstrual status among ballet dancers in training. Br J Obstet Gynaecol 1982;89:507–510.

163 Chumlea WC, Schubert CM, Roche AF, Kulin HE, Lee PA, Himes JH, Sun SS: Age at menarche and racial comparisons in US girls. Pediatrics 2003;111:110–113.

164 Beals, KA, Meyer NL: Female athlete triad update. Clin Sports Med 2007;26: 69–89.

165 Nichols JF, Rauh MJ, Lawson MJ, Ming JI, Barkai HS: Prevalence of the female athlete triad syndrome among high school athletes. Arch Pediatr Adoesc Med 2006;160:137–142.

166 Hoch AZ, Pajewski NM, Moraski L, Carrera GF, Wilson CR, Hoffmann RG, Schimke JE, Gutterman DD: Prevalence of the female athlete triad in high school athletes and sedentary students. Clin J Sport Med 2009;19:421–428.

167 Loucks AB, Heath EM: Induction of low T_3 syndrome in exercising women occurs at a threshold of energy availability. Am J Physiol 1994;226:R817–R823.

168 Loucks AB, Thurma JA: Luteinizing hormone pulsatility is disrupted at a threshold of energy availability in regularly menstruating women. J Clin Endocrinol Metab 2003;88:297–311.

169 Ihle R, Loucks AB: Dose-response relationships between energy availability and bone turnover in young exercising women. J Bone Miner Res 2004;19: 1231–1240.

170 Loucks AB: Refutation of 'the myth of the female athlete triad'. Br J Sports Med 2007;41:55–57.

171 De Souza MJ, Vescovi JD, Willijmas NI, Van Heest JL, Warren MP: Correction of misinterpretation and misrepresentations of the female athlete triad. Br J Sports Med 2007;41:58–59.

172 Klungland-Torstveig M, Sundgot-Borgen J: The female athlete triad exists in both elite athletes and controls. Med Sci Sports Exerc 2005;37:1449–1459.

173 American Psychiatric Association: Eating disorders; in First M (ed): Diagnostic and Statistical Manual of Mental Disorders, ed 4. Washington, American Psychiatric Publishing, 1994 pp 539–550.

174 Practice Committee of the American Society for Reproductive Medicine: Current evaluation of amenorrhea. Fertil Steril 2004;82:266–272.

175 Bianchi ML, Baim S, Bishop NJ, Gordon CM, Hans DB, Langman CB, Leonard MB, Kalkwarf HJ: Official positions of the International Society for Clinical Densitometry (ISCD) on DXA evaluation in children and adolescents. Pediatr Nephrol 2010;25:37–47.

Dr. Alison M. McManus
Institute of Human Performance, University of Hong Kong
Hong Kong, SAR (China)
Tel. +852 2589 0582, Fax +852 2855 1712, E-Mail alimac@hku.hk

Chapter 3

Armstrong N, McManus AM (eds): The Elite Young Athlete.
Med Sport Sci. Basel, Karger, 2011, vol 56, pp 47–58

Nutrition and Elite Young Athletes

Asker Jeukendrup[a] · Linda Cronin[b]

[a]School of Sport and Exercise Sciences, University of Birmingham, Birmingham, [b]Roehampton University, London, UK

Abstract

Nutrition can play an essential role in the health of elite young athletes as well as exercise performance. Children and adolescents need adequate energy intake to ensure proper growth, development, and maturation. In addition, the requirements may further increase with increasing exercise training. There are, however, several metabolic differences that result in slightly different advice for young versus adult athletes. For example, younger athletes generally rely more on fat as a fuel, have smaller glycogen stores and have a limited glycolytic capacity. This would imply reduced carbohydrate requirements but a greater capacity to oxidize fat. There are also differences in thermoregulation, although the exact impact on fluid requirements is not clear. The limited evidence suggests that acute energy and fluid imbalances can be detrimental to performance and there may be benefits of ingesting carbohydrate and fluid during exercise, especially during more prolonged exercise. Exogenous carbohydrate oxidation rates have been reported to contribute more to energy expenditure in children. This may, however, simply be a reflection of the fact that the oxidation of this carbohydrate is not limited by body size, but by absorption. Absorption rates are likely to be similar in children and adults and therefore exogenous carbohydrate oxidation rates should be comparable. The relative contribution will therefore be higher because of the lower absolute intensities in children. There are a large number of questions still unanswered and sports nutrition advice to the elite young athlete is largely extrapolated from the adult population. Therefore, more research is needed in the years to come to give better advice to these young athletes.

Copyright © 2011 S. Karger AG, Basel

For many children and adolescents who are strongly committed to sport, nutrition is not on the radar. However, nutrition is a major component of their training. Nutrition interacts not only with growth and development, but also with recovery, performance, avoiding injury and problems that may arise as a result of deficiencies. Nutrition is important for both health and performance. This chapter addresses some of the main nutritional issues of young athletes and discusses nutrition for children from the age of 6 to 20 years. Where no evidence is available, information on young adults will be used.

Energy Requirements

The growth of pre-pubertal children (between 2 and 10 years) is linear and occurs at a relatively constant rate of 6 cm per year. The median heights and weights for boys and girls are similar, averaging 87 cm and 12 kg at the age of 2 years to 137 cm and 32 kg by the age of 10 years. Even in childhood, boys tend to have slightly greater lean tissue mass and a lower proportion of body fat than girls. Children and adolescents need adequate energy intake to ensure proper growth, development, and maturation. Dietary reference values (DRVs) have been established for various ages. The athletic or very active child or adolescent generally will have needs in excess of this level due to the greater energy expenditure from their higher levels of physical activity. It is difficult to establish a DRV for energy for this group because of very large inter-individual variability. In adolescents in particular the onset of the growth spurt, which is a major impetus for increased energy requirements, is unpredictable. Prolonged inadequate energy intake may result in short stature, delayed puberty, menstrual irregularities or absence, poor bone health and increased risk of injuries [1]. Certain categories of young athletes are more at risk for developing eating disorders like distance runners, jumpers and gymnasts.

It is important to realise that it is impossible to derive estimations of energy expenditure for children based on adult data. It has repeatedly been demonstrated that children are less metabolically efficient during motor activities, resulting in higher energy requirements per kilogram body mass during activities. For example, one study reported that children require 30% more energy during running [2]. There may be several explanations for the higher energy expenditures. First, children have a higher resting metabolic rate, but they also have a disadvantageous stride frequency and stride length (imposed by shorter limbs). Traditionally, it has been stated that children's lower mechanical efficiency would negatively affect the regulation of their body temperature, however this supposition was based upon studies that did not exercise children and adults at the same relative exercise intensity and so children were actually working at a higher exercise intensity than adults, consequently resulting in higher heat production. Similarly, the initial studies did not account for children's shorter leg length (i.e. their higher stride frequency), nor account for how this would affect the metabolic cost of any exercise undertaken. However, if when comparing thermoregulation effects in children and adults relative exercise intensity is calculated by adjusting treadmill speed to stride frequency, the differences between adults' and children's energy expenditure and exercise economy disappear [3]. Thermoregulation in children has been discussed in more detail by Falk and Dotan [4].

It is important to educate children to eat a healthy and balanced diet and to encourage good eating habits. This can reinforce lifelong eating habits that contribute to the overall well-being of children and may enhance performance. On the other hand, any bad habits are difficult to get rid of later in a sporting career and should therefore be avoided. There is an important role for both coach and parents to encourage appropriate eating behaviours, but also to avoid bad habits such as too much attention to body weight (see section on weight management).

Exercise Metabolism in Children

The quality of the muscle – rather than the quantity – is a major determinant of substrate utilisation. Studies in adults clearly show a correlation between mitochondrial density of the muscle and fat metabolism (i.e. the more mitochondria, the higher fat oxidation rates during exercise). There also seems to be a correlation between muscle fibre type and substrate metabolism with higher percentage type I fibres favouring fat metabolism. For obvious reasons, very few studies have investigated muscle composition in children. However, a study by Bell et al. [5] found a similar mitochondrial to myofibrillar volume ratio in children and adults, indicating that with growth and maturation, increases in muscle mass are paralleled by an increase in mitochondria within these fibres. The maximal oxygen uptakes ($\dot{V}O_2$ max) of these children were similar to the $\dot{V}O_2$ max of an average adult (45 ml $\bullet$ kg^{-1} $\bullet$ min^{-1}) and it was argued that the oxidative capacity of children could be further developed later in life when an endurance training programme was followed (or reduced when a sedentary lifestyle was adopted). In one study muscle fibre type composition was determined in a large number of 16-year-olds and reassessed 10 years later when they were biopsied again to determine the muscle fibre type composition [6, 7]. It was concluded that fibre type did not change significantly (~52% type I fibres, 33% type IIA and 15% type IIX). Based on the limited information available it seems fair to conclude that there are no major shifts in muscle fibre type or composition with age, however, mitochondrial density can be increased with specific training.

Even though the phenotypic characteristics of the muscle may be similar in children and adults, there do appear to be differences in substrate utilisation. These differences have been discussed in more detail elsewhere [8] but include a lower glycolytic capacity, a higher oxidative capacity and higher rates of fat oxidation. For more detailed reviews the reader is referred to Riddell [8] and Boisseau and Delamarche [9].

In brief, studies using indirect calorimetry suggest that the proportion of fatty acids to carbohydrates used for energy during exercise is different in children than in adults, possibly due to children's smaller endogenous carbohydrate stores. In fact, the contribution of fatty acid oxidation towards energy production has been reported to be larger for both girls and boys than it is for adults [8, 10–12], suggesting that children are well equipped for sustained aerobic activity, but that their capacity for anaerobic performance may be limited by their maturation status [9, 13]. This difference, however, seems to diminish throughout adolescence, especially in boys [8, 14], suggesting that the hormones associated with puberty (i.e. growth hormone, insulin-like growth factor, sex steroids and catecholamines) play an influential role in controlling the regulation of energy metabolism in children [9]. In fact, pubertal development has long been associated with a period of insulin resistance and reduced insulin-stimulated glucose disposal at rest in pubescent children, when compared to pre-pubertal children and is probably caused by the conservation of carbohydrate stores for the energy requirements of growth. This difference in substrate utilisation in children seems to exist until mid- to late puberty, after which a more 'adult-like metabolic profile' seems to be evident [14]. It has been suggested that as fat metabolism appears to be more dominant in exercising children than in adults, children may possibly have a reduced requirement for dietary carbohydrates, particularly prepubescent children [12, 15].

Protein

In order to support growth and development, children and adolescents have protein requirements that are relatively high compared to adults. The Recommended Daily Allowances (RDAs) for protein in the United States and Canada are displayed in table 1. However, the protein requirements for young elite athletes are likely to be higher. Boisseau et al. [16] studied protein requirements of 14-year-old soccer players, who played 10–12 h per week, using nitrogen balance measurements. The estimated daily protein needed to maintain nitrogen balance was 1.04 $g \cdot kg^{-1} \cdot day^{-1}$. It was suggested that the RDA for protein for these young athletes was 1.40 $g \cdot kg^{-1} \cdot day^{-1}$ (or 75 $g \cdot day^{-1}$ in this group), which would be well above the RDA for non-athletic children (52 $g \cdot day^{-1}$) [17]. However, as is the case with adult athletes [18] this requirement is quite easily met. The study in soccer players was performed in France and the suggested RDA of 1.40 $g \cdot kg^{-1} \cdot day^{-1}$ is still well below the average protein intake by that age group in France (2.07 $g \cdot kg^{-1} \cdot day^{-1}$). In the United States [19] and in Australia protein intake by children and adolescents are generally 2–3 times the RDA (USA) or recommendations in the United Kingdom (table 1) or Australia (not listed). Even in sports where elite young athletes were reported to restrict energy intakes, protein intakes were still between 1.5–2.0 $g \cdot kg^{-1} \cdot day^{-1}$ [1]. Although on the whole protein requirements seem to be no particular concern in young athletes, it is important to be aware that there may be individuals who, perhaps through a

Table 1. Recommended protein intake for boys and girls versus typical intake in USA and Australia

Gender and age		Recommendations			Examples of reported intake, g/day	
		RDA USA and Canada g/kg/day	RDA, g/day	GDA, UK g/day	P intake in USA	P intake in AUS
Males	1–3 years	1.05	13		55	
	4–8 years	0.95	19	20 (4–6 years)	66	64
	9-13 years	0.95	34	28-41 (7–10 years, 11–14 years)	81	75
	14–18 years	0. 85	52	45 (14–16 years)	97	120
	19–30 years	0.80	56	56	109	
Females	1–3 years	1.05	13		55	
	4–8 years	0.95	19	20 (4–6 years)	66	64
	9–13 years	0.95	34	28–41 (7–10 years, 11–14 years)	68	75
	14–18 years	0.85	46	45 (14–16 years)	68	80
	19–30 years	0.80	46	45	72	

These data show that recommendations are exceeded and, at least at the group level, protein intake is more than adequate. RDA data derived from Dietary Reference Intakes (DRIs): Recommended Intakes for Individuals, Macronutrients. Food and Nutrition Board, Institute of Medicine, National Academies, 2005 [17] and Working Group Report. Guideline Daily Amounts (GDA) derived from report of the IGD/PIC Industry Nutrition Strategy Group Technical Working Group on Guideline Daily Amounts (GDAs). Watford, UK. IGD, 2005 [20]. Intake data from references [19] USA and [21] Australia.

combination of energy restriction and a vegetarian diet, have a very low protein intake.

Carbohydrates

It has been shown that carbohydrate ingestion in adults both before and during exercise can delay fatigue and improve endurance performance. Unlike protein which has a quite general recommendation, recommendations for carbohydrate intake highly depend on the intensity, type and duration of exercise that is performed by young athletes. Carbohydrate loading is a technique that is often used by adult athletes to maximize muscle glycogen stores and enhance endurance exercise performance. Glycogen loading is not advised for children [22] but since most events will be shorter and glycolytic capacity is limited, it must be questioned whether such a strategy would be beneficial at all. A relatively high carbohydrate diet is advised but there is probably no need to follow a dedicated glycogen loading regimen.

During exercise in adults carbohydrates can help by maintaining high rates of total carbohydrate oxidation, sparing endogenous muscle glycogen stores and maintaining blood glucose concentrations, particularly in the later stages of exercise [for reviews, see 23, 24]. In addition to these metabolic effects there is also evidence to suggest that carbohydrates may affect central drive (or motivation) too, possibly via oral carbohydrate receptors [25–27].

In contrast, neither glucose consumption before [28] or during [11] exercise has been reported to improve performance time in male adolescents. In fact, in a study by Riddell et al. [11], twelve 10- to 14-year-old boys intermittently drank either water or a 6% glucose drink whilst undertaking 90 min of cycling at 55% peak $\dot{V}O_2$, followed by an all-out performance ride to volitional exhaustion at 90% peak power. Although there was a trend for the glucose solution to improve performance time (occurring in seven of the 12 boys), this finding was not consistent and no significant differences were found in performance between the two drinks (water session: 142 ± 37 s vs. glucose: 177 ± 33 s). Interestingly though, the same study showed that drinking a 3% glucose plus 3% fructose solution did result in cycling time significantly improving by ~40% (202 ± 40 s). Although this finding of an improved performance with a glucose plus fructose drink has also been reported in adult studies [29], the mechanisms may be very different, as the amounts of carbohydrate ingested in these studies were much larger and the exercise duration longer. In addition to enhancing exercise performance in endurance exercise, carbohydrate ingestion has also been shown to increase performance in intermittent, high-intensity exercise [30] and increase explosive strength and speed, as well as shooting skill performance [31] in a basketball skill test.

Furthermore, the subjective rating of perceived exertion (RPE) may also be influenced by carbohydrate ingestion. In another study by Riddell et al. [32], it was reported that when healthy boys aged 13–19 years periodically drank a carbohydrate drink (2% glucose and 4% sucrose), whilst completing a cycle test at 60% $\dot{V}O_2$ max, their subjective rating of exercise intensity was significantly decreased by 1–2 points (RPE scale).

Beneficial effects of carbohydrate ingestion on subjective ratings of perceived exertion have been reported in healthy adults too, although interestingly in the boys the effect occurred after just 60 min of moderate intensity cycling, rather than after 90–120 min, commonly reported in adult studies. This effect occurring earlier in children could be due to be the result of smaller carbohydrate stores in children and therefore their earlier reliance on exogenous carbohydrate. It must be noted, however, that this finding was not reproduced in a more recent study, where ingestion of a 6% carbohydrate-electrolyte solution was found to have no effect on RPE in boys during a 60 min cycling test at ~70% peak $\dot{V}O_2$ [12].

It has been suggested that the ingestion of carbohydrates may alter the substrates used by exercising children. Indeed, Riddell et al. [33] reported that the ingestion of a ^{13}C-labeled glucose solution induced a sparing of endogenous glucose utilization in boys (from 68 to 59% of total energy utilization) and decreased fat utilization (from 32 to 18% of total energy expended). Furthermore, subsequent studies have also reported that children appear to oxidize relatively more exogenous carbohydrate during exercise than do adults [11, 12], despite their lower whole body rate of carbohydrate oxidation and much higher rate of fat oxidation. In fact, one study looking at the effect of pubertal status and age on exogenous carbohydrate oxidation reported that exogenous carbohydrate oxidation contributed to ~30% of the total energy expenditure in the pre-pubertal and early pubertal boys, compared to only ~24% in the mid-to-late pubertal boys. It was suggested that the reliance on exogenous carbohydrate oxidation during exercise is sensitive to pubertal status, rather than just chronological age [12].

51 Shi X, Summers R, Schedl H, Flanagan S, Chang R, Gisolfi C: Effects of carbohydrate type and concentration and solution osmolality on water absorption. Med Sci Sports Exerc 1995;27:1607–1615.

52 Meyer F, Bar-Or O, Salsberg A, Passe D: Hypohydration during exercise in children: effect on thirst, drink preferences, and rehydration. Int J Sport Nutr 1994;4:22–35.

53 Sawka MN, Burke LM, Eichner ER, Maughan RJ, Montain SJ, Stachenfeld NS: American College of Sports Medicine position stand: exercise and fluid replacement. Med Sci Sports Exerc 2007;39:377–390.

54 Climatic heat stress and the exercising child and adolescent. American Academy of Pediatrics Committee on Sports Medicine and Fitness. Pediatrics 2000;106:158–159.

55 Nieper A: Nutritional supplement practices in UK junior national track and field athletes. Br J Sports Med 2005;39:645–649.

56 McDowall JA: Supplement use by young athletes. J Sports Sci Med 2007;6:337–342.

57 O'Dea JA: Consumption of nutritional supplements among adolescents: usage and perceived benefits. Health Educ Res 2003;18:98–107.

58 Petroczi A, Naughton DP, Pearce G, Bailey R, Bloodworth A, McNamee M: Nutritional supplement use by elite young UK athletes: fallacies of advice regarding efficacy. J Int Soc Sports Nutr 2008;5:22.

59 Petroczi A, Naughton DP, Mazanov J, Holloway A, Bingham J: Performance enhancement with supplements: incongruence between rationale and practice. J Int Soc Sports Nutr 2007;4:19.

60 Petroczi A, Naughton DP, Mazanov J, Holloway A, Bingham J: Limited agreement exists between rationale and practice in athletes' supplement use for maintenance of health: a retrospective study. Nutr J 2007;6:34.

61 Geyer H, Parr MK, Koehler K, Mareck U, Schanzer W, Thevis M: Nutritional supplements cross-contaminated and faked with doping substances. J Mass Spectrom 2008;43:892–902.

62 Promotion of healthy weight control practices in young athletes. Pediatrics 2005;116:1557–1564.

63 Manore MM, Kam LC, Loucks AB: The female athlete triad: components, nutrition issues, and health consequences. J Sports Sci 2007;25(suppl 1):S61–S71.

Prof. A.E. Jeukendrup
School of Sport and Exercise Sciences
University of Birmingham
Birmingham B15 2TT (UK)
Tel. +44 0 121 414 4124, Fax +44 0 121 414 4121, E-Mail A.E.Jeukendrup@bham.ac.uk

Chapter 4

Armstrong N, McManus AM (eds): The Elite Young Athlete.
Med Sport Sci. Basel, Karger, 2011, vol 56, pp 59–83

Endurance Training and Elite Young Athletes

Neil Armstrong · Alan R. Barker

Children's Health and Exercise Research Centre, University of Exeter, Exeter, UK

Abstract

Endurance training consists of a structured exercise programme that is sustained for a sufficient length of time with sufficient intensity and frequency to induce an improvement in aerobic fitness. Elite young athletes generally have higher peak oxygen uptakes (peak $\dot{V}O_2$) than their untrained peers largely due to their greater maximal stroke volumes. Trained young athletes have faster $\dot{V}O_2$ kinetic responses to step changes in exercise intensity but whether this is due to enhanced oxygen delivery or increased oxygen utilization by the muscles remains to be explored. Blood lactate accumulation in young athletes during submaximal exercise is lower than in untrained youth and this appears to be due to enhanced oxidative function in the active muscles. No well-designed, longitudinal endurance training studies of elite young athletes have been published. Even in the general paediatric population peak $\dot{V}O_2$ is the only component of aerobic fitness on which there are sufficient data to examine dose-response effects of endurance training. The existence of a maturational threshold below which children are not trainable remains to be proven. The magnitude of training responses is independent of sex. Pre-training peak $\dot{V}O_2$ has a moderate but significant inverse relationship with post-training peak $\dot{V}O_2$ which suggests that elite young athletes are likely to experience smaller increases in peak $\dot{V}O_2$ with further endurance training than untrained youth. Empirical evidence strongly indicates that both trained and untrained young people can benefit from endurance training but the relative intensity of exercise required for optimum benefits is higher than that recommended for adults.

Endurance training consists of a structured exercise programme that is sustained for a sufficient length of time and at sufficient intensity and frequency to induce an improvement in aerobic fitness. Aerobic fitness may be defined as the ability to deliver oxygen to the muscles and to utilize it to generate energy through aerobic metabolism to support muscle activity during exercise.

Peak oxygen uptake (peak $\dot{V}O_2$), the highest rate at which a child or adolescent can consume oxygen during exercise, is widely recognized as the best single indicator of young people's aerobic fitness [1]. Peak $\dot{V}O_2$ limits the rate at which oxygen can be provided during exercise and is therefore a key component of high level performance in many sports (e.g. aspects of cycling and track athletics) but it does not describe fully all aspects of sport-related aerobic fitness [2]. In several sports (e.g. football, hockey, basketball), intermittent exercise and the ability to engage in rapid changes of pace is at least as important as achieving and maintaining maximal aerobic performance. Under these conditions, it is the transient kinetics of $\dot{V}O_2$ which describe the relevant component of aerobic fitness [3]. During sustained exercise lactate accumulates within the muscle and, although output does not match production, some lactate diffuses into the blood where, during submaximal exercise, it accumulates and can be sampled and analysed to provide an estimate of the relative anaerobic and aerobic contribution to the exercise. Blood lactate accumulation is therefore a useful indicator of aerobic fitness with reference to the ability to sustain submaximal exercise as in long distance running [4].

Numerous cross-sectional studies have demonstrated that elite young athletes show higher aerobic fitness than their non-athletic or untrained peers but, although interesting, these data are limited by the inability to establish cause and effect from endurance training. To determine the endurance trainability of children and adolescents (i.e. the extent to which the physiological markers of aerobic fitness change as a result of regular participation in appropriate exercise) requires longitudinal endurance training studies but understanding has been clouded by the paucity of well-designed investigations.

This chapter briefly describes the principal components of aerobic fitness, outlines studies comparing and contrasting the aerobic fitness of trained and untrained youth, and explores the mechanisms underpinning changes in aerobic fitness with endurance training. There are insufficient data to rigorously analyse the effects of endurance training on the aerobic fitness of elite young athletes. Even in the general paediatric population peak $\dot{V}O_2$ is the only component of aerobic fitness on which there are sufficient secure data to examine the dose-response effect of endurance training. The chapter therefore concludes with a systematic review of well-designed studies of the response of peak $\dot{V}O_2$ to endurance training in healthy young people and provides evidence-based recommendations for exercise prescription for the promotion of aerobic fitness during youth.

Peak Oxygen Uptake

Young people's peak $\dot{V}O_2$ has been extensively documented since the pioneering studies of Robinson [5] and Astrand [6] and there is a large and consistent data base on the peak $\dot{V}O_2$ of 8- to 18-year-olds [7]. Sex differences in absolute peak $\dot{V}O_2$ (litres $\bullet$ min^{-1}) are apparent in pre-pubescent children and they increase through adolescence with girls and boys enhancing their peak $\dot{V}O_2$ by about 80 and 150%, respectively, over the age range 8–16 years. When peak $\dot{V}O_2$ is expressed in ratio with body mass (ml $\bullet$ kg^{-1} $\bullet$ min^{-1}) it remains essentially unchanged with age in untrained boys at about 48–50 ml $\bullet$ kg^{-1} $\bullet$ min^{-1} but girls show a decline from approximately 45–35 ml $\bullet$ kg^{-1} $\bullet$ min^{-1} from 8 to 16 years of age.

The reporting of peak $\dot{V}O_2$ in ratio with body mass might be appropriate in the context of sports where body mass is moved but it has clouded the physiological understanding of peak $\dot{V}O_2$ during growth and maturation [8]. Using multi-level modelling, longitudinal studies of both trained [9] and untrained [10] young people have demonstrated that, in addition to age, growth and maturation positively and independently influence peak $\dot{V}O_2$. Maximum heart rate (HR$_{max}$) is independent of sex but from an early age boys appear to benefit from a greater maximal stroke volume (SV$_{max}$), and therefore maximal cardiac output ($\dot{Q}_{max}$), than girls. Whether this is due to differences in heart size or function is unknown. There are data which suggest that adolescent boys have greater arterio-venous oxygen differences than girls, perhaps through their higher haemoglobin concentration, but this remains to be proven. Boys' peak $\dot{V}O_2$ is further augmented compared to girls through their increasingly greater muscle mass as they move through adolescence [7].

Peak $\dot{V}O_2$ of Trained and Untrained Youth

It is well documented that elite young athletes in some sports have higher peak $\dot{V}O_2$ than athletes in other sports and their non-sporting peers. However, as almost all studies report cross-sectional data, whether this is due to initial selection for sport or subsequent training is unknown. Trained young male athletes tend to have greater peak $\dot{V}O_2$ than trained females but this is probably due to the sex differences in peak $\dot{V}O_2$ described earlier, although variations in training volume cannot be ruled out.

The majority of studies have compared the peak $\dot{V}O_2$ of young distance runners involved in a programme of structured training with either the peak $\dot{V}O_2$ of a control group of untrained young people or peak $\dot{V}O_2$ values from the literature. Trained youth have been reported to have significantly higher peak $\dot{V}O_2$ than their untrained peers [11–13]. Focused studies have reported higher peak $\dot{V}O_2$ in trained cyclists [14–16], swimmers [17–19], canoeists and cross-country skiers [20]. Peak $\dot{V}O_2$ values >60 and >50 ml $\cdot$ kg^{-1} $\cdot$ min^{-1} for trained boys and girls, respectively, have been regularly observed.

One investigation reported the mean peak $\dot{V}O_2$ of 14-year-old, male, trained swimmers as 67 ml $\cdot$ kg^{-1} $\cdot$ min^{-1}. Two boys attained a peak $\dot{V}O_2$ >75 ml $\cdot$ kg^{-1} $\cdot$ min^{-1}, about 50% higher than the typical peak $\dot{V}O_2$ of similarly aged, untrained boys [21]. Several papers have also reported lower HRs at a given level of submaximal exercise in trained compared to untrained children [12, 13, 15]. Others have noted similar HRs but higher stroke and cardiac indices in trained young people exercising at the same relative exercise intensities as their untrained peers [14]. Mahon [22] has comprehensively tabulated and described studies comparing the peak $\dot{V}O_2$ of trained and untrained children and published in the period 1973–2006.

We are unaware of any well-designed, intervention studies of training effects on elite child or adolescent athletes but a recent study of elite young adult footballers is worthy of note. Nineteen 18-year-old Norwegian footballers were randomly assigned to either a training group or a control group. As an extension of their normal training programme, which was also followed by the control group, the training group experienced twice weekly intensive interval training over an 8-week period and showed a 10% increase in their peak

$\dot{V}O_2$, whereas the control group's peak $\dot{V}O_2$ remained stable [23].

Mechanisms Underpinning Changes in Peak $\dot{V}O_2$ with Training

According to the Fick equation, $\dot{V}O_2$ is the product of cardiac output and arterio-venous oxygen difference. Maximal arterio-venous oxygen differences exhibited by trained young athletes have not been showed to be different from those of untrained young people [14, 15]. Therefore, training-induced differences in peak $\dot{V}O_2$ appear to be due to increased $\dot{Q}$. There is no convincing evidence to suggest that trained youth have higher HR$_{max}$ than untrained youth. Increased $\dot{Q}$ and enhanced oxygen delivery to the muscles following training must therefore be through increased SV [24, 25]. However, the methodological difficulties of assessing and interpreting a young person's SV and $\dot{Q}$ during exercise are well-documented. Well-designed longitudinal studies are sparse and the extant data must therefore be treated cautiously.

An early study reported greater SV and $\dot{Q}$ in trained young female track athletes than in untrained girls [27] and more recent work with trained young cyclists has confirmed these findings [28]. Eriksson and Koch [29] observed a 12% increase in estimated blood volume and a 17% increase in peak $\dot{V}O_2$ in nine 11- to 13-year-old boys following a 4-month training programme. They concluded that the increase in peak $\dot{V}O_2$ was wholly attributable to an increase in SV$_{max}$ and therefore $\dot{Q}_{max}$. When SV and $\dot{Q}$ are indexed to body surface area, as the stroke and cardiac indices, respectively, the literature is consistent in noting superior values in trained children compared to their age-matched peers [14, 28]. These findings are supported by a longitudinal study in which significant increases in stroke and cardiac indices in both boys and girls were observed following an endurance training programme with no changes noted in control groups [30].

A significant contribution to trained young athletes' enhanced SV might be through a more effective peripheral muscle pump and/or plasma volume expansion increasing venous return but direct supporting evidence is not available. Data on cardiac dimensions are equivocal with some studies observing no differences between trained and untrained youth in left ventricular size and mass [11, 31]. Other studies have reported larger left ventricular dimensions at rest [14, 32] and at maximal exercise [14] in trained youth. Most [31, 32] but not all [13] studies have observed no differences between trained and untrained youngsters in ventricular wall thickness.

Data from longitudinal studies are also inconsistent with some reporting increases in cardiac dimensions following a training programme [30, 32] and others noting no significant training-induced changes [33, 34]. Estimates of shortening fraction and ejection fraction at rest appear to be similar in both trained and untrained children [14, 32]. However, Oyen et al. [35] reported that trained children increase their shortening fraction more during maximal exercise than untrained children. The observed inconsistencies in cardiac dimensions in studies of trained and untrained youth might be due to factors such as differences in age, maturation, training volume, and years of training.

In summary, although the precise mechanisms are still to be elucidated, training-induced increases in peak $\dot{V}O_2$ appear to be primarily a function of enhanced oxygen delivery to the muscles through an increase in maximal SV.

Oxygen Uptake Kinetics

The $\dot{V}O_2$ kinetic response can be defined in relation to a number of exercise domains (moderate, heavy, very heavy, or severe intensity) but rigorously determined data with children and adolescents are only available in the moderate (i.e. exercise below the lactate threshold (T_{LAC})) and heavy (i.e. exercise above the T_{LAC} but below the maximal lactate steady state (MLSS) or critical power) exercise domains.

With a step change in exercise intensity, there is an almost immediate increase in $\dot{V}O_2$ measured at the mouth. This cardiodynamic phase is associated with the increase in $\dot{Q}$ which occurs prior to the arrival at the lungs of venous blood from the exercising muscles and is independent of oxygen consumption at the muscles. The cardiodynamic phase is followed by a rapid exponential increase in $\dot{V}O_2$ (the primary component) that during moderate and heavy intensity exercise drives $\dot{V}O_2$ to a steady state, albeit after an additional slow component of $\dot{V}O_2$ during heavy intensity exercise. The principal parameter of interest in this context is the time constant of the $\dot{V}O_2$ primary component which reflects the kinetics of oxygen consumption at the muscles. The faster the time constant, the smaller the anaerobic contribution to the step changes in exercise intensity. The $\dot{V}O_2$ slow component most likely originates in the exercising muscle and depends upon fibre type distribution and recruitment and the matching of oxygen delivery to the active muscle fibres [3].

Few studies of children's and adolescents' $\dot{V}O_2$ kinetics have involved rigorous collection and analysis of data but the extant literature in the moderate and heavy intensity exercise domains is generally consistent [36, 37]. The time constant of the exponential increase in $\dot{V}O_2$ has been shown to be age-dependent during step changes to both moderate [38] and heavy [39] intensity exercise. Boys have a faster $\dot{V}O_2$ primary component time constant than girls during the transition from rest to heavy intensity exercise [40] but the $\dot{V}O_2$ kinetic response to a step change to moderate intensity exercise is independent of sex [38].

In children and adolescents, peak $\dot{V}O_2$ has not been demonstrated to be related to the $\dot{V}O_2$ primary component time constant during the transition to either moderate [38] or heavy [40] intensity exercise. This is not surprising as peak $\dot{V}O_2$ is largely dependent on oxygen delivery to the muscles whereas young people's $\dot{V}O_2$ kinetics in these exercise domains appear to be primarily related to oxygen utilization by the muscles [3].

$\dot{V}O_2$ Kinetics in Trained and Untrained Youth

Slow $\dot{V}O_2$ kinetics result in a greater depletion of intra-muscular high-energy phosphates and a greater accumulation of hydrogen ions and inorganic phosphate within the muscle, all of which have been implicated in the cause of muscle fatigue. In addition, the aetiology of the $\dot{V}O_2$ slow component has been associated with fatigue occurring in the active muscle fibres during exercise. Therefore a training-induced speeding of the $\dot{V}O_2$ primary component and/or a reduction in the $\dot{V}O_2$ slow component could enhance sport performance. In adults, the $\dot{V}O_2$ primary component time constant has been shown to be shorter and the magnitude of the $\dot{V}O_2$ slow component smaller following training [42].

To date, the effect of training on young people's $\dot{V}O_2$ kinetics has not been investigated with a longitudinal design and the results of cross-sectional comparisons of trained and untrained youth are equivocal. Two very similar studies from the same research group compared the $\dot{V}O_2$ kinetics of trained and untrained swimmers [43, 44]. Both studies determined $\dot{V}O_2$ kinetic parameters during cycle ergometry and compared a group of pre-pubertal male and female swimmers from a local youth swimming team with non-sporting children. They observed no differences between the trained and untrained children in the $\dot{V}O_2$ primary component time constant during the transition to either moderate or very heavy intensity exercise or in the $\dot{V}O_2$ slow component during very heavy exercise.

A more recent study compared the $\dot{V}O_2$ kinetics response to heavy exercise on a cycle ergometer of 11-year-old, trained, female swimmers with a similarly aged untrained group. In agreement with earlier studies, no significant differences in either the $\dot{V}O_2$ primary component time constant or the $\dot{V}O_2$ slow component were noted. However, when the girls' $\dot{V}O_2$ kinetic parameters were determined during arm cranking the trained girls exhibited a significantly shorter $\dot{V}O_2$ primary component time constant than the untrained girls. This emphasises the specificity of training and, in this case, the importance of matching the testing modality with the arm-based training programme. No differences in the magnitude of the $\dot{V}O_2$ slow component were observed. Interestingly, there were no significant differences in peak $\dot{V}O_2$ during arm cranking in the trained and untrained girls suggesting that, in accord with adult data, changes in peak $\dot{V}O_2$ with training are not related to changes in $\dot{V}O_2$ kinetics [45].

Marwood et al. [46] examined the $\dot{V}O_2$ kinetic responses of elite 15-year-old footballers and similarly aged, untrained boys during the transition from rest to moderate intensity exercise on a cycle ergometer. They reported the footballers to have significantly faster $\dot{V}O_2$ primary component time constants than the untrained boys. These results are in conflict with the swimming studies in the same exercise domain but this might be due to differences in experimental rigour, age, maturation, and/or sex of the participants. Although the mode of exercise was not specific to the sport of either group, testing predominantly arm-trained swimmers on a cycle ergometer is likely to have disadvantaged them more than the leg-trained footballers. Or, the elite footballers, drawn from a Premier League Club Academy, might have been more rigorously selected than the swimmers from a local swimming team.

Breese et al. [47] argued that, based on skeletal muscle power-velocity relationships, the recruitment of type II muscle fibres would be enhanced for the same external power output by increasing pedal rate. They therefore investigated the effect of different pedal rates (50 and 115 rpm) at the same external power output on $\dot{V}O_2$ kinetics at the onset of very heavy exercise in 15- to 16-year-old trained and untrained male cyclists.

They reported no significant difference in the $\dot{V}O_2$ primary component time constants at 50 rpm but a significant slowing (~41%) of the $\dot{V}O_2$ kinetics at 115 rpm in the untrained boys which was not replicated by the trained cyclists. No significant differences in the $\dot{V}O_2$ slow component at either pedal cadence were observed.

Mechanisms Underpinning Changes in $\dot{V}O_2$ Kinetics following Training

The evidence that endurance training enhances young people's $\dot{V}O_2$ kinetics is limited to three cross-sectional comparisons of trained and untrained participants and the underlying mechanisms therefore remain speculative. Winlove et al. [45] postulated that the faster $\dot{V}O_2$ kinetics during heavy exercise of trained girls compared to untrained girls could be related to an increased oxygen delivery, greater muscle oxidative capacity or to differences in muscle fibre type distribution or recruitment. However, their finding of no difference between trained and untrained girls in the magnitude of the $\dot{V}O_2$ slow component suggests that muscle fibre type and recruitment patterns are unaffected by training. Furthermore, they reported that $\dot{V}O_2$ kinetics and HR kinetics are not related. As HR kinetics provide an estimate of muscle blood flow kinetics [48], these data suggest that oxygen delivery is not a limiting factor in $\dot{V}O_2$ kinetics. Similarly, the lack of relationship between $\dot{V}O_2$ kinetics and peak $\dot{V}O_2$ in this study supports the view that the predominant mechanism underpinning faster $\dot{V}O_2$ kinetics in trained girls is likely to be enhanced oxygen utilization.

In conflict with Winlove et al.'s [45] observations during heavy cycling exercise, Marwood et al. [46] reported faster $\dot{V}O_2$ kinetics, estimated capillary blood flow kinetics, and HR kinetics during moderate exercise in trained boys. They suggested that this indicated enhanced oxygen delivery to the exercising muscles and that $\dot{V}O_2$ kinetics might therefore normally be limited by oxygen delivery. In support of this hypothesis they also reported higher peak $\dot{V}O_2$ in the elite young footballers. Using the deoxyhaemoglobin signal from near-infra red spectroscopy to interrogate the muscle, Marwood and colleagues hypothesized that the unchanged dynamics of deoxyhaemoglobin and myoglobin between trained and untrained boys during the transition to exercise reflected maintenance of the oxygen delivery-to-oxygen consumption ratio because of similar changes in oxygen delivery and oxygen utilization in the elite young footballers. They therefore concluded that the faster $\dot{V}O_2$ kinetics in the trained boys were due to enhancements in both central (oxygen delivery) and peripheral (oxygen utilization) mechanisms.

On the basis of their observation of trained cyclists having faster $\dot{V}O_2$ kinetics than untrained cyclists while pedalling at 115 rpm but not while pedalling at 50 rpm, Breese et al. [47] speculated that cyclists benefited from specific training effects that enhance the mitochondrial oxygen utilization in type II muscle fibres.

In summary, more research is required to establish whether the speeding of children's and adolescents' $\dot{V}O_2$ kinetics through endurance training is due to enhanced oxygen delivery or increased oxygen utilization, or both. Similarly, whether the effect on the primary mechanism is dependent on the intensity of the step change in exercise and/or the specificity of the mode of exercise in relation to the training programme remains to be proven.

Blood Lactate Accumulation

Lactate is continuously produced in active muscle fibres and exercise-driven increases in the anaerobic re-synthesis of adenosine triphosphate (ATP) result in a greater production of lactate. The amount of lactate produced is a function of the balance between the anaerobic and aerobic metabolism of pyruvate and the higher the aerobic

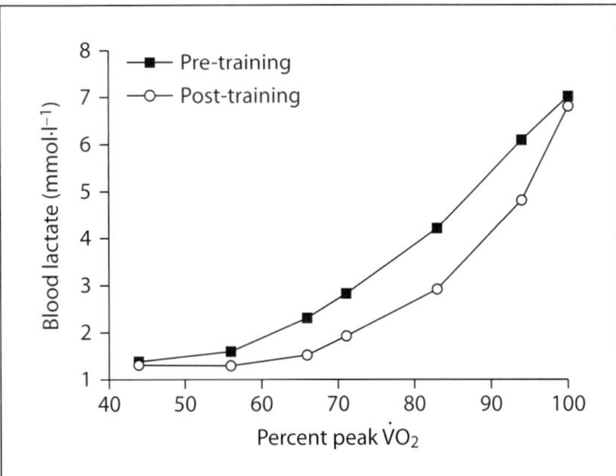

Fig. 1. Blood lactate response to exercise and training. From Armstrong and Welsman [4], by permission of Oxford University Press.

metabolism the lower the muscle lactate production. Lactate metabolism is a dynamic process and while some fibres produce lactate others consume it as an energy source.

During incremental exercise blood lactate accumulation typically increases, as illustrated in figure 1. Initially, there are minimal changes in lactate with the rate of diffusion into the blood being matched by the rate of removal from the blood but, as exercise progresses, an inflection point is reached where blood lactate accumulation begins to rise rapidly with a steep rise to exhaustion. The point at which lactate increases non-linearly during incremental exercise is defined as the T_{LAC} which serves as a useful indicator of aerobic fitness [49].

The literature describing young people's blood lactate responses to exercise is confounded by methodological issues and data need to be interpreted with caution. Sex differences and maturation effects independent of age remain to be substantiated. However, consistent findings are that children accumulate less lactate in the blood during exercise than adults and that there is a negative correlation between T_{LAC} as a percentage of peak $\dot{V}O_2$ and age [4].

Endurance training has been demonstrated to move young people's lactate curve (fig. 1) to the right (i.e. less blood lactate accumulation post-training at the same pre-training exercise intensity or $\dot{V}O_2$). Monitoring blood lactate accumulation therefore provides a sensitive means of detecting increases in aerobic fitness following training in the absence of significant changes in peak $\dot{V}O_2$. Any point on the curve might be used to detect individual responses but conventionally it is changes in T_{LAC} which are monitored. The MLSS (the highest exercise intensity that can be sustained without incurring a progressive accumulation of blood lactate) and fixed blood lactate reference values derived from the MLSS (e.g. 4 mmol•l⁻¹) have been used in sports such as swimming and athletics to monitor the effects of endurance training. However, secure data from children and adolescents are not currently available [4, 49].

Blood Lactate Accumulation in Trained and Untrained Youth

Comparisons between studies are confounded through differences in methodology and T_{LAC} definitions. Nevertheless, the evidence available consistently indicates that compared to untrained young people elite young athletes accumulate less blood lactate at the same relative sub-maximal exercise intensity [4]. Some studies have reported T_{LAC} in trained young people to occur at a higher percentage of peak $\dot{V}O_2$ than others have reported for untrained youngsters [50, 51]. Other studies have reported that the running speed corresponding to a blood lactate accumulation of 4 mmol•l⁻¹ increases following a training programme [52, 53]. Blood lactate accumulation has been observed to be lower in trained runners compared with similarly aged, untrained children [13]. Intervention studies have suggested that high intensity exercise training results in a decrease in blood lactate accumulation during subsequent sub-maximal exercise [54, 55]. This appears not to be the case following less intense exercise training [29, 56].

The ventilatory threshold (T_{vent}, a non-invasive surrogate for T_{LAC}) has been reported to occur at a higher percentage of peak $\dot{V}O_2$ in 11-year-old elite runners (71%) compared with less-talented runners (67%) and untrained children (61%) of comparable age [57]. However, two well-designed intervention studies with 10- to 11-year-olds observed no significant increases in the % of peak $\dot{V}O_2$ at which T_{vent} occurred following 8 weeks of training [58, 59].

Mechanisms Underpinning Changes in Blood Lactate Accumulation with Training

No study has specifically investigated the potential mechanisms underlying the training-induced reduction in blood lactate accumulation in young people. However, adult data suggest that a reduction in blood lactate accumulation during sub-maximal exercise following endurance training is due to increased oxidative capacity in the exercising muscles [60, 61]. Alternatively, changes in locomotion economy (the oxygen cost at a fixed level of sub-maximal exercise) following training might have clouded our understanding of the training-induced reduction in blood lactate accumulation during submaximal exercise. Intuitively, one would expect locomotion economy to improve with training (practice) but the extant data are mixed. Trained cyclists have been shown to have superior cycling economy than untrained cyclists [62], but well-controlled endurance training studies have reported no change in cycling economy following cycling training despite significant increases in peak $\dot{V}O_2$ [54, 63]. Similarly, in walking and running, some well-controlled endurance training studies have not observed changes in economy [64, 65] and others have reported significant increases in economy [66].

Only one study has attempted to directly investigate training-induced changes in children's oxidative capacity. Eriksson et al. [55] analyzed the effects of cycle training for 20–50 min, 3 days per week, for 6 weeks on five 11-year-old boys' muscle metabolism. They reported a 29% increase in the activity of the oxidative enzyme succinate dehydrogenase and postulated that the observed smaller lactate production per unit of glycogen broken down resulted from a greater oxidative capacity of the muscle. However, the hypothesized increase in oxidative capacity, which might have been offset by a simultaneous training-induced increase in the glycolytic enzyme phosphofructokinase, did not have a glycogen-sparing effect or produce lower muscle lactate during sub-maximal exercise following training. Nevertheless, blood lactate accumulation tended to be lower during submaximal exercise following training. Eriksson et al. [55] suggested that the lower blood lactate accumulation might have resulted from a greater extraction of lactate by other tissues or from a different rate of production and utilization by the different fibre types in the exercising muscle.

In summary, data from adults suggest that an increase in oxidative capacity is the primary mechanism underlying a reduction in blood lactate accumulation during subsequent submaximal exercise. However, the role in young people of a potential reduction in lactate diffusion from the muscles to the blood and/or an enhanced lactate clearance from the blood remains to be investigated.

Peak $\dot{V}O_2$ and Endurance Training

Factors to be considered in designing an endurance training study with children and adolescents include, age and maturation of the participants, recruitment of experimental and control groups, pre-training fitness and habitual physical activity (HPA) of the participants, adherence to the training programme, the outcome measure and its determination, and the exercise prescription (mode, frequency, intensity, and duration of exercise, and programme length).

There are insufficient data in the literature to investigate evidence-based, dose-response relationships between endurance training and aerobic fitness in young athletes. In the paediatric population, the only component of aerobic fitness which has been rigorously analysed is peak $\dot{V}O_2$. This section will therefore focus on well-designed and executed endurance training studies which have examined the effect of structured endurance training on healthy young people's peak $\dot{V}O_2$.

Method of Review

Relevant studies were located through computer searches of PubMed, Sport Discus, and personal databases, supplemented with an extensive search of bibliographies of accessed publications and previous reviews. Studies were only included in the analysis if they satisfied the following criteria:

- Published in the peer-reviewed literature
- Participants were normal, healthy young people
- Participants were aged 8.0–17.9 years
- Included both an experimental group and a control group
- Used appropriate statistical procedures
- Provided a clear training prescription in terms of frequency, intensity, duration and programme length
- Used directly determined peak $\dot{V}O_2$ as the criterion measure

Sixty-nine studies were located but only 21 met the criteria listed above and they are summarized in tables 1 and 2. Table 1 describes studies of participants aged 8.0–10.9 years and table 2 describes studies of participants aged 11.0–17.9 years. Table 3 lists eight other studies which, although they do not satisfy the criteria applied, are worthy of note and comment.

Methodological Issues

Although the studies included in tables 1 and 2 satisfied rigorous criteria, there are methodological issues which need to be noted to provide context for the extant data. Endurance training studies with young people are very demanding and participants are volunteers rather than randomly selected children and adolescents. Sample sizes are generally small with an inevitable effect on the statistical power of the study. Participants in experimental and control groups tend to be recruited from different classes in the same school or from different schools in the same area. In the 21 studies tabulated, experimental group size varied from 8 to 37 with an average of 15 participants. Control group size varied from 7 to 37 with an average of 12 participants. In 67% of the studies the experimental and control group sizes were uneven. Most of the tabulated studies do not refer to participant drop-out rates and/or adherence to the training programme. Those that do generally report high compliance and attendance rates with two studies [64, 79] reporting no drop-outs although one study [68] reported a 63% attrition rate.

Most of the tabulated studies used the same mode of exercise in the criterion peak $\dot{V}O_2$ test as in the training programme but there are exceptions where predominantly running programmes were assessed using cycle ergometry or vice versa [30, 63, 70, 71, 73]. Although intuitively one might hypothesise that specificity of training and testing would be likely to maximise observed endurance training-induced changes in young people's peak $\dot{V}O_2$ the supporting evidence is not convincing. The largest, significant percentage increase in peak $\dot{V}O_2$ recorded in tables 1 and 2 occurred when a running training programme was assessed using cycle ergometry [30].

To record and maintain training intensity, some studies meticulously and electronically monitored the HR of all participants during the training sessions [54, 58, 64, 70–73, 79]. Others monitored randomly selected participants [30,

Table 1. Endurance training and peak oxygen uptake: studies with participants under 11 years of age

Study	Participants		Training protocol		
	experimental (E)	control (C)	frequency (per week)	intensity	duration
Lussier and Buskirk [67]	n = 16 11 B 5 G, 10.3 years	n = 10 9 B 1 G, 10.5 years	4	92% max HR	45 min
Gilliam and Freedson [68]	n = 11 B and G, 8.5 years	n = 12 B and G, 8.5 years	4	HR at 165 beats·min^{-1}	25 min
Becker and Vaccaro [59]	n = 11 B, 9.6 years	n = 11 B, 10.0 years	3	50% of the way between AT and peak VO_2	40 min
Savage et al. [69]*	E_1 n = 12 B, 8.0 years E_2 n = 8 B, 8.5 years	n = 10 B, 9.0 years	3	E_1 85% max HR E_2 68% max HR	2.4–4.8 km
McManus et al. [70]*	E_1 n = 12 G, 9.3 years E_2 n = 11 G 9.8 years	n = 7 G, 9.6 years	3	E_1 80–85% max HR E_2 max sprints	E_1 20 min E_2 8–16 min
Welsman et al. [71]*	E_1 n = 18 G, 10.1 years E_2 n = 17 G, 10.2 years	n = 16 G, 10.2 years	3	E_1 80% max HR E_2 75–80% max HR	20 min 20–25 min
Tolfrey et al. [72]*	n = 12 B, 10.6 years n = 14 G, 10.6 years	n = 10 B, 10.3 years n = 9 G, 10.5 years	3	80% max HR	30 min
Williams et al. [73]*	E_1 n = 13 B, 10.1 years E_2 n = 12 B, 10.1 years	n = 14 B, 10.1 years	3	E_1 80 – 85% max HR E_2 max sprints	E_1 20 min E_2 6–8 min
Mandigout et al. [63]*	n = 18 B, 10.7 years n = 17 G, 10.5 years	n = 28 B, 10.5 years n = 22 G, 10.5 years	3	75–80% max HR continuous 90% max HR interval	15–20 min continuous 60–90 min interval
Baquet et al. [65]*	n = 13 B n = 20 G 9.5 years	n = 10 B n = 10 G 9.9 years	2	80–95% max HR	30 min

length (weeks)	type	Peak $\dot{V}O_2$ (litres·min^{-1})			Peak $\dot{V}O_2$ (ml·kg^{-1}·min^{-1})		
		pre	post	change (%)	pre	post	change (%)
12	continuous running and games	E 1.76	1.96	11.4	55.6	59.4	6.8**
		C 1.83	1.96	7.1	53.1	53.9	1.5
12	enhanced PE programme	E 1.29	1.34	3.9	43.4	42.9	−1.2 NS
		C 1.34	1.40	4.5	40.5	40.9	1.0
8	continuous cycling	E –	–	–	39.0	47.0	20.5 NS
		C –	–	–	41.7	44.0	5.5
10	interval running	E$_1$ –	–	–	55.9	58.5	4.7**
		E$_2$ –	–	–	52.2	54.6	4.6 NS
		C –	–	–	57.0	55.7	−2.3
8	E$_1$ continuous cycling E$_2$ interval running	E$_1$ 1.30	1.43	10.0	45.4	48.7	7.3**
		E$_2$ 1.54	1.67	8.4	48.3	50.3	4.1**
		C 1.49	1.46	−2.0	44.9	43.8	−2.4
8	E$_1$ continuous cycling E$_2$ aerobics and circuit training	E$_1$ 1.76	1.79	1.7	51.8	52.2	0.7 NS
		E$_2$ 1.58	1.61	1.9	47.0	47.8	1.7 NS
		C 1.72	1.72	0.0	46.2	45.9	−0.6
12	continuous cycling	EB 1.60	1.66	3.8	46.6	47.2	1.3 NS
		EG 1.36	1.54	13.2	39.3	42.4	7.9 NS
		CB 1.62	1.65	1.9	50.7	50.3	−0.1
		CG 1.52	1.52	0.0	44.7	43.0	−3.8
8	E$_1$ continuous cycling E$_2$ interval running	E$_1$ 1.80	1.93	7.2	54.7	57.5	5.1 NS
		E$_2$ 1.84	1.91	3.8	54.8	56.2	2.6 NS
		C 1.92	1.97	2.6	56.4	56.7	0.5
13	continuous and interval running aerobic activities	EB 1.70	1.84	8.2	47.2	49.2	4.2**
		EG 1.30	1.57	20.7	38.6	41.9	8.5**
		CB 1.60	1.70	6.2	46.1	45.5	−1.3
		CG 1.40	1.50	7.4	39.6	39.5	0.2
7	interval running	E 1.54	1.68	9.1	43.9	47.5	8.2**
		C 1.62	1.62	0.0	46.2	45.3	−1.9

Table 1. Continued

Study	Participants		Training protocol		
	experimental (E)	control (C)	frequency (per week)	intensity	duration
Obert et al. [30]	n = 9 B, 10.5 years n = 10 G, 10.4 years	n = 9 B, 10.7 years n = 7 G, 10.7 years	3	80% max HR continuous 90% max HR interval	60 min
McManus et al. [58]	E_1 n = 10 B 10.4 years E_2 n = 10 B 10.4 years	n = 15 B 10.5 years	3	E_1 85% max HR E_2 max sprints	20 min
Gamelin et al. [74]*	n – 22 12 B 10 G, 9.8 years	n – 16 7 B 9 G, 9.3 years	3	100 120% of maximal aerobic velocity (80–90% max HR)	30 min
Obert et al. [75]	n = 25 14 B 11 G	n = 25 13 B 12 G	3	100–130% of maximal aerobic velocity	25–30 min

B = Boys; G = girls; AT = anaerobic threshold; HR = heart rate; *maturity assessed; ** indicates significantly different from pretraining value (p ≤ 0.05) ; NS indicates not significantly different from pretraining value (p ≥ 0.05).

63, 68, 78], used self-monitoring [69], or did not objectively monitor training intensity [59, 66, 67, 76, 77]. To ensure that all individuals exercised at the same intensity over the same duration three studies from the same research group [65, 74, 75] based their training programme on percentages of maximal aerobic velocity (MAV), where MAV is the lowest velocity allowing peak $\dot{V}O_2$ to be elicited during a graded exercise test [86].

Genetic Influences on Training Peak $\dot{V}O_2$

Genetic influences on the responsiveness of peak $\dot{V}O_2$ to endurance training are not well-understood. Evidence suggests that some individuals are high responders to training whereas others are almost non-responders, with a whole range of response phenotypes between these two extremes [87]. Specific candidate genes have been identified that might account for individual differences in young people's responsiveness to endurance training [88–90] but few paediatric endurance training studies have investigated the issue. In adults, it has been estimated that almost half the change in peak $\dot{V}O_2$ following an endurance training programme is due to heritability [91] and limited evidence suggests that this might also be the case with young people. One of the papers described in table 3, studied nine male pairs of monozygotic twins, aged 11–14 years, with one boy from each twin pair undergoing 6 months of endurance training, and reported a heritability estimate of 45% for the adaptability of peak $\dot{V}O_2$ [53].

In order to 'minimize the genetic effects of trainability between subjects', two studies from

length (weeks)	type	Peak $\dot{V}O_2$ (litres·min^{-1})			Peak $\dot{V}O_2$ (ml·kg^{-1}·min^{-1})		
		pre	post	change (%)	pre	post	change (%)
13	continuous and interval running	EB –	–	–	44.1	50.9	15.4**
		EG –	–	–	40.9	44.2	8.1**
		CB –	–	–	51.5	50.3	–2.3
		CG –	–	–	42.4	42.6	0.5
8	E_1 continuous cycling	E_1 1.65	1.72	4.2	47.0	50.7	7.8**
	E_2 interval cycling	E_2 1.76	1.96	11.4**	45.5	50.7	11.4**
		C 1.59	1.57	–0.1	44.7	45.4	–0.2
7	interval running	E –	–	–	51.6	54.1	4.8**
		C –	–	–	49.9	48.7	–2.4
8	interval running	E –	–	–	51.6	55.0	6.6**
		C –	–	–	50.3	50.5	–0.4

the same research group [64, 78] employed a design in which participants acted as their own controls with peak $\dot{V}O_2$ being determined 12/13 weeks prior to training, immediately before, and at the termination of the training programme. In the first study [64], a significant increase in peak $\dot{V}O_2$ was reported following 12 weeks' training but in the second study [78] no significant changes in peak $\dot{V}O_2$ were observed between the control and experimental groups following 13 weeks' training despite the use of a higher training intensity.

The variability of peak $\dot{V}O_2$ responses to endurance training might be clearer if studies noted the range of responses in addition to the standard deviation but this is seldom reported. For example, Williams et al. [73] trained 25 boys using continuous cycle ergometry or sprint interval running and reported non-significant increases in peak $\dot{V}O_2$ of 7.2 and 3.8%, respectively. However, the range of responses in peak $\dot{V}O_2$ varied from –9.8 to 25.3% in the cycle group and –6.1 to 16.4% in the running group illustrating the wide variation in response rates and implying the possibility of individual genetic differences in responses to endurance training.

Baseline Peak $\dot{V}O_2$ and Habitual Physical Activity

Elite young athletes tend to have higher peak $\dot{V}O_2$ than their untrained peers so, an important question is whether additional training will have a similar effect on increasing peak $\dot{V}O_2$ in young people with high baseline values as with those with low levels of aerobic fitness. In adults,

Table 2. Endurance training and peak oxygen uptake: studies with participants 11 years of age and above

Study	Participants		Training protocol		
	experimental (E)	control (C)	frequency (per week)	intensity	duration
Massicotte and Macnab [54]	3 groups n = 9 B in each, 12.5 years	n = 9 B, 12.5 years	3	E_1 HR at 170–180 beats·min⁻¹ E_2 HR at 150–160 beats·min⁻¹ E_3 HR at 130–140 beats·min⁻¹	12 min
Stewart and Gutin [76]	n = 13 B, 10–12 years	n = 11 B, 10–12 years	4	90% of max HR	14–21 min
Burkett et al. [66]	n = 10 G, 15.6 years	n = 9 G, 15.6 years	5	70% of max HR continuous 90% of max HR interval	started at 9.7 km·week⁻¹ up to 32.2 km·week⁻¹
Mahon and Vaccaro [77]	n = 8 B, 12.4 years	n = 8 B, 12.3 years	4	70–80% max HR continuous 90–100% peak VO_2, 135% HR at VT interval	20–30 min continuous 100–800 m (from 1.5 to 2.5 km) interval
Rowland and Boyajian [64]*	n = 13 B, n = 24 G, 10.9–12.8 years	n = 13 B, n = 24 G, 10.9–12.8 years	3	HR at 153–184 beats.min⁻¹	20–30 min
Rowland et al. [78]*	n = 9 B, n = 20 G, 11.8 years	n = 9 B, n = 20 G, 11.8 years	3	85–90% max HR	30 min
Stoedefalke et al. [79]*	n = 20 G, 13.6 years	n = 18 G, 13.7 years	3	75–85% max HR	20 min

B = Boys; G = girls; VT = ventilatory threshold; HR = heart rate; *maturity assessed; ** indicates significantly different from pre-training value ($p \leq 0.05$); NS = not significantly different from pre-training value ($p \geq 0.05$).

length (weeks)	type	Peak $\dot{V}O_2$ (litres·min⁻¹)			Peak $\dot{V}O_2$ (ml·kg⁻¹·min⁻¹)		
		pre	post	change (%)	pre	post	change (%)
6	continuous cycling	E_1 2.00	2.30	15.0	46.7	51.8	10.8**
		E_2 1.80	1.90	5.6	47.4	48.0	1.3 NS
		E_3 1.70	1.80	5.9	46.6	48.2	3.4 NS
		C 2.00	1.90	−5.0	45.7	44.2	−3.3
8	interval running	E −	−	−	49.8	49.5	−0.6 NS
		C −	−	−	48.4	49.2	1.7
20	continuous and interval running	E −	−	−	45.1	49.4	9.3**
		C −	−	−	43.2	43.2	0.0
8	continuous and interval running	E 1.87	2.04	9.1	45.9	49.4	7.6**
		C 1.77	1.84	4.0	45.4	45.9	1.1
12	aerobic circuit training distance running/walking games, basketball	E 2.02	2.24	10.9	44.7	47.6	6.5**
		C 1.96	2.02	0.1	44.3	44.7	0.9
13	aerobic dance, step aerobics' distance running, circuit activities	EB 2.15	2.29	6.5	45.4	48.2	6.1 NS
		EG 1.81	1.97	8.8	43.9	46.1	5.0 NS
		CB 2.08	2.15	3.4	45.3	45.4	0.2
		CG 1.46	1.81	24.0	43.7	43.9	0.4
20	treadmill running, cycle and rowing ergometry, stair stepping, aerobic dance	E 2.25	2.32	3.1 NS	−	−	−
		C 2.39	2.45	2.5	−	−	−

Table 3. Endurance training and peak oxygen uptake: other studies of note

Study	Participants		Training protocol		
	experimental (E)	control (C)	frequency (per week)	intensity	duration
Weber et al. [80]	3 groups E_1 n = 4 B, 10.0 years E_2 n = 4 B, 13.0 years E_3 n = 4 B, 16.0 years	C_1 n = 4 B, 10.0 years C_2 n = 4 B, 13.0 years C_3 n = 4 B, 16.0 years	3	162 beats·min⁻¹ to max HR	1 mile run max effort, stepping 8.5 min, cycling duration unspecified hockey/rugby training duration unspecified
Stransky et al. [81]	n = 16 G, 15.8 years	n = 14 G, 15.9 years	4	unknown	12,800 yards/week
Kobayashi et al. [82]	n = 7 B, 9.7 years at onset, 14.7 years at conclusion	n = 43 B, 13.2 years at onset, 15.2 at conclusion	4–5	unknown	1–1.5 h
Docherty et al. [83]	2 groups E_1 n = 11 B, 12.4 years E_2 n = 12 B, 12.4 years	n = 11 B, 12.4 years	3	E_1 high velocity/ low resistance E_2 low velocity/ high resistance	2 × 20 s all-out at an unspecified number of stations
Rotstein et al. [52]	n = 16 B, 10.8 years	n = 12 B, 10.8 years	3	unknown	45 min
Weltman et al. [84]*	n = 16 B, 8.2 years	n = 10 B, 8.2 years	4	unknown	45 min
Obert et al. [85]*†	n = 5 G, 9.3 years	n = 9 G, 9.3 years	10	HR at 170–180 beats·min⁻¹	60–90 min
Danis et al. [53]*	n = 9 B, 11–14 years	n = 9 B, 11–14 years	3	75–97% of peak $\dot{V}O_2$	60 min

B = Boys; G = girls; HR = heart rate; *maturity assessed; † peak $\dot{V}O_2$ determined on a swim bench; ** indicates significantly different from pre-training value (p ≤ 0.05); NS = not significantly different from pre-training value (p ≥ 0.05); *** significance not reported here because of lack of control group in early years of study.

length (weeks)	type	Peak $\dot{V}O_2$ (litres$\cdot$min^{-1})			Peak $\dot{V}O_2$ (ml$\cdot$kg$^{-1}\cdot$min^{-1})		
		pre	post	change (%)	pre	post	change (%)
10	running, stepping, cycling, hockey, rugby	E_1 1.59	1.96	23.5**	–	–	–
		E_2 2.19	2.49	14.2 NS	–	–	–
		E_3 2.95	3.55	20.5**	–	–	–
		C_1 1.58	1.77	11.8	–	–	–
		C_2 2.18	2.51	16.0	–	–	–
		C_3 2.95	3.03	3.2	–	–	–
7	swim training	E 2.45	2.80	14.3	41.6	48.3	16.1**
		C 2.46	2.50	1.6	42.9	42.9	0.0
260	endurance running, soccer, swimming	E 1.29	3.13	14.3	47.5	63.2	33.0***
		C 1.91	2.61	3.7	45.0	49.1	9.1
4	isokinetic resistance training	E_1 1.90	2.31	21.6	46.2	54.7	18.4**
		E_2 2.06	2.43	18.0	47.0	55.1	17.2**
		C 2.12	2.22	4.7	47.0	49.0	4.3
9	interval running, aerobic activities, games	E –	–	–	54.2	58.6	8.1**
		C –	–	–	57.1	58.3	2.1
14	resistance training	E 1.39	1.66	19.4	46.8	53.2	13.7**
		C 1.48	1.44	−2.7	54.6	51.7	−5.3
52	swimming	E 0.79	1.10	38.0	26.2	33.8	29.0**
		C 0.69	0.78	13.0	24.7	24.9	0.0
24	continuous and interval running	E 2.08	2.37	13.9**	52.1	57.5	10.4**
		C 2.10	2.32	10.5**	54.0	55.4	2.6

it is well-established that there is an inverse relationship between the pre-training $\dot{V}O_{2max}$ and the amount that it will increase with endurance training [92] but in youth the data are equivocal.

In their review of the literature, Pate and Ward [93] analyzed 15 studies of 8- to 17-year-olds and concluded that 'children apparently can increase their maximal aerobic power with systematic training regardless of their initial $\dot{V}O_2$ max level. It may be that the initial fitness level per se does not affect trainability; the initial level of habitual activity may be a more important factor' [p. 47]. In contrast, another review analyzed 18 studies of pre-pubertal children and concluded that the mean improvement in peak $\dot{V}O_2$ for individuals with high baseline peak $\dot{V}O_2$ was lower than for those with low initial peak $\dot{V}O_2$ [94]. More recently, Mahon [22] compared baseline peak $\dot{V}O_2$ with training-induced percentage changes in peak $\dot{V}O_2$ from 21 studies of children and adolescents and concluded that there is a small but significant inverse relationship between the two variables.

Three of the tabulated studies directly addressed this issue. Mandigout et al. [63] observed a significant negative relationship between baseline peak $\dot{V}O_2$ and percentage change in peak $\dot{V}O_2$ following training. Tolfrey et al. [72] reported a similar finding although in this case the relationship accounted for only 9% of the variance in peak $\dot{V}O_2$ over time and once the training-induced changes in peak $\dot{V}O_2$ were scaled to account for differences in body size the changes were no longer significant. Rowland and Boyajian [64] observed no relationship between pre-training peak $\dot{V}O_2$ and training response.

As with all analyses reported here, one should compare the results of studies using different training volumes with caution but analysis of the 21 studies described in tables 1 and 2 reveals a significant negative relationship between pre-training peak $\dot{V}O_2$ and the training-induced percentage change in peak $\dot{V}O_2$ (fig. 2). This suggests that elite young athletes with higher baseline

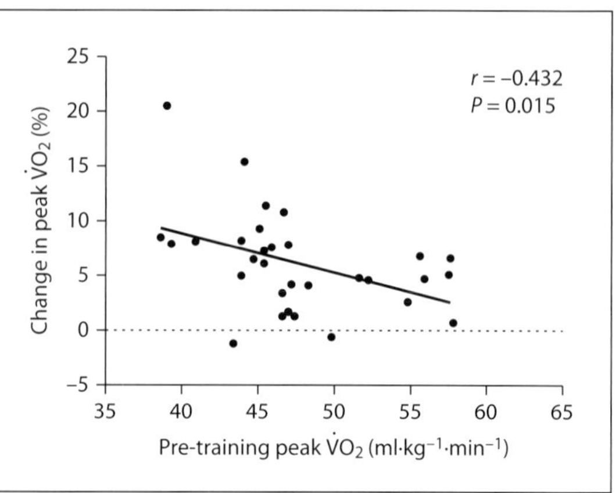

Fig. 2. Relationship between pre-training peak $\dot{V}O_2$ and percentage change in peak $\dot{V}O_2$ with training. Data from studies described in tables 1 and 2.

levels of aerobic fitness are likely to experience smaller percentage increases in peak $\dot{V}O_2$ following training than young people less fit at the onset of a training programme.

Pate and Ward [93] suggested that HPA might be an important factor when assessing the influence of training on peak $\dot{V}O_2$ and others [95] have proposed high levels of HPA as an explanation for blunted training responses in children. Two of the tabulated studies investigated the relationship between HPA and changes in peak $\dot{V}O_2$. Tolfrey et al. [72] estimated HPA using continuous HR monitoring over 4 days but reported no relationship between HPA and changes in peak $\dot{V}O_2$ with training. In contrast, Rowland and Boyajian [64] used a parent questionnaire to estimate HPA and reported a significant negative relationship (r = –0.35) between level of HPA and percentage training-induced increase in peak $\dot{V}O_2$. However, in a more recent review, the same author [96, p. 209] concluded that, the idea that the higher HPA levels of children might 'pre-train young subjects has been largely discounted.' Empirical evidence shows that the view that HPA might influence the effect of endurance training on peak $\dot{V}O_2$ is untenable as data unequivocally demonstrate that children and adolescents very rarely (if ever) experience the volume of HPA necessary to enhance peak $\dot{V}O_2$ [97] and that young people's HPA is not related to their peak $\dot{V}O_2$ [98].

Sex Effects on the Peak $\dot{V}O_2$ Response to Endurance Training

There is no credible evidence to suggest that the peak $\dot{V}O_2$ response to endurance training is dependent on sex. Data extracted from the studies described in tables 1 and 2 show significant increases in peak $\dot{V}O_2$ in 59% of male experimental groups and 73% of female experimental groups. The average increase in peak $\dot{V}O_2$ with endurance training is 6.7% (range –0.6 to 20.5%) in male groups and 5.9% (range 0.7–9.3%) in female groups. Five studies specifically investigated sex differences in peak $\dot{V}O_2$ responses to endurance training and concluded that training-induced changes were independent of sex [63–65, 72, 78]. Similar conclusions have been reached in earlier reviews of the extant literature [94, 99, 100].

Age and Maturation Effects on the Peak $\dot{V}O_2$ Response to Endurance Training

Gilliam and Freedson [68] introduced an enhanced physical education programme into the lifestyles of 8-year-olds over a period of 12 weeks and on observing no significant changes in a range of physiological variables including peak $\dot{V}O_2$ they concluded that, 'a maturational threshold exists whereby pre-pubescent children are unable to elicit physiologic changes in response to exercise training' [p. 76]. Katch [101] subsequently proposed that there is one critical time period in a child's life (a trigger point) below which the effects of training will be minimal, or will not occur at all. He suggested that 'this trigger phenomenon is the result of modulating effects of hormones that initiate puberty and influence functional development and subsequent organic adaptations' [p. 241]. More recently, Rowland [102] re-visited Katch's trigger hypothesis, examined the extant data and concluded that although there are some 'tantalizing clues' that hormonal responses at puberty are critical for the enhancement of peak $\dot{V}O_2$ there are insufficient data to accept or reject the trigger hypothesis.

In a study which is often used to support the trigger hypothesis, Kobayashi et al. [82] followed a group of 7 boys from the age of 9.7 to 15.8 years and determined their peak $\dot{V}O_2$ annually. The boys trained for 1–1.5 h per day, four or five times per week throughout the period of observation although the intensity of training was not reported. Peak $\dot{V}O_2$ increased slowly until 1 year prior to peak height velocity (PHV) after which it was found to increase above the normal amount attributable to age and growth. A major limitation of this study, however, was that measurements of peak $\dot{V}O_2$ for the control group did not begin until after the age of PHV.

In a conflicting report, Weber et al. [80] studied 12 pairs of identical twins, four sets aged 10 years, four sets aged 13 years, and four sets aged 16 years. One twin from each set followed a 10-week training programme as outlined in table 3. Significant changes in peak $\dot{V}O_2$ were observed in the 10- and 16-year-old twins but not in the 13-year-olds. This was interpreted by the authors to demonstrate that children are less trainable around the age of puberty. In a similar investigation, Danis et al. [53] trained one from each of nine pairs of 11- to 14-year-old monozygotic male twins as described in table 3 and reported significant increases in peak $\dot{V}O_2$ in the pre-pubertal twins but not in the pubertal twins.

Additional insights into the effect of age and maturation on the response of peak $\dot{V}O_2$ to training might be gained by comparing the outcomes of studies in table 1 (participants under 11 years) with those of table 2 (participants 11 years and above). Nine of the 14 studies in table 1 (i.e. 64%) reported a significant increase in peak $\dot{V}O_2$ with an average increase of 6.7% whereas four of the seven studies in table 2 (i.e. 57%) reported an increase in peak $\dot{V}O_2$ with an average increase of 5.5%. Nine studies in table 1 verified the pre-pubertal status of their participants and six of them (i.e. 67%) reported significant increases in peak $\dot{V}O_2$. In the studies which applied a sufficient stimulus to increase peak $\dot{V}O_2$, the magnitude of the average increase in the table 1 studies was 7.7% compared to an average increase in peak $\dot{V}O_2$ of 8.6% in the table 2 studies.

The magnitude of the reported increase in peak $\dot{V}O_2$ with training is less than would be expected on the basis of adult studies but studies which have directly investigated the peak $\dot{V}O_2$ response of children and adults to the same relative training intensity have not reported significantly different responses to training. In a study described in table 1, Savage et al. [69] trained 8 men and 8 pre-pubertal boys using low-intensity exercise and 12 men and 12 pre-pubertal boys followed the same high-intensity training programme. Significant increases in peak $\dot{V}O_2$ were limited to the high-intensity training groups but did not differ between men and boys. Another study involved 8 girls, aged 12.7 years, following the same 14-week training programme as 8 young women aged 19.6 years. The rate and magnitude of increases in peak $\dot{V}O_2$ were identical in both groups [103]. Empirical training studies therefore suggest that the existence of a maturational threshold below which children are not trainable remains to be proven.

Exercise Prescription

Training programmes depend upon the mode, frequency, duration, and intensity of exercise and programme length and each of these elements needs to be considered in the development of an optimal training programme for young people.

In this section, we will interrogate the studies described in tables 1 and 2 and refer to relevant studies described in table 3 in order to tease out an evidence-based exercise prescription to improve the peak $\dot{V}O_2$ of healthy youth.

Mode of training
Training programmes which have significantly increased young people's peak $\dot{V}O_2$ have involved a variety of modes of exercise including cycling [54, 58, 70], running [30, 51, 62, 64–67, 69, 70, 74, 75, 77], swimming [81, 85], aerobic activities including circuit training [62, 64] and resistance training [83, 84]. It can therefore be concluded that exercise using large muscle groups, regardless of mode of exercise, has the potential to increase peak $\dot{V}O_2$. Of the well-controlled studies, those basing their training programme on running have been more successful than cycling-based programmes. Both continuous- [54, 58, 65, 70] and interval- [58, 65, 69, 70, 74, 75] based training programmes have been shown to enhance peak $\dot{V}O_2$ but those studies which incorporated both interval and continuous running [30, 62, 66, 77] have been the most consistently successful.

Frequency and Duration of Training
With two exceptions, the frequency of training of all the studies described in tables 1 and 2 was 3–4 sessions per week. One study [66] employed five sessions per week and another [65] two sessions per week. Both of these investigations reported significant increases in peak $\dot{V}O_2$, i.e. 9.3 and 8.2%, respectively. The duration of sessions varied from 12 to 90 min with most studies in the range of 20–40 min per session. Interestingly, the study employing session durations of 12 min reported a significant increase in peak $\dot{V}O_2$ only in the high-intensity group [54] which might indicate the importance of training volume (interaction between intensity and duration). In general, training sessions of 40–60 min duration have been the most successful in increasing peak $\dot{V}O_2$.

Intensity of Training
The intensity of exercise appears to be crucial and of the 10 studies which used a training stimulus of 85–90% of HR_{max} 8 induced significant increases in peak $\dot{V}O_2$. Two studies have specifically addressed training intensity. Savage et al. [69] observed a significant increase in peak $\dot{V}O_2$ in boys who trained at 85% of HR_{max} but no increase in peak $\dot{V}O_2$ in boys who trained at 70% of HR_{max}. Similarly, Massicotte and MacNab [54] compared boys who trained for 12 min, three times per week, for 6 weeks at intensities of 66–72% HR_{max}, 75–80% HR_{max}, and 88–93% of HR_{max}. Only the highest intensity training group significantly improved their peak $\dot{V}O_2$. It should, however, be noted that in both these studies the duration of exercise was the same for all groups and the boys in the higher intensity groups therefore experienced greater training volumes. Nevertheless, the popular assertion that children have a 'blunted' response to endurance training compared to adults [22] might be explained by adults being able to enhance their peak $\dot{V}O_2$ with a lower relative training intensity than children and adolescents. Most longitudinal training studies with young people have not applied a high enough exercise intensity to induce optimum responses in peak $\dot{V}O_2$.

Training Programme Length
The length of training programmes ranged from 6 to 20 weeks but no clear inferences on optimal length of programme can be drawn from the available data. For example, Stoedefalke et al. [79] trained post-menarchal girls for 20 weeks without inducing an increase in peak $\dot{V}O_2$, whereas Massicotte and MacNab [54] demonstrated a 10.8% increase in peak $\dot{V}O_2$ in boys after 6 weeks of training.

A swim training study [85] is worthy of note because of the high frequency (10 sessions per week) and programme length (52 weeks) although the study is limited by the small sample size (5 girls in the experimental group). To maintain consistency between training and assessment mode the pre- and post-test assessments were carried out using a swim bench and the 29% increase in peak $\dot{V}O_2$ was striking. This study highlights the potential improvement in peak $\dot{V}O_2$ which can result from long-term, specific training programmes. Given the inconsistency of programmes lasting 7–8 weeks in inducing significant increases in peak $\dot{V}O_2$, it seems prudent to recommend a minimum training programme length of 12 weeks.

Exercise Prescription Recommendation
Based on the evidence presented in tables 1 and 2, an appropriate training programme for increasing the peak $\dot{V}O_2$ of children and adolescents should include a mixture of continuous and interval exercise using large muscle groups, for a minimum of 3–4 sessions of 40–60 min per week, for a minimum length of 12 weeks. Critically important, the intensity of the sessions should be in the range 85–90% of HR_{max} which is generally higher than the exercise stimulus used in most published studies. These recommendations, which are described in table 4, have been adopted by the International Olympic Committee in its consensus statement on 'Training the Elite Child Athlete' [104].

Conclusions

Despite the limitations of cross-sectional analyses, the evidence that elite young athletes have greater peak $\dot{V}O_2$ (in litres $\cdot$ min^{-1}) than their untrained peers is convincing, and the difference in peak $\dot{V}O_2$ appears to be due to greater maximal SV and therefore maximal $\dot{Q}$ in trained youngsters. Although sparse, the extant data suggest that the $\dot{V}O_2$ kinetic response to step changes in exercise intensity can be enhanced by endurance training. However, the published literature is restricted to cross-sectional studies of trained and untrained youth and can only provide limited insights into the mechanisms underlying the response of $\dot{V}O_2$

Table 4. Exercise prescription for improvement of peak oxygen uptake

Mode	Mixture of continuous and interval training using large muscle groups
Frequency	minimum 3–4 sessions per week
Duration	40–60 min
Intensity	85–90% maximum heart rate
Programme length	minimum length 12 weeks

kinetics to training. Whether oxygen delivery or oxygen utilization is the primary influence on the trainability of $\dot{V}O_2$ kinetics during childhood and adolescence remains an intriguing but unanswered question.

The extant data demonstrate that blood lactate accumulation in elite young athletes during submaximal exercise is lower than in untrained children and adolescents and that T_{LAC} occurs at a higher percentage of peak $\dot{V}O_2$ in trained young people. The reduced blood lactate accumulation in elite young athletes appears to be due to training-induced, increased oxidative capacity in the exercising muscles. However, the potential effects of decreased lactate diffusion into the blood and increased removal from the blood remain to be explored fully.

Rigorous studies of training interventions with young athletes are sparse. In the healthy paediatric population, peak $\dot{V}O_2$ is the only measure of aerobic fitness on which there is sufficient data to analyse dose-response relationships with

endurance training. Genetic influences on the response of peak $\dot{V}O_2$ to endurance training during youth are not well understood but extrapolation from adult studies and the few paediatric data suggest a heritability estimate of about 45–50% for the adaptability of peak $\dot{V}O_2$. There is no evidence to indicate that the peak $\dot{V}O_2$ response to endurance training is dependent on sex. The existence of a trigger point below which children are not trainable remains to be proven. Baseline (or pre-training) peak $\dot{V}O_2$ appears to have a moderate but significant inverse relationship with post-training peak $\dot{V}O_2$. This suggests that young athletes with higher initial levels of aerobic fitness will therefore experience smaller percentage increases in peak $\dot{V}O_2$ following endurance training than their untrained peers. However, empirical evidence suggests that both trained and untrained youth can benefit from endurance training. The critical variable appears to be training intensity which, for optimum benefits, should be held in the range 85–90% of HR_{max}.

References

1 Armstrong N, Welsman J: Assessment and interpretation of aerobic fitness in children and adolescents. Exerc Sports Sci Rev 1994;22:435–476.

2 Armstrong N, Welsman JR: Aerobic fitness: what are we measuring? in Tomkinson GR, Olds TS (eds): Pediatric Fitness. Basel, Karger, 2007, pp 5–25.

3 Armstrong N, Barker AR: Oxygen uptake kinetics in children and adolescents: a review. Pediatr Exerc Sci 2009; 21:130–147.

4 Armstrong N, Welsman JR: Aerobic fitness; in Armstrong N, Van Mechelen W (eds): Paediatric Exercise Science and Medicine, ed 2. Oxford, Oxford University Press, 2008, pp 97–108.

5 Robinson S: Experimental studies of physical fitness in relation to age. Arbeitsphysiologie 1938;10:251–323.

6 Astrand PO: Experimental Studies of Physical Working Capacity in Relation to Sex and Age. Copenhagen, Munksgaard, 1952.

7 Armstrong N, McManus AM, Welsman JR: Aerobic fitness; in Armstrong N, Van Mechelen W (eds): Paediatric Exercise Science and Medicine, ed 2. Oxford, Oxford University Press, 2008, pp 269–282.

8 Welsman JR, Armstrong N: Statistical techniques for interpreting body size-related exercise performance during growth. Pediatr Exerc Sci 2000;12:112–127.

9 Baxter-Jones A, Goldstein H, Helms P: The development of aerobic power in young athletes. J Appl Physiol 1993;75:1160–1167.

10 Armstrong N, Welsman JR: Peak oxygen uptake in relation to growth and maturation in 11–17 year old humans. Eur J of Appl Physiol 2001;85:546–551.

11 Rowland TW, Unnithan VB, MacFarlane NG, Gibson NG, Paton JY: Clinical manifestations of the athlete's heart in prepubertal male runners. Int J Sports Med 1994;15:515–519.

12 Mayers N, Gutin B: Physiological characteristics of elite prepubertal cross-country runners. Med Sci Sports 1979;11:172–176.

13 van Huss WD, Evans SA, Kurowski T, Anderson DJ, Allen R, Stephens K: Physiological characteristics of male and female age-group runners; in Brown EW, Branta CF (eds): Competitive Sports for Children and Youth. Champaign, Human Kinetics, 1988, pp 143–158.

14 Nottin S, Vinet A, Stecken F, N'Guyen ID, Ounissi F, Lecoq AM, Obert P: Central and peripheral cardiovascular adaptations to exercise in endurance-trained children. Acta Physiol Scand 2002;175:85–92.

15 Rowland TW, Wehnert M, Miller K: Cardiac responses to exercise in competitive child cyclists. Med Sci Sports Exerc 2000;32:747–752.

16 Unnithan VB, Rowland TW, Cable NT, Raine N: Cardiac responses in elite male junior cyclists; in Armstrong N, Kirby BJ, Welsman JR (eds): Children and Exercise. London, Spon, 1997, pp 501–506.

17 Cunningham DA, Enyon RB: The working capacity of young competitive swimmers, 10–16 years of age. Med Sci Sports 1973;5:227–231.

18 Holmer I: Oxygen uptake during swimming in man. J Appl Physiol 1980;33:502–509.

19 Nomura T: Maximal oxygen uptake of age group swimmers. Swim Tech 1979;15:105–109.

20 Wells CL, Scrutton EW, Archibald LD, Cooke WP, De La Mothe JW: Physical working capacity and maximal oxygen uptake of teenaged athletes. Med Sci Sports 1973;5:232–238.

21 Armstrong N, Davies B: An ergometric analysis of age group swimmers. Br J Sports Med 1981;15:20–26.

22 Mahon AD: Aerobic training; in Armstrong N, Van Mechelen W (eds): Paediatric Exercise Science and Medicine, ed 2. Oxford, Oxford University Press, 2008, pp 513–529.

23 Helgerud J, Engen LC, Wisloff U, Hoff J: Aerobic endurance training improves soccer performance. Med Sci Sports Exerc 2001;33:1925–1931.

24 Armstrong N, Welsman J: Young People and Physical Activity. Oxford, Oxford University Press, 1997.

25 Bar-Or, O: Trainability of the prepubescent child. Phys Sports Med 1989;17:65–82.

26 Warburton DER, Nettlefold L, McGuire KA, Bredin SSD: Cardiovascular function; in Armstrong N, Van Mechelen W (eds): Paediatric Exercise Science and Medicine, ed 2. Oxford, Oxford University Press, 2008, pp 77–96.

27 Raven PB, Drinkwater BL, Horvath SM: Cardiovascular responses of young female track athletes during exercise. Med Sci Sports 1973;4:205–209.

28 Rowland TW, Unnithan V, Fernhall B, Baynard T, Lange C: Left ventricular responses to dynamic exercise in young cyclists. Med Sci Sports Exerc 2002;34:637–642.

29 Eriksson BO, Koch G: Effect of physical training on hemodynamic response during submaximal and maximal exercise in 11–13-year-old boys. Acta Physiol Scand 1973;87:27–39.

30 Obert P, Mandigout S, Nottin S, Vinet A, N'Guyen D, Lecoq A-M: Cardiovascular responses to endurance training in children: effect of gender. Eur J Clin Invest 2003;33:199–208.

31 Telford RD, McDonald IG, Ellis LB, Chennells MHD, Sandstrom ER, Fuller PJ: Echocardiographic dimensions in trained and untrained 12-year-old boys and girls. J Sport Sci 1988;6:49–57.

32 Obert P, Stecken F, Courteix D, Lecoq AM, Guenon P: Effect of long-term intensive endurance training on left ventricular structure and diastolic function in prepubertal children. Int J Sports Med 1998;19:149–154.

33 Geenen DL, Gilliam TB, Crowley D, Moorehead-Steffans C, Rosenthal A: Echocardiographic measures in 6- to 7-year-old children after an 8-month exercise program. Am J Cardiol 1982;49:1990–1995.

34 George KP, Gates PE, Tolfrey K: Impact of aerobic training upon left ventricular morphology and function in pre-pubescent children. Ergonomics 2005;48:1378–1389.

35 Oyen E-M, Scuster S, Brode PE: Dynamic exercise echocardiography of the left ventricle in physically trained children compared to untrained healthy children. Int J Cardiol 1990;29:29–33.

36 Barstow TJ, Schuermann B: $\dot{V}O_2$ kinetics effects of maturation and aging; in Jones AM, Poole DC (eds): Oxygen Uptake Kinetics in Sport, Exercise and Medicine. London, Routledge, 2004, pp 331–352.

37 Fawkner SG, Armstrong N: Oxygen uptake kinetic response to exercise in children. Sports Med 2003;33:651–669.

38 Fawkner SG, Armstrong N, Potter CR, Welsman JR: Oxygen uptake kinetics in children and adults after the onset of moderate intensity exercise. J Sports Sci 2002;20:319–326.

39 Fawkner SG, Armstrong N: Longitudinal changes in the kinetic response to heavy intensity exercise. J Appl Physiol 2004;97:460–466.

40 Fawkner SG, Armstrong N: Sex differences in the oxygen uptake kinetic response to heavy intensity exercise in prepubertal children. Eur J Appl Physiol 2004;93:210–216.

41 Breese BC, Williams CA, Barker AR, Welsman JR, Fawkner SG, Armstrong N: Longitudinal changes in the oxygen uptake response to heavy intensity exercise in 14–16 year old boys. Pediatr Exerc Sci 2010;22:314–325.

42 Jones AM, Koppo K: Effect of training on $\dot{V}O_2$ kinetics and performance; in Jones AM, Poole DC (eds): Oxygen Uptake Kinetics in Sport, Exercise and Medicine. London, Routledge, 2004, pp 373–398.

43 Obert P, Cleuziou C, Candau R, Courteix D, Lecoq A-M, Guenon P: The slow component of oxygen uptake kinetics during high-intensity exercise in trained and untrained prepubertal children. Int J Sports Med 2000;21:31–36.

44 Cleuzoiu C, Lecoq AM, Candau R, Courteix D, Guenon P, Obert P: Kinetics of oxygen uptake at the onset of moderate and heavy exercise in trained and untrained prepubertal children. Sci Sports 2002;17:291–296.

45 Winlove MA, Jones AM, Welsman JR: Influence of training status and exercise modality on pulmonary oxygen uptake kinetics in pre-pubertal girls. Eur J Appl Physiol 2010;108:1169–1179.

46 Marwood S, Roche D, Rowland TW, Garrard M, Unnithan VB: Faster pulmonary oxygen uptake kinetics in trained versus untrained male adolescents. Med Sci Sports Exerc 2010;42:127–134.

47 Breese BC, Barker AR, Armstrong N, Williams CA: Effect of pedal rate on pulmonary oxygen uptake kinetics during high intensity cycling in adolescent boys; in Baquet G, Berthoin S (eds): Children and Exercise XXV. London, Routledge, 2010, pp 131–134.

48 MacPhee SL, Shoemaker JK, Paterson DH, Kowalchuk JM: Kinetics of oxygen uptake, leg blood flow, and muscle deoxygenation are slowed in the upper compared with lower region of the moderate-intensity domain. J Appl Physiol 2005;99:1822–1834.

49 Pfitzinger P, Freedson P: Blood lactate responses to exercise in children. 2. Lactate threshold. Pediatr Exerc Sci 1997;9:299–307.

50 Rusko H, Rahkila P, Karvinen E: Anaerobic threshold, skeletal muscle enzymes and fiber composition in young female cross-country skiers. Acta Physiol Scand 1980;108:263–268.

51 Fernhall B, Kohrt W, Burkett LN, Walters S: Relationship between the lactate threshold and cross-country run performance in high school male and female runners. Pediatr Exerc Sci 1996;8:37–47.

52 Rotstein A, Dotan R, Bar-Or O, Tenebaum G: Effect of training on anaerobic threshold, maximal aerobic power, and anaerobic performance of preadolescent boys. Int J Sports Med 1986;7:281–286.

53 Danis A, Kyriazis Y, Klisssouras V: The effect of training in male prepubertal and pubertal monozygotic twins. Eur J Appl Physiol 2003;89:309–318.

54 Massicote DR, Macnab RBJ: Cardiorespiratory adaptations to training at specific intensities in children. Med Sci Sports 1974;6:242–246.

55 Eriksson BO, Gollnick PD, Saltin B: Muscle metabolism and enzyme activities after training in boys 11–13 years old. Acta Physiol Scand 1973;87:485–497.

56 Ekblom B: Effect of physical training in adolescent boys. J Appl Physiol 1969;27:350–355.

57 Gutin B, Mayers N, Levy JA, Herman MV: Physiological and echocardiographic studies of age-group runners; in Brown EW, Branta CF (eds): Competitive Sports for Children and Youth. Champaign, Human Kinetics, 1988, pp 117–128.

58 McManus AM, Cheung CH, Leung MP, Yung TC, Macfarlane DJ: Improving aerobic power in primary school boys: a comparison of continuous and interval training. Int J Sports Med 2005;26:781–786.

59 Becker DM, Vaccaro P: Anaerobic threshold alterations caused by endurance training in children. J Sports Med Phys Fitness 1983;23:445–449.

60 Mogensen M, Bagger M, Pedersen PK, Fernstrom M, Sahlin K: Cycling efficiency in humans is related to low UCP3 content and to type 1 fibres but not to mitochondrial efficiency. J Physiol 2006;571:669–681.

61 Holloszy JO: Biochemical adaptations in muscle-effects of exercise on mitochondrial oxygen uptake and respiratory enzyme activity in skeletal muscle. J Biol Chem 1967;242:2278–2282.

62 Gatch W, Byrd AW: Endurance training and cardiovascular function in 9-and 10-year-old boys. Arch Phys Med Rehabil 1979;60:574–577.

63 Mandigout S, Lecoq A-M, Coutreix D, Guenon P, Obert P: Effect of gender in response to an aerobic training programme in prepubertal children Acta Paediatr 2001;90:9–15.

64 Rowland TW, Boyajian A: Aerobic response to aerobic exercise training in children. Pediatr 1995;96:654–658.

65 Baquet G, Berthoin S, Dupont G, Blondel N, Fabre C, Van Praagh E: Effects of high intensity intermittent training on peak $\dot{V}O_2$ in prepubertal children. Int J Sports Med 2002;23:439–444.

66 Burkett LN, Fernhall B, Walters SC: Physiological effects of distance running training on teenage females. Res Q Exerc Sport 1985;56:215–220.

67 Lussier L, Buskirk ER: Effects of an endurance training regime on assessment of work capacity in pre-pubertal children. Ann NY Acad Sci 1977;30:734–747.

68 Gilliam TB, Freedson P: Effects of a 12 week school physical fitness program on peak $\dot{V}O_2$, body composition and blood lipids in 7 to 9 year old children. Int J Sports Med 1980;1:73–78.

69 Savage MP, Petratis M, Thomson WH, Berg K, Smith JL, Sady SP: Exercise training effects on serum lipids of pre-pubescent boys and adult men. Med Sci Sports Exerc 1986;18:197–204.

70 McManus AM, Armstrong N, Williams CA: Effect of training on the aerobic power and anaerobic performance of prepubertal girls. Acta Paediatr 1997;86:456–459.

71 Welsman JR, Armstrong N, Withers S: Responses of young girls to two modes of aerobic training. Br J Sports Med 1997;31:139–142.

72 Tolfrey K, Campbell IG, Batterham AM: Aerobic trainability of pre-pubertal boys and girls. Pediatr Exerc Sci 1998;10:248–263.

73 Williams CA, Armstrong N, Powell J: Aerobic responses of pre-pubertal boys to two modes of training. Br J Sports Med 2000;34:168–173.

74 Gamelin F-X, Bacquet G, Berthoin S, Thevenet D, Nourry C, Nottin S, Bosquet L: Effect of high intensity intermittent training on heart rate variability in pre-pubescent children. Eur J Appl Physiol 2009;105:731–738.

75 Obert P, Nottin S, Bacquet G, Thevenet D, Gamelin F-X, Berthoin S: Two months of endurance training does not alter diastolic function evaluated by TDI in 9- to 11-year-old boys and girls. Br J Sports Med 2009;43:132–135.

76 Stewart KJ, Gutin B: Effects of physical training on cardiorespiratory fitness in children. Res Q 1976;47:110–120.

77 Mahon AD, Vaccaro P: Ventilatory threshold and $\dot{V}O_2$ changes in children following endurance training. Med Sci Sports Exerc 1989;21:425–431.

78 Rowland TW, Martel L, Vanderburgh P, Manos T, Charkoudian N: The influence of short-term aerobic training on blood lipids in healthy 10–12 year old children. Int J Sports Med 1996;17:487–492.

79 Stoedefalke K, Armstrong N, Kirby BJ, Welsman JR: Effect of training on peak oxygen uptake and blood lipids in 13- to 14-year old girls. Acta Paediatr 2000;89: 1290–1294.

80 Weber G, Kartodihardjo W, Klissouras V: Growth and physical training with reference to heredity. J Appl Physiol 1976;40: 211–215.

81 Stransky AW, Mickelson RJ, van Fleet C, Davis R: Effects of a swimming training regime on hematological, cardiorespiratory and body composition changes in young females. J Sports Med Phys Fitness 1979;19:347–354.

82 Kobashyi K, Kitamura K, Miura M, Sodeyama H, Murase Y, Miyashita M: Aerobic power as related to body growth and training in Japanese boys: a longitudinal study. J Appl Physiol 1978;44:666–672.

83 Docherty D, Wenger HA, Collis ML: Effects of resistance training on aerobic and anaerobic power in young boys. Med Sci Sports Exerc 1987;19:389–392.

84 Weltman A, Janney C, Rians CB, Strand K, Berg B, Tippett S, Wise J, Cahill BR, Katch FI: The effects of hydraulic resistance strength training in pre-pubertal males Med Sci Sports Exerc 1986;18: 629–638.

85 Obert P, Courteix D, Lecoq A-M, Guenon P: Effect of long-term intense swimming training on the upper body peak oxygen uptake of pre-pubertal girls. Eur J Appl Physiol 1996;73:136–143.

86 Billat V, Koralsztein JP: Significance of the velocity at $\dot{V}O_2$ max and time to exhaustion at this velocity. Sports Med 1996;22:90–108.

87 Bouchard C, Dionne FT, Simoneau JA, Boulay MR: Genetics of aerobic and anaerobic performances. Exerc Sports Sci Rev 1992;20:27–58.

88 Ranikinen T, Bray MS, Hagberg JM, Peruse L, Roth SM, Wolfarth B, Bouchard C: The human gene map for performance and health-related fitness phenotypes: the 2005 update. Med Sci Sports Exerc 2006;38:1863–1888.

89 Rivera MA, Dionne FT, Simoneau JA, Perusse L, Chagnon M, Chagnon Y, Gagnon J, Leon AS, Rao DC, Skinner JS, Wilmore JF, Bouchard C: Muscle-specific creatine kinase gene polymorphism and $\dot{V}O_2$ max in the HERITAGE Family Study. Med Sci Sports Exerc 1997;23: 1311–1317.

90 Rivera MA, Perusse L, Simoneau JA, Gagnon J, Dionne FT, Leon AS, Skinner JS, Wilmore JH, Province M, Rao DC, Bouchard C: Linkage between a specific muscle CK gene marker and $\dot{V}O_2$ max in the HERITAGE Family Study. Med Sci Sports Exerc 1999;31:698–701.

91 Bouchard C, Rankinen T: Individual differences in response to regular physical activity. Med Sci Sports Exerc 2001;33: S446–S451.

92 Rowell LB: Human Cardiovascular Control. Oxford, Oxford University Press, 1993.

93 Pate RR, Ward DS: Endurance exercise trainability in children and youth; in Grana WA, Lombardo JA, Sharkey BJ, Stone EJ (eds): Advances in Sport Medicine and Fitness. Chicago, Year Book Medical Publishers, 1990, pp 37–55.

94 Bacquet G, Van Praagh E, Berthoin S: Endurance training and endurance fitness in young people. Sports Med 2003; 33:1127–1143.

95 Krahenbuhl GS, Skinner JS, Kohrt WM: Developmental aspects of maximal aerobic power in children. Exerc Sports Sci Rev 1985;13:502–538.

96 Rowland TW: Children's Exercise Physiology. Champaign, Human Kinetics, 2005.

97 Armstrong N, Welsman JR: Patterns of physical activity in European children with reference to methods of assessment. Sports Med 2006;36:1067–1086.

98 Armstrong N, Fawkner SG: Aerobic fitness; in Armstrong N (ed): Paediatric Exercise Physiology. Edinburgh, Churchill-Livingstone, 2006, pp 161–188.

99 Pfeiffer KA, Lobelo F, Ward DS, Pate RR: Endurance trainability of children and youth; in Hebestreit H, Bar-Or O (eds): The Young Athlete. Oxford, Blackwell, 2007, pp 84–95.

100 Le Mura LM, von Dullivard SP, Carlonas R, Andreacci J: Can exercise training improve maximal aerobic power ($\dot{V}O_2$ max) in children: a meta-analytic review. J Exerc Physiol 1999;2:1–22.

101 Katch VL: Physical conditioning of children. J Adolesc Health 1983;3:241–246.

102 Rowland TW: The 'trigger hypothesis' for aerobic trainability: a 14-year follow-up. Pediatr Exerc Sci 1997;9:1–9.

103 Eisenman PA, Golding LA: Comparison of effects of training on $\dot{V}O_2$ max in girls and young women. Med Sci Sports 1975;7:136–138.

104 Mountjoy M, Armstrong N, Bizzini L, Blimkie C, Evans J, Gerrard D, Hangen J, Knoll K, Micheli L, Sangenis P, Van Mechelen, W: IOC consensus statement: 'training the elite child athlete'. Clin J Sports Med 2008;18:122–123.

Prof. Neil Armstrong
Executive Suite, Northcote House
The Queen's Building, University of Exeter
Exeter, EX4 4QJ (UK)
Tel. +44 1392263006, Fax +44 1392263008, E-Mail N.Armstrong@exeter.ac.uk

Armstrong N, McManus AM (eds): The Elite Young Athlete.
Med Sport Sci. Basel, Karger, 2011, vol 56, pp 84–96

High-intensity and Resistance Training and Elite Young Athletes

Sébastien Ratel

Clermont Université, Université Blaise Pascal, EA 3533, Laboratoire de Biologie des Activités Physiques et Sportives, Clermont Ferrand, France

Abstract
Although in the past resistance and high-intensity exercise training among young children was the subject of numerous controversies, it is now well-documented that this training mode is a safe and effective means of developing maximal strength, maximal power output and athletic performance in youth, provided that exercises are performed with appropriate supervision and precautions. Muscular strength and power output values measured from vertical jump and Wingate anaerobic tests are higher in elite than in non-elite young athletes and normal children, and the specific training effects on maximal power output normalised for body size are clearly more distinct before puberty. At present, there is no scientific evidence to support the view that high-intensity and/or resistance training might hinder growth and maturation in young children. Pre-pubertal growth is not adversely affected by sport at a competitive level and anthropometric factors are of importance for choice of sport in children. However, coaches, teachers and parents should be aware that unsupervised high-intensity and resistance training programmes involving maximal loads or too frequently repeated resistance exercises increase the risk of injury. Resistance training alone is an effective additional means of developing athletic performance throughout planned youth sports training programmes. Strategies for enhancing the effectiveness and safety of youth resistance and high-intensity exercise training are discussed in this chapter.

Copyright © 2011 S. Karger AG, Basel

Because of the increasing demands for high performance many young children are, more than ever, exposed to high-intensity and resistance training regimens as part of their planned sports programme from an early age. Short-burst activities associated with resistance exercises on weight machines or with free weights are used by young athletes to enhance their muscle performance. However, although physicians, parents, coaches and teachers should promote healthy activity, resistance and high-intensity exercise training at a young age could predispose young children to risks of injury, stunted growth or psychological difficulties. On that basis, a number of important questions have been asked. What are the implications of young athletes performing high-intensity and resistance training programmes involving short-burst activities and resistive loads? Can high-intensity and resistance training increase the muscle strength, short-term muscle power and athletic performance of young athletes? Is resistance training safe and should young athletes be exposed to this mode of training? What is the benefit-to-risk ratio when young athletes are exposed to high-intensity and resistance exercises? At what age should we introduce young athletes to high-intensity resistance training programmes? This chapter will address these questions.

Terminology

For the purpose of this chapter, the term 'resistance training' will be defined as any programme of exercise, which uses one or several training methods in an attempt to enhance health, fitness and sports performance. Methods include (1) progressive exercises using body mass, such as push-ups and pull-ups, (2) free weights or weight machines to provide resistance, and (3) various devices which provide accommodating resistance such as isokinetic, pneumatic and hydraulic machines or friction-loaded and air-braked ergometers (i.e. cycle or rowing ergometers). High-intensity exercises are defined as any exercise that exceeds the maximal power of the oxidative metabolism, the likes of which are met in resistance efforts and sustained all-out sprints. In this chapter, the elite young athlete is considered to be one who undergoes specialized training, receives expert coaching and is exposed early to competition [1]. The terms 'pre-pubescent' and 'child' will refer to girls and boys prior to the development of secondary sex characteristics, roughly defined as up to the age of 11 years for girls and up to age 13 years for boys. The terms 'pubescent' and 'adolescent' will be applied to girls aged 12–18 years and boys aged 14–18 years. The term 'youth' will include the years of childhood and adolescence.

Effectiveness of Resistance Training

In the past, several studies supported the contention that resistance training was ineffective for young children. For instance, in a frequently cited report, Vrijens [2] showed no significant strength improvement in the upper arm and the thigh for pre-pubertal children undergoing training sessions three times a week for 8 weeks. Only the post-pubertal group exhibited distinct strength improvements in all investigated muscles, along with larger cross-sectional areas in the upper arm and the thigh. Vrijens [2] concluded that strength development in response to resistance training was clearly related to sexual maturation, and that resistance training was ineffective before puberty possibly due to insufficient levels of circulating androgens. However, in this study, the training intensity was moderate (on average 70% of 1 repetition maximum, RM) and the overall volume per session was very low (only one set of exercises). The ineffectiveness of resistance training was also supported in pre-pubescent boys by Docherty et al. [3]. These authors indicated that pre-pubescent children did not experience significant improvements in isokinetic leg flexion and extension strength after a resistance training programme that consisted of three sessions a week for 4–6 weeks. However, both the low training volume per session and the short duration of the training programme may have compromised the results of the study. Therefore, although the aforementioned studies suffered from several methodological weaknesses (i.e. an inappropriate training programme in terms of intensity, frequency and duration and in some cases, a lack of systematic control for growth and/or learning), resistance training was not recommended in pre-pubertal children as it was believed to be ineffective in terms of strength improvements [2].

During the last two decades, a number of learned society position papers [4–8] and review articles [9–20] have refuted early claims that resistance training is ineffective in children. Compelling evidence indicates that pre-pubertal children may increase their muscle strength as long as resistance training programmes are well-designed and supervised. One of the earliest well-controlled clinical studies supporting the beneficial effects of resistance training in children was carried out by Sewall and Micheli [21]. Eighteen pre-pubertal children underwent a progressive resistance training programme on weight machines three times per week for 9 weeks. The children involved in training had a mean increase of 43% in upper and lower extremity strength measurements whereas strength in the control group increased by 9%. Similar findings were reported by Weltman et al. [22] in pre-pubescent boys following a hydraulic resistance training programme that consisted of three sessions a week for 14 weeks. The authors found significant improvements of 18–37% in the isokinetic strength of knee/elbow flexor and extensor muscles compared with control group values. It was concluded that resistance training using hydraulic resistance equipment was both safe and effective in prepubescent children.

Compared to the aforementioned studies, Ramsay et al. [23] reported similar gains in maximum isometric and isokinetic strength values of various muscles in pre-pubertal boys, despite a longer training programme of 20 weeks requiring participation thrice weekly. Surprisingly, Faigenbaum et al. [24], who studied the effects of various resistance training protocols using child-sized weight machines in pre-pubertal children, reported strength gains of up to 74% in leg extension and chest press exercises after only 8 weeks of training.

The degree of variability in strength gains may be related to differences in training volume (i.e. the total amount of work performed per training session and per week). It seems that high-volume training programmes (i.e. 3 sets of 10–15 repetitions per exercise with a moderate load, 2–3 sessions a week, and a training duration of 8–14 weeks) result in greater gains in muscular strength than lower volume training programmes [24]. In this respect, isometric strength measurements of elbow flexor and extensor muscles were found to be greater in 11-year-old elite swimmers as compared with age-matched non-elite counterparts for whom the training volume was less [25]. Also, the specificity of training and testing could be of great importance for explaining the differences in strength gains in children.

It was recently shown in young soccer players that combining a resistance training programme with soccer-specific training significantly improved the maximal strength of leg and arm muscles and athletic performance (i.e. vertical jump height and 30 m sprint) more than a resistance training programme alone [26]. Furthermore, the combination of a resistance training programme with plyometrics significantly improved various selected strength variables in 12-year-old children [27]. Bencke et al. [25] also highlighted the specificity of training and/or testing by showing no significant difference in isometric elbow flexor and extensor strength between young elite and non-elite gymnasts, handball and tennis players for whom isometric arm strength, measured at an angle of 90°, is likely to be less decisive in their sports practice than for elite swimmers.

Some studies also showed that pre- and early-pubertal children make similar (if not greater) relative strength gains as compared with post-pubescent children and adults, but usually demonstrate smaller absolute strength gains following resistance training [10, 12, 28]. There are apparently no or only small sex-related differences in response to resistance training among pre- and early-pubertal elite and non-elite athletes [12, 18, 27, 29, 30]. However, further studies are required before definitive conclusions can be drawn on the interaction effect of sex and training.

Effectiveness of High-intensity Exercise Training

While some studies have failed to demonstrate any positive effects of resistance training on anaerobic power development in young children [31], others have reported significant effects of high-intensity exercise training [32–34]. For instance, Grodjinovsky et al. [32] showed significant short-term leg power improvements for 11- to 13-year-old boys undergoing repeated sprint training sessions three times a week for 6 weeks

(5% in subjects trained on a cycle ergometer and 4% in subjects trained during sprint-running). More precisely, the training of the running group consisted of three 40 m sprints followed by three sprints of 150 m during the first 2 weeks. Then, the number of runs was progressively increased every 2 weeks in order to maintain adequate training intensity. The training session of the 'cycle ergometer group' consisted initially of three 8 s all-out cycling bouts followed by three 30 s all-out rides. The number of rides was subsequently increased as described above.

The effectiveness of high-intensity sprint-type training programmes was also supported in pre-pubescent girls by McManus et al. [33]. These authors indicated that 10-year-old girls experienced significant improvements in short-term leg cycling power (10%) after sprint running training that consisted of three sessions a week for 8 weeks, compared with control subjects who demonstrated no significant changes. Similar findings were reported by Diallo et al. [34] in 12- to 13-year-old soccer players after a plyometric training programme of 3 sessions per week for 10 weeks including various dynamic exercises (jumping, bouncing and skipping drills). These authors showed that children significantly increased their short-term leg-cycling power (12%) and jumping and sprint running performances (vertical and horizontal jumps; 20, 30 and 40 m sprints). Furthermore, Kasabalis et al. [35] showed that vertical jump and Wingate anaerobic test scores were higher in elite young male volleyball players than in non-elite young athletes, and the specific training effects of anaerobic power ($W \cdot kg^{-1}$ body mass) were more pronounced at the age of 10–11 years (15%) than at the age of 15–16 years (4%). Significantly higher anaerobic power values ($W \cdot kg^{-1}$ body mass) were also reported by Bencke et al. [27] in elite 11-year-old athletes (swimmers, gymnasts, tennis players and handball players) as compared with normal values.

In summary, there is clear evidence that young children can increase their muscular strength and short-term muscle power above and beyond growth and maturation by participating in a supervised resistance and high-intensity sprint-type training programme based on weight machines or all-out activities. Overall, strength improvements of 10–40% have been obtained in children following short-term (<20 weeks) resistance training programmes [12], although gains of up to 74% have been observed [24]. However, muscle power gains following high-intensity sprint-type training exercises were clearly lower (5–12%). This is certainly related to the non-specific training of short-burst activities on a target muscle as can be the case in more specific resistance training programmes on weight machines. Although the frequency, duration and intensity of training continue to be debated in search of an optimal programme, children develop significantly more strength on weight machines after higher-repetitions training programmes with moderate loads than following lower-repetitions training programmes with heavier loads [36, 37]. Also, it appears that a training frequency of twice a week is sufficient to induce strength improvements in young athletes [24]. However, more frequent and specific training sessions are likely to induce significantly greater muscle strength and anaerobic power values as observed in elite young athletes.

Physiological Mechanisms for Strength Development

Although factors related to strength development following resistance training have been thoroughly investigated in adults [38, 39], few studies have evaluated the mechanisms responsible for strength gains in young people. Numerous factors including muscle hypertrophy, neural drive, motor unit synchronisation and psychological drive may contribute to strength development following resistance training [38, 39]. However, the relative contribution of each of these factors could be different according to age, gender and maturity status.

In an attempt to determine the contribution of muscle hypertrophy to increased strength in children, several studies have included morphological measurements in the evaluation of training-induced strength gains [22, 23, 25, 40–42]. These studies have used either indirect techniques such as anthropometry or direct methods such as soft-tissue roentgenography [2], computed tomography [23, 41] and magnetic resonance imaging [40]. Collectively, the results from these studies show that resistance training programmes during the pre-adolescent period do not induce significant muscle hypertrophy [2, 22, 23, 42]. However, some studies have challenged this conclusion and suggest that muscle hypertrophy may occur among pre-pubescent children following resistance training [40, 41]. For instance, Mersch and Stoboy [40] reported more significant quadriceps cross-sectional area improvements (4–9%) in two pre-pubertal monozygotic twin boys undergoing 10 weeks of maximal isometric training of knee extensors as compared with their control twin. Similar findings were reported by Fukunaga et al. [41] in a cohort of 52 pre-pubescent Japanese boys and girls. Twelve weeks of isometric resistance training (three 10-second maximal contractions, twice per day, 3 days weekly) resulted in increased cross-sectional areas (8%) of elbow flexors as measured by ultrasonic methods. This increment was attributed to significant increases in muscle and bone areas in the trained group whereas in the control group, this was due to an increase in fat area. Interestingly, the increment of muscle cross-sectional area after training was significantly correlated with the skeletal age. Therefore, even though it is as yet premature to draw definitive conclusions, these two studies do present the prospect that muscle hypertrophy is possible during the pre-pubertal period.

According to Fukunaga et al. [41], the increase of muscle area in response to resistance training in pre-pubertal children would be about 50% of that observed in adults. As suggested by Faigenbaum [15] and Faigenbaum et al. [8], more intensive training programmes, longer training durations and more sensitive measuring techniques may be required to uncover the potentially greater effects of resistance training for muscle hypertrophy in prepubescent athletes. Hence, muscle hypertrophy could be more frequently observed in young elite athletes. Nevertheless, this is speculative as, to the best of my knowledge, no studies have been devoted to compare muscle morphology between elite and non-elite young athletes. For children in advanced puberty, the strength gains could be explained by a greater muscle hypertrophy contribution because of increased circulating levels of growth and gonadal hormones [15].

While muscle hypertrophy still remains the subject of some controversy, neurological adaptations following high-intensity and resistance training are more evident in pre-pubertal children [22, 23, 42, 43]. For instance, Ozmun et al. [42] addressed this issue in a study aiming to examine the effects of 8 weeks of resistance training on muscular strength of elbow flexors in pre-pubescent boys and girls. Significant isotonic (23%) and isokinetic (28%) strength gains were observed without concomitant changes in arm circumference or skinfolds measurements. While these results are disposed to show that the strength gains are not due to muscle hypertrophy, the greater amplitude of electromyographic signals (17%) reported in the trained children, suggests a significantly increased neuromuscular activation. Similarly, Weltman et al. [22] ascribed indirectly the strength gains to neural adaptations following 14 weeks of resistance training in pre-pubertal boys and girls since no modification in body circumferences or skinfold measurements were observed. However, such interpretation should be made with caution since neural adaptations were inferred from the lack of muscle hypertrophy as determined by anthropometry, which is well known to induce a systematic bias as compared with reference methods (i.e. magnetic resonance imaging), especially in pre-pubertal children [44]. Furthermore, as indicated by Folland and Williams [39], any increase in specific strength (scaled for muscle size) can be explained not only by neurological adaptations, but also by some morphological adaptations such as increases in tendinous stiffness and/or the angle of muscle pennation.

To the best of my knowledge, only two studies have addressed more directly the neurological changes in pre-pubertal children following resistance training. Using the interpolated twitch technique, Ramsay et al. [23] showed in pre-pubescent children that 10 weeks of resistance training significantly increased motor unit activation of the elbow flexors (9%) and knee extensors (12%), and a supplementary training of 10 weeks resulted in much smaller gains of only 3 and 2%, respectively. This study demonstrates that neurological adaptations occur predominantly in the early phase of training. Furthermore, using surface electromyography, Ozmun et al. [42] showed that 8 weeks of resistance training significantly improved the neuromuscular activation of elbow flexors in pre-pubertal children.

Other potential factors, which may explain increases in muscle strength, include changes in the intrinsic contractile characteristics of muscle. Specifically, Ramsay et al. [23] showed that resistance training could result in increased elbow flexor and knee extensor evoked twitch torque without concomitant changes in muscle cross-sectional area, thereby suggesting adaptations in muscle excitation-contraction coupling. Furthermore, Mero et al. [45] have pointed out that the greater fast-twitch fibre distribution in the more powerful elite young athletes aged 11–13 years (sprinters, weightlifters and tennis players) could be related to their event-specific training that consisted of more fast force production. Although speculative, it is also likely that training-induced strength gains are attributed, in some measure, to improved motor skill coordination, especially in more complex multi-joint actions [11], and to developmental changes in muscle

fibre architecture as the angle of muscle pennation [8, 19]. Furthermore, alterations in central inhibitory influences should be considered to explain the increased muscle strength following resistance training [8].

Although it is not simple to quantify the relative contribution of muscle and neurological adaptations in strength gains, it appears that resistance training in pre-pubertal children is principally attributed to neurological adaptations and modestly, if at all, to muscle hypertrophy. Although speculative, muscle hypertrophy can be more frequently observed in elite young athletes as they are often engaged in more intensive resistance training programmes than non-elite young athletes. In elite and non-elite pubescent children, the strength gains can be largely explained by muscle hypertrophy, due to greater levels of circulating androgenic hormones.

Reversibility of Strength Gains in Youth

Resistance training-induced strength gains can be partially or completely lost if the training stimulus is insufficient or abolished [46]. Only a few studies have investigated the effects of detraining on muscle strength following resistance training in young children [21, 24, 26, 47–49]. This statement is all the more surprising when young elite athletes undergo short- or long-term periods of reduced training or inactivity, due to training design, injuries, travel plans or decreased motivation.

Some evidence indicates that training-induced strength gains are significantly reversible when resistance training programmes are slowed down or interrupted. For instance, over 9 weeks of detraining, Sewall and Micheli [21] reported significant decreases of 1.4% a week on average compared to post-training results in various isometric strength measures in pre-pubertal children. A significant decline was also reported by Faigenbaum et al. [24] over 8 weeks of detraining. However, the magnitude of decline was clearly greater (3% per week). More recently, Ingle et al. [26] provided further evidence that the strength gains achieved during a 12 week complex training programme (resistance training + plyometrics) in early pubertal boys regressed rapidly towards control values after 12 weeks of detraining. According to Guy and Micheli [16], the magnitude of the decline appears to be dependent on the amplitude of training-induced strength gains, level of inactivity, and duration of detraining. Maturational and growth-related changes in muscle size could also justify the degree of reversibility as the loss of muscle strength might be completely or partially covered by natural muscular hypertrophy-induced strength gains during growth [10, 11]. In elite young athletes, the decline in muscle strength could be faster as their muscle strength level was found to be higher than in non-elite young athletes [27]. However, this is speculative and further studies are required before definitive conclusions can be drawn on this issue.

The amount of training required to maintain or at least slow the loss of exercise-induced adaptations in young athletes has yet to be determined. In one study involving six pre-pubertal boys, a maintenance training programme of once a week was not enough to sustain gains achieved during progressive resistance training of 20 weeks [47]. Conversely, DeRenne et al. [48] showed in a group of pubescent baseball players that resistance training once a week was as effective as twice a week in maintaining training-induced strength gains. Others observed that 8 weeks of reduced training including only soccer practice could maintain muscle power gains made previously by 10 weeks of plyometric training in pre-pubescent soccer players [34].

Therefore, more information is warranted before specific maintenance training guidelines can be made for children and adolescents according to their level of sports practice. For performance reasons, young athletes should participate in maintenance training programmes during the sports season [15]. Although available data are limited, it also appears in pre-pubertal children the decline in training-induced strength gains during the detraining period is mainly due to changes in the level of neuromuscular activation and motor skill coordination [11, 47]. Furthermore, because of the resistance training-induced possible gains in muscle size during the pubertal period [2], the mechanisms responsible for the loss of strength during detraining in adolescents could be attributed, in addition to neuromuscular adaptations, to muscle loss.

Potential Effects on Growth and Maturation

The question of how resistance and high-intensity exercise training could influence the growth process and maturation has challenged researchers for numerous years. To address this question, most studies have investigated growth-associated changes in stature in elite and non-elite young athletes in comparison with control subjects [18, 22–24, 50]. From these studies, it appears that resistance training in pre-pubescent children does not hinder stature, at least for training durations of 8–20 weeks [18, 22–24]. However, we need to be cautious with this interpretation since the average growth rate in stature before the pubertal period is around 5 cm per year, and short-term training durations (<20 weeks) are insufficient to reflect any possible effect of resistance training on stature [17]. To respond conveniently to this question, the impact of a resistance training programme on the growth rate should be investigated over several years until the achievement of final stature.

At the present time, only Sadres et al. [51] have demonstrated in a 21-month intervention that resistance training in pre-pubescent boys significantly improved muscle strength compared to control group values without having adverse effects on stature. Such results could be unexpected as pre-pubertal female gymnasts, whose training involves high-impact and heavy resistive loads, have a slower growth rate compared with control children [52, 53]. However, this assertion does not seem to be related to the training itself but is rather the result of selection because of a morphological advantage of athletes in this sport [52, 53]. This finding was confirmed in elite pre-pubertal and early pubertal athletes competing at a national level in swimming, tennis, team handball and gymnastics [50]. Damsgaard et al. [50] have shown that genetic factors, stature attained 2–4 years before starting the sport, as well as maturation status, were decisive factors for stature attained between 9 and 13 years of age. Interestingly, the authors failed to demonstrate any significant influence from the type of sport and number of training hours on maturation and the stature attained. This strongly suggests that selection of sport in children is dependent on anthropometrical factors, and that the sport itself is of lesser importance. This does not exclude, however, that the form of training as well as nutrition could play a role in attained stature. Therefore, at present, there is no scientific evidence to support the argument that resistance and high-intensity exercise training under appropriate supervision might hinder growth and maturation in young elite and non-elite athletes.

Injury Risks

One of the reasons that restricted children and adolescents from performing high-intensity and resistance training programmes was the presumed high risks of injuries associated with weight machines, free weights, body weight activities and repeated all-out activities inducing muscle fatigue. In particular, it was claimed that resistance training programmes led to injuries of epiphyseal plates, cartilage, ligaments or muscles. However, compelling evidence in athletic or non-athletic children and adolescents does not support this conviction provided that appropriate resistance-training guidelines are properly followed (cf. next section).

For instance, Sewall and Micheli [21] reported no injuries in 18 pre-pubescent children undergoing progressive resistance training sessions on weight machines three times a week for 9 weeks. Similar findings were reported in a study by Weltman et al. [22] examining the effectiveness and safety of a 14-week hydraulic resistance training programme in 26 pre-pubertal males. Using biphasic musculoskeletal scintigraphy before and after the programme, these authors found no evidence of damage to epiphyses, bone or muscle. Only one strength training-related injury was reported (left shoulder pain). It was concluded that short-term, supervised resistance training using hydraulic resistance equipment is safe and effective in pre-pubescent children. The safety of resistance training programmes was also confirmed by Lillegard et al. [33] in pre-pubescent compared to early post-pubescent males and females. The 52 subjects involved in the 12-week resistance training programme were exposed to approximately 1,872 h during which only one injury (a minor strain of a shoulder muscle) occurred. This minor injury was considered incidental because of the high exercise-to-injury ratio and the low severity of the injury. As the training loads on weight machines are often set at selected percentages of the 1 RM, Faigenbaum et al. [48] also considered whether 1 RM strength testing may be potentially injurious to young athletes. Under close supervision by qualified professionals, 32 girls and 64 boys between 6 and 13 years performed a 1 RM test on upper- and lower-body exercises using child-size weight training machines. No injuries occurred over the study period, and the testing protocol was well tolerated by the volunteers. Faigenbaum et al. [54] concluded that young children can safely perform 1 RM strength tests provided that careful precautions are properly followed. To my knowledge, no studies have been devoted to analyse the prevalence of injuries in young elite athletes. However, as young elite athletes receive expert coaching, it is likely that they are no more exposed to risks of injury than non-elite young athletes who are under close supervision.

While not related to injury per se, it has been shown that intensive eccentric exercise induced muscle damage is clearly less in young children compared with adults [55, 56]. For instance, Soares et al. [55] reported that children appeared to suffer less damage compared with young adults after a weight training protocol, based on measurements of soreness, creatine kinase activity, and isometric strength. In the same way, it has been shown that pre-pubertal boys experienced less severe symptoms of damage than men after intensive plyometric exercise [56]. Less muscle damage in pre-pubertal children may be explained by their greater flexibility leading to less over extension of sarcomeres during eccentric exercise, fewer fast-twitch muscle fibres, and perhaps more varied habitual physical activity patterns [56].

Therefore, it appears that the risks of injury associated with resistance and high-intensity exercise training programmes during youth are no greater than those associated with other sports and recreational activities common to this age group [16, 20]. However, this is based on the understanding that a given high-intensity and resistance training programme is appropriately prescribed and supervised as indicated in youth resistance training guidelines.

Youth Resistance Training Guidelines

Many position papers [5, 6, 8] and review articles [9, 15, 19, 57] have established youth resistance training guidelines designed to improve muscular strength and athletic performance, and concomitantly reduce the risks of injury in young children.

Overall, youth resistance-training guidelines point out that:

(1) Programmes should be instructed and supervised by qualified professionals who have an understanding of the guidelines and who have practical experience working with young children. It is important that coaches, trainers and teachers speak at a level that children and adolescents understand. All exercises must be clearly explained and appropriately demonstrated to young children. It is also important that children are prepared psychologically and physically to comply with coaching instructions and undergo the stress of intensive training programmes. However, elite young athletes appear to be more willing to invest effort into practice and competition than their non-elite peers [58]. Therefore, they seem to be less exposed to physical and psychological constraints associated with high-intensity resistance efforts.

(2) A 5- to 10-min warm-up period of light aerobic and stretching exercises is necessary before each training session. Dynamic warm-up procedures are likely to be effective in children to engage them to listen to instructions [19]. Furthermore, dynamic warm-up protocols of sufficient intensity have been shown to enhance aerobic and anaerobic performance in children and teenagers [59, 60].

(3) Initial training sessions should be directed toward the development of a proper technique on a variety of ergometers and strength-building exercises, using light loads (<50% 1 RM). Beginning a resistance training programme for children with a single set of 13–15 repetitions per exercise not only allows for positive changes in muscle performance, but provides an opportunity for each child to experience success and feel good about his/her own performance.

(4) Exercises, including body weight, rubber tubing, medicine balls, free weights and child-sized ergometers, should be recommended to avoid any risks of injuries [61]. It is important to include multi-joint exercises in the workout programmes because these promote the use of co-ordinated movements. Exercises strengthening

the core musculature should be also incorporated into the training programmes. The muscular development should be symmetrical, ensuring an appropriate muscle balance around joints [1].

(5) As the muscle adapts to the resistance-training load, the exercise-induced stimulus need to be increased progressively over time (i.e. approximately 5–10%). This can be made by increasing the resistance, the number of repetitions or the number of sets. The training load on weight machines can be set at selected percentages of the 1 RM. However, 1 RM tests must be begun using an adequate warm-up, an individualized progression of loads and under close and competent supervision. The best approach may be to first establish the repetition training range (i.e. 10–15), and then by trial and error determine the maximum load that can be handled for the prescribed range [15]. On friction-loaded cycle ergometers, the work load could be calculated as a function of body mass, lean body mass or lean leg volume.

(6) For specific sports/athletic events, where strength is a key determinant of performance, a training frequency of 2–3 nonconsecutive days per week is necessary, as resistance training programmes of only once per week may result in suboptimal adaptations [62].

(7) As muscle sensitivity to fatigue was found to be less in children as compared with adults [55, 56, 63–66], shorter rest intervals than those commonly used by adults may be used with children when performing repeated bouts of high-intensity resistance exercise. However, such recommendations should be taken with caution in adolescents for whom muscle sensitivity to fatigue is clearly greater than in pre-pubertal children [67–69].

(8) Finally, resistance training programmes should be considered as part of a planned youth sports programme. Goals should be realistic and established according to the physical and psychological capacities of each child athlete.

Conclusions

It is now well documented that resistance training based on weight machines or high-intensity sprint-type activities is a safe and effective means of developing muscle strength, muscle power and athletic performance in child and adolescent athletes provided that exercises are performed with appropriate supervision and precautions. While some studies showed strength improvements of 10–40% in young children following resistance training programmes on weight machines, others reported short-term muscle power gains of 5–12% following repeated all-out running or cycling activities. This difference in the amplitude of muscle strength and power gains can be attributed to the amount and specificity of training programmes as well as biological age. Elite young athletes were found to be stronger and more powerful than their non-elite young counterparts. Vertical jump and Wingate anaerobic test scores were found to be higher in elite young athletes, and the specific training effects of anaerobic power were clearly more pronounced at the age of 10–11 years than at the age of 15–16 years.

At present, there is no scientific evidence to support the view that resistance and high-intensity exercise training might hinder growth and maturation in young children. It appears that selection of sport is dependent on anthropometrical factors, and that the sport itself is of lesser importance. However, coaches, teachers and parents should be aware that unsupervised high-intensity resistance training programmes involving maximal loads or too frequently repeated resistance exercises increase the risks of injury, which could slow down the progression of children. Resistance training alone has not to be a proxy but rather an additional means of developing muscle power and athletic performance throughout planned youth sports training programmes.

References

1 Mountjoy M, Armstrong N, Bizzini L, Blimkie C, Evans J, Gerrard D, Hangen J, Knoll K, Micheli L, Sangenis P, Van Mechelen W: IOC consensus statement: 'Training the elite child athlete'. Br J Sports Med 2008;42:163–164.

2 Vrijens F: Muscle strength development in the pre- and post-pubescent age. Med Sport 1978;11:244–246.

3 Docherty D, Wenger HA, Collis ML, Quinney HA: The effects of variable speed resistance training on strength development in prepubertal boys. J Hum Mov Stud 1987;13:377–382.

4 Golan R, Falk B, Hoffman J, Hochberg Z, Ben-Sira D, Barak Y: Resistance training for children and adolescents; in Chan KM, Micheli LJ (eds): Sports and Children. Hong Kong, Williams & Wilkins, 1998, pp 265–270.

5 Stratton G, Jones M, Fox KR, Tolfrey K, Harris J, Maffulli N, Lee M, Frostick SP: BASES position statement on guidelines for resistance exercise in young people. J Sports Sci 2004;22:383–390.

6 American College of Sports Medicine: ACSM's Guidelines for Exercise Testing and Prescription, ed 7. Lippincott, Williams & Wilkins, 2006.

7 American Academy of Pediatrics Council on Sports Medicine and Fitness, McCambridge TM, Stricker PR: Strength training by children and adolescents. Pediatrics 2008;121:835–840.

8 Faigenbaum AD, Kraemer WJ, Blimkie CJ, Jeffreys I, Micheli LJ, Nitka M, Rowland TW: Youth resistance training: updated position statement paper from the National Strength and Conditioning Association. J Strength Cond Res 2009; 23:S60–S79.

9 Webb DR: Strength training in children and adolescents. Pediatr Clin North Am 1990;37:1187–1210.

10 Blimkie CJ: Resistance training during pre- and early puberty: efficacy, trainability, mechanisms, and persistence. Can J Sport Sci 1992;17:264–279.

11 Blimkie CJ: Resistance training during preadolescence: issues and controversies. Sports Med 1993;15:389–407.

12 Falk B, Tenenbaum G: The effectiveness of resistance training in children: a meta-analysis. Sports Med 1996;22:176–186.

13 Payne VG, Morrow JR Jr, Johnson L, Dalton SN: Resistance training in children and youth: a meta-analysis. Res Q Exerc Sport 1997;68:80–88.

14 Blimkie CJR, Sale DG: Strength development and trainability during childhood; in Van Praagh E (ed): Pediatric Anaerobic Performance. Champaign, Human Kinetics, 1998, pp 193–224.

15 Faigenbaum AD: Strength training for children and adolescents. Clin Sports Med 2000;19:593–619.

16 Guy JA, Micheli LJ: Strength training for children and adolescents. J Am Acad Orthop Surg 2001;9:29–36.

17 Falk B, Eliakim A: Resistance training, skeletal muscle and growth. Pediatr Endocrinol Rev 2003;1:120–127.

18 Malina RM: Weight training in youth-growth, maturation, and safety: an evidence-based review. Clin J Sport Med 2006;16:478–487.

19 Behm DG, Faigenbaum AD, Falk B, Klentrou P: Canadian Society for Exercise Physiology position paper: resistance training in children and adolescents. Appl Physiol Nutr Metab 2008; 33:547–561.

20 Faigenbaum AD, Myer GD: Resistance training among young athletes: safety, efficacy and injury prevention effects. Br J Sports Med 2010;44:56–63.

21 Sewall L, Micheli LJ: Strength training for children. J Pediatr Orthop 1986;6: 143–146.

22 Weltman A, Janney C, Rians CB, Strand K, Berg B, Tippitt S, Wise J, Cahill BR, Katch FI: The effects of hydraulic resistance strength training in prepubertal males. Med Sci Sports Exerc 1986;18:629–638.

23 Ramsay JA, Blimkie CJ, Smith K, Garner S, MacDougall JD, Sale DG: Strength training effects in pre-pubescent boys. Med Sci Sports Exerc 1990;22:605–614.

24 Faigenbaum AD, Westcott WL, Micheli LJ, Outerbridge AR, Long CJ, LaRosa-Loud R, Zaichkowsky LD: The effects of strength training and detraining on children. J Strength Cond Res 1996;10:109–114.

25 Bencke J, Damsgaard R, Saekmose A, Jørgensen P, Jørgensen K, Klausen K: Anaerobic power and muscle strength characteristics of 11 years old elite and non-elite boys and girls from gymnastics, team handball, tennis and swimming. Scand J Med Sci Sports 2002;12: 171–178.

26 Christou M, Smilios I, Sotiropoulos K, Volaklis K, Pilianidis T, Tokmakidis SP: Effects of resistance training on the physical capacities of adolescent soccer players. J Strength Cond Res 2006;20: 783–791.

27 Ingle L, Sleap M, Tolfrey K: The effect of a complex training and detraining programme on selected strength and power variables in early pubertal boys. J Sports Sci 2006;24:987–997.

28 Pfeiffer R, Francis R: Effects of strength training on muscle development in pre-pubescent, pubescent and post-pubescent males. Phys Sports Med 1986; 14:134–143.

29 Blimkie C: Age- and sex-associated variation in strength during childhood: Anthropometric, morphologic, neurological, biomechanical, endocrinologic, genetic and physical activity correlates; in Gisolfi C, Lamb D (eds): Perspectives in Exercise Science and Sports. Indianapolis, Benchmark, 1989, pp 99–163.

30 Lillegard WA, Brown EW, Wilson DJ, Henderson R, Lewis E: Efficacy of strength training in prepubescent to early postpubescent males and females: effects of gender and maturity. Pediatr Rehabil 1997;1:147–157.

31 Docherty D, Wenger HA, Collis ML: The effects of resistance training on aerobic and anaerobic power of young boys. Med Sci Sports Exerc 1987;19:389–392.

32 Grodjinovsky D, Inbar O, Dotan R, Bar-Or O: Training effect on the anaerobic performance of children as measured by the Wingate anaerobic test; in Borg K, Eriksson BO (eds): Children and Exercise. Part IX. Baltimore, University Park Press, 1980, pp 139–145.

33 McManus AM, Armstrong N, Williams CA: Effect of training on the aerobic power and anaerobic performance of prepubertal girls. Acta Paediatr 1997;86: 456–459.

34 Diallo O, Dore E, Duche P, Van Praagh E: Effects of plyometric training followed by a reduced training programme on physical performance in pre-pubescent soccer players. J Sports Med Phys Fitness 2001;41:342–348.

35 Kasabalis A, Douda H, Tokmakidis SP: Relationship between anaerobic power and jumping of selected male volleyball players of different ages. Percept Mot Skills 2005;100:607–614.

36 Faigenbaum AD, Westcott WL, Loud RL, Long C: The effects of different resistance training protocols on muscular strength and endurance development in children. Pediatrics 1999;104:e5.

37 Faigenbaum AD, Loud RL, O'Connell J, Glover S, O'Connell J, Westcott WL: Effects of different resistance training protocols on upper-body strength and endurance development in children. J Strength Cond Res 2001;15:459–465.

38 Gabriel DA, Kamen G, Frost G: Neural adaptations to resistive exercise: mechanisms and recommendations for training practices. Sports Med 2006;36:133–149.

39 Folland JP, Williams AG: The adaptations to strength training: morphological and neurological contributions to increased strength. Sports Med 2007;37:145–168.

40 Mersch F, Stoboy H: Strength training and muscle hypertrophy in children; in Oseid S, Carlsen K (eds): Children and Exercise. Part XIII. Champaign, Human Kinetics, 1989, pp 165–182.

41 Fukunaga T, Funato K, Ikegawa S: The effects of resistance training on muscle area and strength in pre-pubescent age. Ann Physiol Anthropol 1992;11:357–364.

42 Ozmun JC, Mikesky AE, Surburg PR: Neuromuscular adaptations following pre-pubescent strength training. Med Sci Sports Exerc 1994;26:510–514.

43 Blimkie CJR, Ramsay J, Sale D, MacDougall D, Smith K, Garner S: Effects of 10 weeks of resistance training on strength development in prepubertal boys; in Oseid S, Carlsen K (eds): Children and Exercise. Part XIII. Champaign, Human Kinetics, 1989, pp 183–197.

44 Tonson A, Ratel S, Le Fur Y, Cozzone P, Bendahan D: Effect of maturation on the relationship between muscle size and force production. Med Sci Sports Exerc 2008;40:918–925.

45 Mero A, Jaakkola L, Komi PV: Relationships between muscle fibre characteristics and physical performance capacity in trained athletic boys. J Sports Sci 1991;9:161–171.

46 Mujika I, Padilla S: Detraining: loss of training-induced physiological and performance adaptations. 1. Short term insufficient training stimulus. Sports Med 2000;30:79–87.

47 Blimkie C, Martin J, Ramsay J, Sale D, MacDougall D: The effects of detraining and maintenance weight training on strength development in prepubertal boys. Can J Sport Sci 1989;14:102P.

48 DeRenne C, Hetzler R, Buxton B, Ho K: Effects of training frequency on strength maintenance in pubescent baseball players. J Strength Cond Res 1996;10:8–14.

49 Tsolakis CK, Vagenas GK, Dessypris AG: Strength adaptations and hormonal responses to resistance training and detraining in pre-adolescent males. J Strength Cond Res 2004;18:625–629.

50 Damsgaard R, Bencke J, Matthiesen G, Petersen JH, Müller J: Is pre-pubertal growth adversely affected by sport? Med Sci Sports Exerc 2000;32:1698–1703.

51 Sadres E, Eliakim A, Constantini N, Lidor R, Falk B: The effect of long-term resistance training on anthropometric measures, muscle strength, and self concept in pre-pubertal boys. Pediatr Exerc Sci 2001;13:357–372.

52 Bass S, Bradney M, Pearce G, Hendrich E, Inge K, Stuckey S, Lo SK, Seeman E: Short stature and delayed puberty in gymnasts: influence of selection bias on leg length and the duration of training on trunk length. J Pediatr 2000;136:149–155.

53 Caine D, Lewis R, O'Connor P, Howe W, Bass S: Does gymnastics training inhibit growth of females? Clin J Sport Med 2001;11:260–270.

54 Faigenbaum AD, Milliken LA, Westcott WL: Maximal strength testing in healthy children. J Strength Cond Res 2003;17:162–166.

55 Soares JMC, Mota P, Duarte JA, Appell HJ: Children are less susceptible to exercise-induced muscle damage than adults: a preliminary investigation. Pediatr Exerc Sci 1996;8:361–367.

56 Marginson V, Rowlands AV, Gleeson NP, Eston RG: Comparison of the symptoms of exercise-induced muscle damage after an initial and repeated bout of plyometric exercise in men and boys. J Appl Physiol 2005;99:1174–1181.

57 Hass CJ, Feigenbaum MS, Franklin BA: Prescription of resistance training for healthy populations. Sports Med 2001;31:953–964.

58 Toering TT, Elferink-Gemser MT, Jordet G, Visscher C: Self-regulation and performance level of elite and non-elite youth soccer players. J Sports Sci 2009;3:1–9.

59 Faigenbaum AD, Bellucci M, Bernieri A, Bakker B, Hoorens K: Acute effects of different warm-up protocols on fitness performance in children. J Strength Cond Res 2005;19:376–381.

60 Faigenbaum A, Kang J, McFarland J, Bloom J, Magnatta J, Ratamess N, Hoffman J: Acute effects of different warm-up protocols on anaerobic performance in teenage athletes. Pediatr Exerc Sci 2006;17:64–75.

61 Kilding AE, Tunstall H, Kuzmic D: Suitability of FIFA's 'the 11' training programme for young football players – impact of physical performance. J Sci Med Sport 2008;7:320–326.

62 Faigenbaum AD, Milliken LA, Loud RL, Burak BT, Doherty CL, Westcott WL: Comparison of 1 and 2 days per week of strength training in children. Res Q Exerc Sport 2002;73:416–424.

63 Ratel S, Williams CA, Oliver J, Armstrong N: Effects of age and mode of exercise on power output profiles during repeated sprints. Eur J Appl Physiol 2004;92:204–210.

64 Ratel S, Duché P, Williams CA: Muscle fatigue during high-intensity exercise in children. Sports Med 2006;36:1031–1065.

65 Faigenbaum AD, Ratamess NA, McFarland J, Kaczmarek J, Coraggio MJ, Kang J, Hoffman JR: Effect of rest interval length on bench press performance in boys, teens, and men. Pediatr Exerc Sci 2008;20:457–469.

66 De Ste Croix MB, Deighan MA, Ratel S, Armstrong N: Age- and sex-associated differences in isokinetic knee muscle endurance between young children and adults. Appl Physiol Nutr Metab 2009;34:725–731.

67   Ratel S, Bedu M, Hennegrave A, Doré E, Duché P: Effects of age and recovery duration on peak power output during repeated cycling sprints. Int J Sports Med 2002;23:397–402.

68   Zafeiridis A, Dalamitros A, Dipla K, Manou V, Galanis N, Kellis S: Recovery during high-intensity intermittent anaerobic exercise in boys, teens, and men. Med Sci Sports Exerc 2005;37:505–512.

69   Dipla K, Tsirini T, Zafeiridis A, Manou V, Dalamitros A, Kellis E, Kellis S: Fatigue resistance during high-intensity intermittent exercise from childhood to adulthood in males and females. Eur J Appl Physiol 2009;106:645–653.

Dr. Sébastien Ratel
Laboratoire de Biologie des Activités Physiques et Sportives
(BAPS, EA 3533), UFR STAPS, Université Blaise Pascal
BP 104
FR–63172 Aubière (France)
Tel. +33 04 73 40 54 86, Fax +33 04 73 40 74 46, E-Mail Sebastien.RATEL@univ-bpclermont.fr

Armstrong N, McManus AM (eds): The Elite Young Athlete.
Med Sport Sci. Basel, Karger, 2011, vol 56, pp 97–105

Overtraining and Elite Young Athletes

Richard Winsley · Nuno Matos

Children's Health and Exercise Research Centre, University of Exeter, Exeter, UK

Abstract

In comparison to adults, our knowledge of the overtraining syndrome in elite young athletes is lacking. The evidence indicates an incidence rate of ~20–30%, with a relatively higher occurrence seen in individual sport athletes, females and those competing at the highest representative levels. The most commonly reported symptoms are similar to those observed in overtrained adult athletes: increased perception of effort during exercise, frequent upper respiratory tract infections, muscle soreness, sleep disturbances, loss of appetite, mood disturbances, shortness of temper, decreased interest in training and competition, decreased self-confidence, inability to concentrate. The association between training load and overtraining is unclear, and underlines the importance of taking a holistic approach when trying to treat or prevent overtraining in the young athlete so that both training and non-training stressors are considered. Of particular relevance to the issue of overtraining in the elite young athlete are the development of a unidimensional identity, the lack of autonomy, disempowerment, perfectionist traits, conditional love, and unrealistic expectations. Overtraining syndrome is a complex phenomenon with unique and multiple antecedents for each individual; therefore, an open-minded and comprehensive perspective is needed to successfully treat/prevent this in the young athlete.

Nearly a century ago, Hill [1] wrote that muscle soreness, stiffness, nervous exhaustion, metabolic disturbances and sleeplessness were all seen in the chronically fatigued athlete, all symptoms that have since become associated with overtraining. Since this time much research has focused on the overtrained athlete, but due to the complexity of this phenomenon, the detection, management and prevention of overtraining remains a real challenge.

A common misperception is that overtraining (OT) is simply an issue about excessive training loads. In support of this viewpoint, the evidence shows that in the quest for improved performance, training loads have increased in parallel. For example, the Olympic swimmer Mark Spitz, winner of 7 gold medals in the 1972 Olympics, trained by swimming around 9 km per day, but within 20 years the average college swimmer had exceeded this training load [2] and a number of Olympic sports have reported a 20% increase in training loads in recent years [3]. Thus, for those who are, or strive to become, an elite athlete, this comes with the expectation that it will be achieved, often in a dose-response manner, by doing even more training; yet this has led some athletes to train so much that they have ended up overtrained [4]. If the young athlete finds themselves embroiled in a 'more is better' culture, propagated by the coaches, athletes and family that surround them, this may ultimately prove destructive and impair the

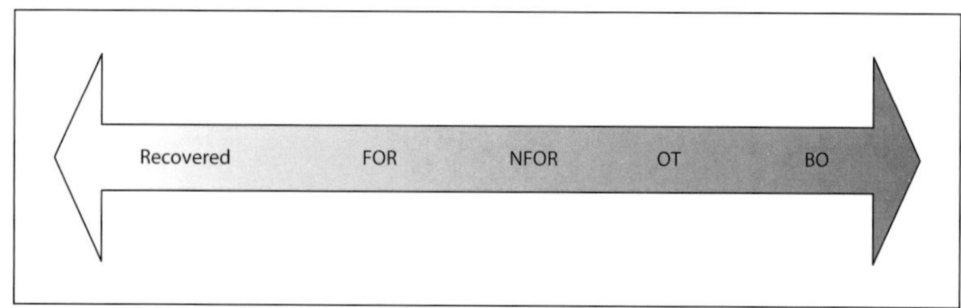

Fig. 1. Overtraining continuum. FOR = Functional overreaching; NFOR = non-functional overreaching; OT = overtraining; BO = burnout.

potential athlete's chances of becoming an elite performer.

Current understanding of OT is largely based on adult data and experience, with relatively little known about this condition in the young elite athlete. However, the available evidence suggests that OT is an issue for young athletes and an awareness of its multi-dimensional nature, will, it is hoped, mean that elite selection will be based on merit and not attrition.

What Is Overtraining?

What exactly is OT and how is it defined? Unfortunately, no agreed single definition of OT exists, something which in its own right has hampered understanding the phenomenon, and a number of alternative definitions are used. This lexicon of definitions has arisen because OT is not a single entity but, as some argue, rather a continuum of related and progressive conditions [5–7] (fig. 1).

Overtraining and overreaching (OR) arise when there is an imbalance between training fatigue and/or non-training stressors and recovery. More specifically, OR is an accumulation of training and non-training stressors that result in a short-term decrement in performance taking from days to several weeks to recover, whilst OT is an accumulation of training and non-training stressors that have detrimental long-term effects on performance and a recovery period that may

take several weeks to months [6]. These definitions imply that the difference between OR and OT is seen in the duration of the performance loss and in the amount of time needed to recover and restore performance, but not in the type or duration of the stressors [8].

Overreaching and Overtraining

Athletes deliberately overload their bodies with physical training so that in the following recovery period, supercompensatory adaptations arise resulting in enhanced physical condition and performance [9]. Indeed, the sensitive management of the balance between overload and recovery on micro to macro scales underpins the science and practice of periodisation, thus many coaches argue that OR is a natural part of the training and supercompensation process. Functional overreaching (FOR) describes the period after an intense overload has been experienced, in which the athlete will be fatigued and there is a short-term decrement in performance, but after a few days or weeks, that recovery is complete and performance/fitness is enhanced. In contrast non-functional overreaching (NFOR) is characterized by stagnation or decrease of performance and a recovery period that lasts weeks to months [6]. If the NFOR becomes severe or protracted, there is the risk of the athlete progressing into a state of OT [6].

Although the position statement of the European College of Sports Sciences [6] provided needed clarity over the issue of OR, it failed to give guidance over the duration of each stage. This has made it difficult to distinguish the stage which the athlete is in and also, when does FOR become NFOR or ultimately OT [10]?

Overtraining Syndrome

It is important to note that the definition of overtraining has varied depending on the author or researcher, and that it can be used to describe a process, an outcome or both. Overtraining can be viewed as the process by which sport and non-sport specific stressors combine to negatively affect the athlete, but it can also be considered an outcome because of the long-lasting decrement in performance, mood disturbances, fatigue and /or depression [8]. In light of the wide range of physiological, psychological symptoms and performance decrements reported by the affected athletes, this condition is increasingly being defined as the OT syndrome [11, 12].

Burnout

Burnout and OT syndrome are terms often used interchangeably as both share many similarities. Foremost, they share diagnostic characteristics such as performance loss, mood disturbances and chronic exhaustion [13, 14]. Whereas OT research has traditionally investigated the maladaptive responses to excessive training [15], burnout research has focused primarily on psychosocial factors such as high external pressure, lack of control and feelings of entrapment [16, 17]. However, researchers do acknowledge that non-training stressors are important factors when studying the OT phenomenon [12] and that OT may be an antecedent to burnout [7] which makes the boundaries between these two phenomena blurred.

Burnout denotes a negative emotional reaction to sport participation, and while it is known that overtrained athletes can still maintain their motivation to keep training, a burned-out athlete will commonly have no motivation to pursue his/her activity [14]. Repeated episodes of OT appear to increase the risk of burnout, with the motivation to continue training being the essential factor to differentiate between the seriousness of the OT episode and the likelihood of dropout [18]. In contrast to the progressive model of OT presented in figure 1, Richardson et al. [12] eloquently argue that burnout should not be seen as the end stage of the OT continuum but as a parallel condition arising from different antecedents; OT syndrome being the state of physical exhaustion arising from a prolonged imbalance between sports-related stressors and recovery, but burnout when the resulting exhaustion is primarily due to emotional factors.

Other definitions used include staleness – initial failure of the body to cope with the psychological and physiological demands of training [7] – and unexplained underperformance syndrome (UPS) [19]. In an attempt to simplify the definition and criteria for the diagnosis of OT, Budget et al. [19] tried to reduce all the discordant OT terms into a single umbrella term – UPS – arguing that the term OT infers that causative factors exist, which often can be difficult to prove. Recently, Kellman [20] has focused more on the recovery aspects of athletes' training, arguing that the main cause of overtraining is the lack of recovery between practice sessions. Under Kellman's definition, to be overtrained is to experience underrecovery. The problem with this concept is that it ignores training loads as a potential causative factor and with its focus on physical recovery this disregards psychological recovery.

Although there is no consensus about the terminology and definitions of the condition, what is clear is that this is a complex phenomenon with multiple presenting characteristics and stages. As with any condition with a continuum of seriousness, it is important to identify athletes who are at the beginning of this process (NFOR) from those who are at more advanced stages (OT), as recovery is suggested to be quicker if dealt with when the athlete is NFOR [6].

What Is the Incidence of the Overtraining Syndrome in Young Athletes?

Little is known about the incidence of NFOR or OT in young athletes and many questions remain unanswered: How common is it? At what age can it start? Are there differences in prevalence between different sports, between team and individual type sports, between the sexes? Is it a problem restricted to elite performers or is it evident at lower representative levels?

Even in adults there are few empirical data of prevalence rates. The studies that have been performed frequently used few participants, often case studies, have employed different definitions of OT, making generalisations difficult. With these caveats in mind, the incidence of OT in elite long-distance runners has been reported at 60% and 64% in females and males, respectively [21]. The rate dropped to 33% in non-elite women runners, a difference attributed to the greater training distance performed by the elite runners [22]. In Collegiate athletes, the yearly incidence of overtraining averaged 10% in wrestlers [22] and 7–31% in swimmers [11, 23]. Twenty-eight percent of US Olympic athletes reported being OT in the 90 days prior to the Atlanta games [24].

One of the largest surveys of adolescent athletes was performed by Raglin et al. [18] who assessed 231 young swimmers (14.8 ± 1.4 years) across four different countries (Japan, USA, Sweden and Greece), finding that 35% reported staleness at least once. Earlier data [25] showed that 31% of adolescent distance runners reported being overtrained but with the average episode lasting about 3 weeks, suggesting that the young athletes were actually NFOR rather than OT. Kentta et al. [5] investigated the prevalence of staleness in elite Swedish athletes (16–20 years) finding that 37% of the athletes had reported staleness at least once in their sport careers and that the incidence was greater in individual sports (48%) compared to team sports (30%). The prevalence of burnout (assessed using the Eades Burnout Inventory) in elite young Swedish athletes (n = 980, 17.5 ± 1.0 years), across 29 different sports was investigated by Gustafsson et al. [26]. Their findings indicated that 11% of individual sport and 5% of team sport athletes reported the highest levels of burnout scores in regard to negative self-concept of athletic ability; devaluation by coach and teammates; psychological withdrawal/devaluation and emotional/physical exhaustion. A recent survey of 376 English young athletes, mean age 15.1 ± 2.0 years (range 11–18 years) [Winsley and Matos, unpubl. data], indicated that 29% had been either NFOR or OT at least once in their sporting careers. There was a higher prevalence in individual sports than in team sports (37 vs. 17%) and in females than males (36 vs. 26%). This study intentionally surveyed young athletes from international down to club standard and although a higher incidence was seen in international (45%) and national (37%) level athletes, approximately 20% of subnational level young athletes also reported being NFOR/OT, suggesting that this is not just an issue specific to the elite child athlete.

What Are the Signs and Symptoms of Overtraining Syndrome in Young Athletes?

Although underperformance is regarded as the main characteristic of an OT athlete, it is not clear how much performance has to drop to confidently indicate a state of OT. To complicate things further, performance decrements can be the result of either OT or other precipitating factors such as family problems, school work, or exams [11, 12]. As a consequence much research has been conducted with the intention of trying to identify valid markers of OT, which could be used as both a diagnostic tool and as an early warning mechanism.

Herein though lies the problem. Fry et al.'s [13] review listed more than 90 different symptoms that are reported by overtrained athletes spanning performance, physiological and psychological factors. Recent reviews by Urhausen and Kindermann [27] and Richardson et al. [12] reiterate the multitude of presenting symptoms but acknowledge that due to the large inter-individual variability of the symptoms themselves, just how difficult it is to diagnose an individual athlete with OT; which paradoxically is the whole point.

The evidence suggests that the signs and symptoms reported in young athletes are similar to the ones found in the adult population. The commonly identified symptoms include increased perception of effort during exercise, frequent upper respiratory tract infections (URTI), muscle soreness, sleep disturbances, feelings of muscular heaviness, loss of appetite and mood disturbances [3, 5, 18]. Additional symptoms reported by young athletes during OT episodes are: increased conflicts with family, partner, coach or friends; decreased interest in training and competition; increased frustration with training; decreased self-confidence; inability to concentrate on a particular task; short temper, depression, sadness, and elevated levels of perceived stress [28]. Clearly, the individual nature of the symptomatology makes profiling a suspected overtrained young athlete difficult.

What Are the Risk Factors of Overtraining Syndrome in Young Athletes?

Richardson et al. [12] provide an excellent summary of the proposed risk factors which range from training issues, situational and environmental stressors, people issues, athletes' physical condition, athletes' beliefs and attitudes, all of which may conspire to push the athlete into a state of OT. Rather than exhaustively repeat that which has been written on the topic in adults – although those involved with elite young athletes should make themselves familiar with these possible risk factors –, it would be better to concentrate on those that might be particularly important for young elite athletes.

Is Training Load the Principal Cause of Overtraining in Young Athletes?

The importance of training load in the aetiology of OT has been endorsed by many authors [8, 29] and numerous adult studies have used increments in training load as the main variable to induce a state of OT/NFOR [30–32]; but this narrow view of the condition may mean that alternative contributors are not investigated and that interventions are focused on mistaken factors.

The degree to which training load is a precursor for OT in young athletes remains unclear. Raglin et al. [18] reported that 'stale' swimmers aged 13–18 years had a training load 10.8% higher than 'healthy' swimmers; however, other studies have reported no relationship between the prevalence of burnout and training load [26]. Clearly, for some OT young athletes, an excessive training load and inadequate rest is indeed the principal reason underlying why they are overtrained, but it would be amiss to think that training load is the only reason for every case of OT and therefore alternative factors/stressors should also be considered [5, 12, 33].

Single Identity

Coakley [16] argued that the time and training demands of the elite young athlete means that they have little or no opportunity to develop a normal, multifaceted identity – as such they become defined by their sport and their sport defines them. Young overtrained or burned out athletes frequently report that sport is the most important thing in their lives and that the amount of time that these individuals dedicate to other activities outside their sport is limited – suggesting the development of a unidimensional identity [16, 34]. Kentta et al. [5], for example, found that 20% of the young overtrained athletes in their study devoted less than 5 h a week to activities outside their sport, and for approximately 40% of these athletes, sport was the only thing (schooling and family aside) in their lives. Identities are claimed and constructed through social relationships experienced throughout life [35], therefore if sport/training provides the sole opportunity for social interaction, it is unsurprising that the young athlete may develop a single identity. Self esteem, identity and self-worth become intertwined and become dependent on sporting success. This is fine when success is forthcoming, but can lead to stress and anxiety when failure/injury are present, possibly contributing to the development of OT. Furthermore, because of their unidimensional identity and lack of alternative avenues in life, some young athletes report that despite having negative experiences and low motivation they continue in their sport, in a scenario referred to as entrapment [36].

The development of self-complexity and multiple identities has been shown to provide a cushion or outlet for the stress related to training and appears to dampen the swings in self-belief/doubt arising from their sport performance – resulting in a more balanced and better coping young athlete [16]. As such, those working with elite young athletes should help provide the opportunities and time for the development of a multi-dimensional identity in the athletes in their care.

Conditional Love, Meeting Expectations and Misperceptions

Wishing to meet parents/coaches expectations, and the anxiety this creates has been frequently mentioned by young athletes as an aggravating factor for OT. The child wishes to meet adults'

expectations through showing their dedication to training and in the achievement of sporting success. If they fail to meet the standards that they perceive are expected of them this can result in increased training, feelings of guilt and threatened self-esteem – all contributory factors for OT or burnout. Additionally, if a 'more-is better' culture pervades the young athlete's training environment, it may also result in a destructive conditional association; if the child gets or perceives to get more praise, acknowledgement, and love by training more and more. This drives the young athlete to keep training excessively, which can ultimately put them at risk of OT [12]. Likewise, there may be pressure to carry on training/competing even whilst tired or injured, combined with the fear of admitting to being so [37], which may push young athletes to continue despite physical/emotional risks.

These forces become internalized and start to be manifested through the young person's identity traits. Of course it is difficult to say whether the athlete's personality is simply a reflection of the parental, sporting and societal influences to which they have been exposed or whether these are innate traits, but certain characteristics seem to be common within OT athletes. A perfectionist tendency in particular is frequently reported in burnt-out young athletes [38] which leads to the belief that more training/practice is required to achieve or sustain perfection and a greater level of self-admonishment if they are not meeting these performance ideals.

It must be remembered that the coaches/parents are not always the villains, as conditional love can be a misperception by the child; the adults supporting and loving the child unconditionally irrespective of what they achieve in their sport. Finally, many young athletes are acutely aware of the sacrifices and commitment their parents/coaches are making for them and do not want to let them down [16]. Thus, misunderstanding and misplaced guilt act to further reinforce the pressure on the child to train.

Lack of Autonomy

A common pattern in the narratives described by adult athletes who experienced OT or burnout as a young elite athlete is the following: the young athlete shows talent/aptitude in a particular sport and achieves early success; the opportunity to become an elite young athlete presents itself and the child agrees; from this point forward the young athlete's life is controlled by adults (coach/parents) in a effort to achieve these goals. Although this is often done with the best intentions and well meaning, the control that the adults assume for managing the young athlete's training programme, competition schedules, travel plans, diet, free time, school work load, disempowers the child leaving them frustrated, impotent and stressed [12, 16]. In a recent study of 96 junior elite athletes, reduced self-determination was observed in those suffering from burnout [39]. These young athletes reported greater external regulation over their lives, were more extrinsically motivated, and consequently felt they had less self-determination over their actions, causing them stress and anxiety. Reduced autonomy and perceptions of powerlessness are directly related to the unidimensionality issue discussed previously, but are also expressed through control over the minutiae of the young athlete's life by adults. Coakley [16] entitled it psychodoping, whereby the young athlete is made dependent on others and discouraged from asking critical questions about why they are participating, what they are doing and how their sporting existence is tied into the rest of their lives. The disenfranchisement of the young athlete even pervades the 'treatment/cure' for OT; the child is assumed not to be coping and therefore is given coping strategies to help [17], but the real issue lies with a lack of self-determination and powerlessness over their lives and not in being able to cope with a system that is enforced on to them. Ensuring that young athletes are involved in the decision-making processes affecting their lives, on both a micro and macro scale, is important [37] and opportunities for this dialogue to occur should be given.

Prevention and Recovery

Because OT is a multidimensional entity any treatment/recovery strategies also need to take a holistic approach [12, 40]. This holistic style will shape not just the questions that are asked but also an appreciation of the interconnectivity of the issues. For example, if competition overload is identified as a concern, on a superficial level by simply cutting down the number of matches/events should resolve the problem as the child gets more rest. But it is important to go deeper and consider whether the young athlete is ever involved in the decision-making process in setting the competition schedule? What is the impact on their school workload and can they cope with this disruption? Has the schedule denied opportunities for socialization outside of the sport and thus potentially fostered the development of a single identity?

Firstly, the adults and the young athlete must reflect and try to identify potential causes, whether training or non-training related. There must also be the maturity and openness by all to accept that they may be the source of the problem, and be willing to change accordingly. Asking such fundamental questions can be difficult both for adults and young athletes, but if these issues go unresolved because of denial and/or power inequities, then any recovery/prevention plan will be a façade and not deal with the root cause of the problem.

In no particular order and by no means exhaustive, the following suggestions may help a coach to start to build a rounded profile of the young athlete, and address the issues pertinent to OT:

- Meet the parents – ask about their motivations for helping the child, their opinion toward sport, their aspirations for the child, their own sporting experiences, how involved do they wish to be? Then ask the young athlete and then ask yourself the same questions.

Measured score = true score + error. (1)

The 'error' can be caused by technological or biological sources, and attributed to the participant (e.g. motivation, biological variability), the test (e.g. compliance with the protocol requirements), or the instrumentation used (e.g. calibration) [8]. The lower the magnitude of the 'error', the closer the 'measured' score reflects the participants' 'true' score. To fully appreciate the likely value of the 'true' score, the magnitude of the 'error' score must be known by the exercise physiologist to make a meaningful interpretation of the test data.

While there is debate as to which statistical test best represents the magnitude of 'error' for a given measurement [9, 10], there is a consensus that Pearson's correlation coefficient provides a limited measure of reliability as it examines the association between two variables and does not address the 'error' magnitude. In contrast, limits of agreement analysis [10] or the typical error score [9] allow researchers to quantify the main components of reliability: (1) systematic mean bias, which scrutinises for a learning or fatigue effect over repeated tests, and (2) within-subject variation, which captures the 'error' expected for an individual's test score. A test with a low within-subject variation (high reliability) will allow small but worthwhile improvements in fitness or performance to be recognised. The 'error' can be expressed in absolute or percentage terms, and with their corresponding confidence limits (68 or 95%) established, allow interpretation of an athlete's test data. This is essential if the objective is to quantify physical fitness or performance longitudinally and/or scrutinise the efficacy of an altered training regime.

Aerobic Fitness

Aerobic fitness is concerned with the ability of the body to consume oxygen and utilize this in the contracting muscle for oxidative adenosine triphosphate (ATP) production. The principal parameters of aerobic fitness are:

- Maximal $\dot{V}O_2$ ($\dot{V}O_{2max}$)
- Oxygen cost of exercise (exercise economy)
- Blood lactate threshold
- Maximal lactate steady state (MLSS)

The collective measurement of these parameters permits a comprehensive assessment of aerobic fitness in young athletes, although this will depend on the objectives of the assessment and predictive power of sporting performance. For example, a comprehensive test battery is likely to be more useful for endurance athletes, whereas for athletes involved in team sports a measurement of $\dot{V}O_{2max}$, or a sport-specific aerobic fitness test, is likely to provide sufficient information regarding the general fitness of the athlete. However, it should be noted that in some team sports a more in-depth assessment of aerobic fitness may be more informative from a performance perspective. For example, following 8 weeks of interval training, several parameters of aerobic fitness ($\dot{V}O_{2max}$, blood lactate threshold and running economy) increased concomitantly with improvements in soccer performance (distance covered, number of sprints and ball 'involvements') in junior players [11].

Maximal Oxygen Uptake

Maximal oxygen uptake ($\dot{V}O_{2max}$) represents the highest rate at which oxygen can be utilized for oxidative metabolism during whole-body exercise, and is recognized as the best single measure of aerobic fitness [12]. Functionally, $\dot{V}O_{2max}$ represents the limit of the respiratory, cardiovascular and muscular systems to transport and utilize oxygen during exercise, and is therefore an important determinant of performance.

Direct Measurement of Maximal Oxygen Uptake
The conventional paradigm for $\dot{V}O_{2max}$ determination requires that during exercise close to

exhaustion, in a well-motivated participant, $\dot{V}O_2$ will no longer increase linearly with the exercise intensity, but display a plateau [13, 14]. In reality, however, the $\dot{V}O_2$ profile at exhaustion may remain linear, accelerate or decelerate (plateau) with respect to exercise intensity during an exercise test in young people [15]. It is well documented that only ~20–40% of untrained children and adolescents display a $\dot{V}O_2$ plateau [16], which is comparable to data collected in trained adolescents during running, cycling and rowing exercise [17]. Rivera-Brown et al. [18] observed that a $\dot{V}O_2$ plateau is more common in adolescent runners using a discontinuous exercise protocol (85%) compared to a continuous exercise protocol (54%), suggesting the choice of exercise protocol may be an important consideration when measuring $\dot{V}O_{2max}$ in young athletes. However, in this study the highest $\dot{V}O_2$ achieved across the two protocols was not different, indicating the athletes had reached their aerobic ceiling in both tests.

Due to the consistent failure to observe a $\dot{V}O_2$ plateau during maximal exercise in both young athletes and non-athletes, it has become conventional to use the term peak $\dot{V}O_2$ in this population. However, tests using exercise intensities above those required to elicit $\dot{V}O_{2max}$ following an initial incremental exercise test to exhaustion, suggest that a peak $\dot{V}O_2$ score is reflective of a young person's true $\dot{V}O_{2max}$ [15, 19]. The reliability of determining peak $\dot{V}O_2$ in trained adolescent runners and cyclists has been reported to be high in treadmill (intra-class correlation coefficient [ICC] = 0.88–0.97), cycling (ICC = 0.86–0.97) and rowing (ICC = 0.90–0.98) exercise [17]. Paterson et al. [20] reported a coefficient of variation of 3.4% for $\dot{V}O_{2max}$ determination in trained athletic boys aged 11–15 years.

As the majority of trained (and untrained) children and adolescents fail to satisfy the traditional plateau criterion, secondary 'objective' criteria have been proposed to verify a 'maximal' response [21–23]. These include:

- Heart rate $\geq$200 beats·min^{-1} during treadmill exercise or $\geq$195 beats·min^{-1} during cycling or a heart rate within 85–95% of age predicted maximum
- Respiratory exchange ratio (RER) $\geq$1.00
- Blood lactate accumulation $\geq$6 mmol$\cdot$l^{-1}

A recent study, however, has demonstrated that the use of secondary criteria may result in the acceptance of a sub-maximal peak $\dot{V}O_2$ or falsely reject a true $\dot{V}O_{2max}$ measurement in untrained children [15]. The authors called for secondary objective criteria to be abandoned and championed the use of a subsequent (follow-up) test involving exercise intensities above those required to elicit $\dot{V}O_{2max}$ following the initial incremental test to confirm the measurement of a true $\dot{V}O_{2max}$ (fig. 1). The composite $\dot{V}O_2$ profile from both tests can then be used to reveal the plateau criterion within a single testing session.

Despite the availability of many exercise protocols to determine $\dot{V}O_{2max}$ in the young athlete [24], there is strong evidence to suggest that peak $\dot{V}O_2$ is a stable measure of aerobic fitness and protocol independent [15, 19, 25, 26]. However, considerable differences in peak $\dot{V}O_2$ can be observed across exercise ergometers, with treadmill exercise producing a ~8–10, ~15 and ~33% higher peak $\dot{V}O_2$ compared to cycling, rowing and swim bench ergometers, respectively [17, 27]. In contrast, when adolescent athletes are tested in their specific training mode, cyclists and runners often record their highest peak $\dot{V}O_2$ on a cycle ergometer or treadmill respectively, presumably reflecting their sport-specific adaptations [19]. This, however, is not the case for swimmers, who record their lowest peak $\dot{V}O_2$ on the modality specific swim bench, compared to cycling and treadmill exercise, presumably because of the smaller muscle mass involved in arm exercise [27].

The choice of protocol will ultimately depend on whether additional information is required from the test. If only a measure of $\dot{V}O_{2max}$ is desired, a continuous incremental exercise protocol

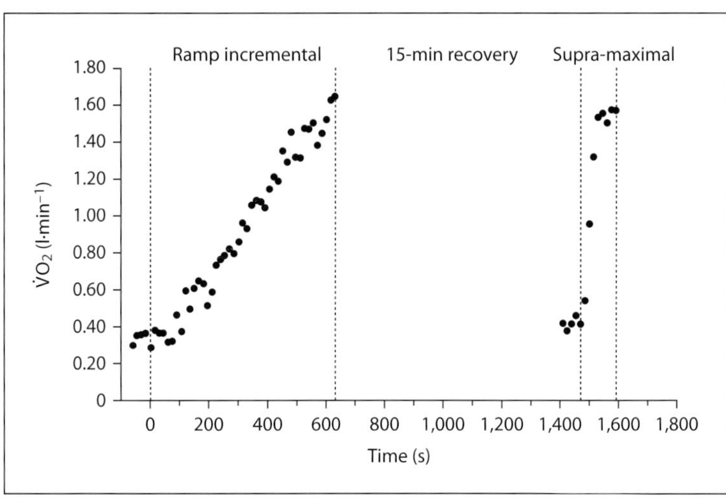

Fig. 1. The $\dot{V}O_2$ response in a 9-year-old boy during a ramp incremental and supra-maximal cycle test separated by 15 min of recovery. The vertical dotted lines represent the start and end of the incremental and supra-maximal bouts. The highest $\dot{V}O_2$ from the ramp test was 1.65 litres·min^{-1} and despite a 5% increase in power output during the subsequent supra-maximal bout, the highest $\dot{V}O_2$ recorded was 1.57 litres·min^{-1}.

employing either a ramp function [15, 26] or 1 min stages [26] allow its determination in a short period of time (typically 8–12 min). In some sports such as cycling, a measure of maximum power output, not $\dot{V}O_{2max}$, is considered a more relevant determinant of performance and should be included as a main outcome measure from a ramp incremental test [28]. Similar to $\dot{V}O_{2max}$ determination, maximum power output during incremental exercise has good to excellent reliability in trained adolescent cyclists (ICC = 0.82–0.92) [17]. If sub-maximal parameters of aerobic function (e.g. exercise economy, blood lactate threshold) are of interest, a discontinuous, incremental exercise protocol where power output or running velocity is increased in 3-min stages is required to allow steady-state determination of $\dot{V}O_2$ and blood lactate [29, 30].

As $\dot{V}O_{2max}$ is heavily correlated with body size, the absolute $\dot{V}O_{2max}$ score of an individual must be adjusted for body size before interpretation. This is typically achieved using the ratio standard method with body mass (i.e. ml·kg^{-1}·min^{-1}). However, the ratio standard method has been heavily criticized due to its failure to create a 'size-free' $\dot{V}O_{2max}$ measure [31]. As an alternative, allometric scaling techniques may allow a more appropriate method to adjust $\dot{V}O_{2max}$ for body size, although normative data are not as readily available as for the ratio standard technique.

Allometric scaling of $\dot{V}O_{2max}$ may also be more relevant for some sporting performances. For example, performance during a soccer specific fitness test (Hoff test) correlates best with peak $\dot{V}O_2$ adjusted for body mass using an exponent of 0.75 in adolescent players [32]. Likewise, Pettersen et al. [33] found adjusted peak $\dot{V}O_2$ using 0.67 and 0.75 scaling exponents (i.e. ml·kg$^{-0.67}$·min^{-1} and ml·kg$^{-0.75}$·min^{-1}) to be better predictors of running performance compared to the ratio standard method in 8- to 17-year-old boys and girls. In contrast, Nevill et al. [34] concluded that the ratio standard method was the best predictor of 1 mile running speed in 12-year-old boys. Given this discrepancy, it may be prudent to analyse and interpret data using both the ratio standard and allometric methods when monitoring young athletes.

Field-Based Estimation of Maximal Oxygen Uptake

Although a valid and reliable measurement of $\dot{V}O_{2max}$ can be obtained only in the laboratory setting, its measurement requires expensive equipment and technical expertise, which may be impractical for use with large groups of young athletes. Therefore, field-based tests which are easy to administer in large groups and require little equipment, may offer a practical alternative.

In particular, the 20-metre shuttle running test has increased in popularity since its introduction in 1982 [35]. The test can be conducted indoors as this demands little space, controls for environmental conditions, and avoids pacing strategies compared to time- and distance- based running tests [see Ref. 36 for details]. However, despite child and adolescent participants providing an acceptable effort based on maximum heart rate responses during the 20-metre shuttle test [37], a recent review based on the outcome of 15 studies (n = 795), found only a moderate criterion validity of $R^2 = 0.51$ (range 0.21–0.77) for the 20-metre shuttle test predicting peak $\dot{V}O_2$ in untrained minors [38]. We are unaware of any validity or reliability data for the 20-metre shuttle test in young athletes, and given their poor to moderate validity in untrained minors, the use of such tests in young athletes may be of limited value. However, such tests are commonly used to monitor aerobic fitness in sports such as basketball, netball and cricket [39–41].

While general field-based tests for assessing aerobic fitness may have limited application to young athletes, sports-specific field tests are available. Chamari et al. [32] found a modified version of the Hoff test, where under-15-years-old male soccer players were required to cover as much distance as possible over a 290-metre lap whilst dribbling a football through, between and around cones, and jumping over hurdles in a 10-min period, to correlate significantly with laboratory determined peak $\dot{V}O_2$ using an exponent of 0.75 (r = 0.68). In addition, the Hoff test was sensitive to 8 weeks of interval training, as the increase in distance covered in the modified Hoff test (10%) was similar to the improvement in peak $\dot{V}O_2$ (12%). In contrast to the Hoff test, the Bangsbo endurance test [42], which involves players performing 40 bouts of alternate maximal intensity running for 15 s and low-intensity 'recovery' runs for 10 s over a 160-metre circuit (total test time = 16.5 min), was not associated with laboratory-determined peak $\dot{V}O_2$ in soccer players aged 17.5 ± 1.1 years [43].

Despite the attractiveness of sports-specific field tests for predicting maximal or peak $\dot{V}O_2$ in young athletes (soccer players), their predictive power is low to moderate, and hence should not be considered a replacement for its determination in a laboratory setting. This poor relationship may reflect, in part, the high skill proficiency needed to perform several of the tests.

Exercise Economy

Exercise economy, the oxygen cost to exercise at a given velocity or power output, is an important determinant of performance in endurance-based events (e.g. running, cycling and swimming). An individual with a better exercise economy will, at any given velocity or power output, be operating at a lower percentage of their $\dot{V}O_{2max}$. There is evidence to suggest running economy is an important determinant of middle distance running performance (e.g. 800–5,000 m) in trained children and adolescents [44–46]. The importance of running economy to performance may act independent of $\dot{V}O_{2max}$ (although a high $\dot{V}O_{2max}$ is still important) as improvements in running performance and running economy have been shown to occur in the absence of changes in peak $\dot{V}O_2$ [47, 48]. Likewise, the oxygen cost of swimming has been reported to be an important predictor of swim performance (50–1,000 m) and national ranking in adolescent swimmers, whereas peak $\dot{V}O_2$ has not [49].

To establish the oxygen cost of exercise, steady-state conditions are required. This is typically

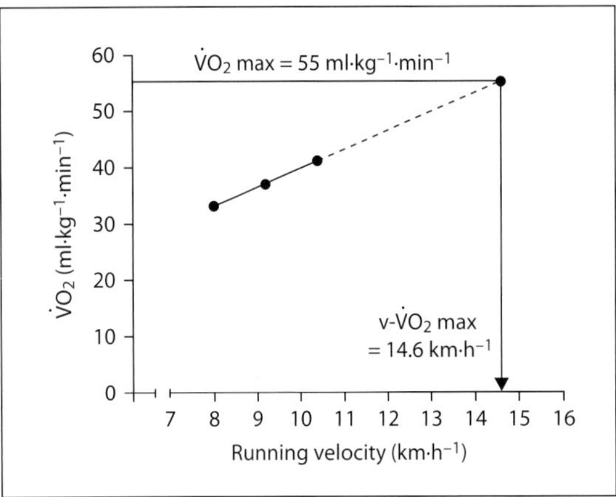

Fig. 2. Determination of the v-$\dot{V}O_{2max}$ in an athletic boy. The relationship between sub-maximal $\dot{V}O_2$ and running velocity was determined over three velocities (8.0, 9.2 and 10.4 km·h^{-1}) and the linear relationship (solid line) was extrapolated (dotted line) to the boy's $\dot{V}O_{2max}$ to yield his v-$\dot{V}O_{2max}$. Figure created using data from Krahenbuhl and Pangrazi [94].

achieved by measuring the $\dot{V}O_2$ amplitude between the 2nd and 3rd min of a 3-min stage during a discontinuous, incremental protocol. Due to the presence of the $\dot{V}O_2$ slow component during exercise above the blood lactate threshold, the accurate assessment of exercise economy can only be obtained during sub-blood lactate threshold intensities (e.g. classified as moderate intensity exercise).

A useful application of establishing the oxygen cost of exercise is to calculate the velocity (or power output) corresponding to $\dot{V}O_{2max}$ (v–$\dot{V}O_{2max}$). That is, the sub-maximal relationship between $\dot{V}O_2$ and velocity is extrapolated via linear regression to $\dot{V}O_{2max}$, providing a 'functional' velocity that corresponds to an individual's $\dot{V}O_{2max}$ (fig. 2). Studies by Cole et al. [45] and Almarwaey et al. [29] indicate that the v-$\dot{V}O_{2max}$ is one of the strongest predictors of middle distance running in trained adolescents, surpassing the independent contributions of running economy and $\dot{V}O_{2max}$.

Blood Lactate Threshold and Maximal Lactate Steady State

Although the accumulation of lactate within the blood represents a complicated balance of physiological processes relating to its efflux from the muscle, and oxidation at various bodily regions, its measurement provides a powerful marker of sub-maximal aerobic fitness. Conventionally this is achieved by identifying the lactate threshold – the point at which blood lactate initially increases above baseline levels during a discontinuous incremental exercise test consisting of 3 min stages [30]. Likewise, a common strategy for endurance-based athletes (e.g. runners, rowers) is to establish their blood lactate profile by plotting blood lactate against velocity or power output during a discontinuous incremental protocol. Improvements in aerobic fitness are characterised by a lower blood lactate at a given velocity or power output, or the ability to attain a higher velocity or power output for a given fixed blood lactate concentration (i.e. typically 2.0–6.0 mmol•l^{-1}). Blood lactate profiling is also used to monitor and assess aerobic fitness in swimmers. A typical test involves the swimmer completing seven 200-metre swims which increase in intensity ranging from ~70 to 100% of their 200 m maximum swimming velocity, with ~5–6 min recovery provided between each stage. Heart rate is recorded immediately upon completion of the stage, and capillary blood lactate is sampled within the first minute of the recovery period [50].

Due to the invasive nature of determining the blood lactate threshold (i.e. repeat capillary blood sampling), one of its non-invasive estimates, the gas exchange threshold (GET) or ventilatory threshold (T_{vent}), may also be employed to monitor sub-maximal aerobic fitness in young athletes [20]. During incremental exercise, the lactate threshold can be estimated as showed in figure 3 [12]:

- GET – non-linear increase in $\dot{V}CO_2$ relative to $\dot{V}O_2$,

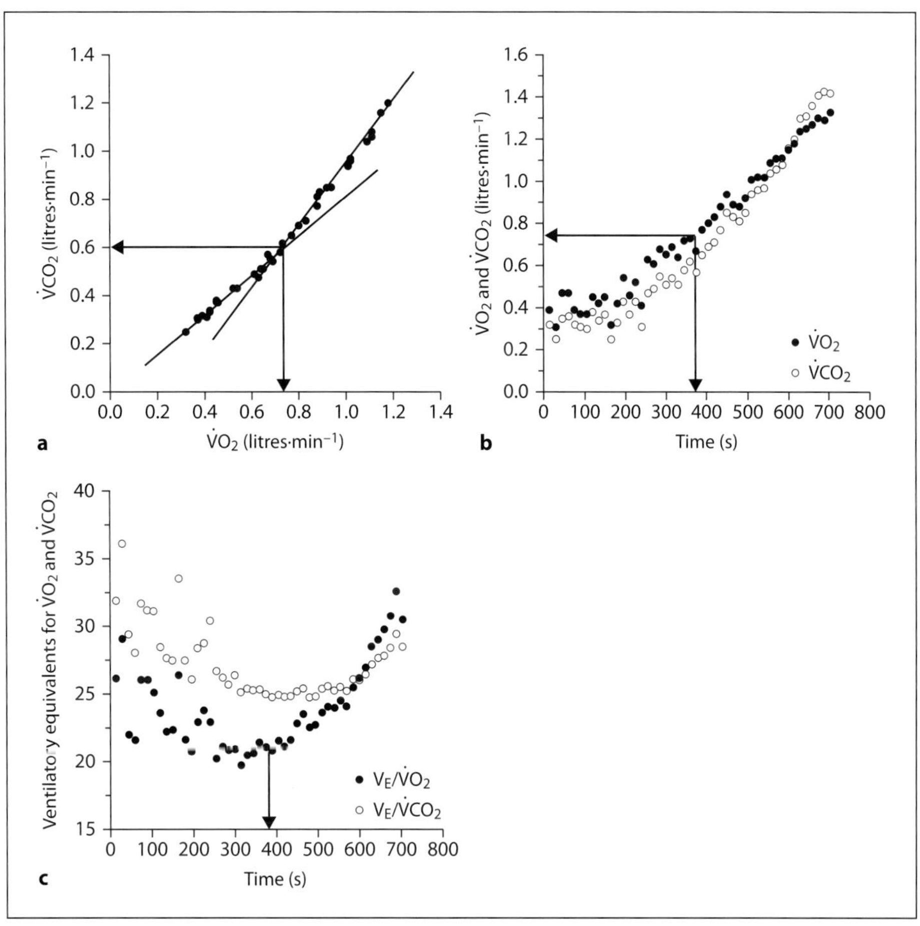

Fig. 3. Identification of the GET (**a, b**) and T_{vent} (**c**) in a 9-year-old child during a ramp test to exhaustion. In **a**, the v-slope method was employed with the resultant $\dot{V}O_2$ at the GET shown also in **b**. In **c**, the ventilatory threshold is shown and occurred at a similar time to the GET (see **b**).

- T_{vent} – an increase in the ventilatory equivalent for oxygen ($\dot{V}_E/\dot{V}O_2$) without an increase in the ventilatory equivalent for carbon dioxide ($\dot{V}_E/\dot{V}CO_2$).

The validity of using the GET or T_{vent} to estimate the blood lactate threshold appears acceptable as a strong correlation has been established between the T_{vent} and lactate threshold in 10- to 11-year-old boys when expressed as an absolute $\dot{V}O_2$ (r = 0.91) and as a percentage of $\dot{V}O_{2max}$ (r =

0.82) [51]. The GET and T_{vent} also have good reproducibility with both trained and untrained children, with a coefficient of variation of ~5–8% [20, 52].

Establishing the blood lactate threshold (or its non-invasive equivalents) is likely to be important from a performance perspective, as the T_{vent} expressed as an absolute $\dot{V}O_2$, percentage of $\dot{V}O_{2max}$, or as a running velocity, correlates (r = 0.77–0.78) with middle distance running performance in

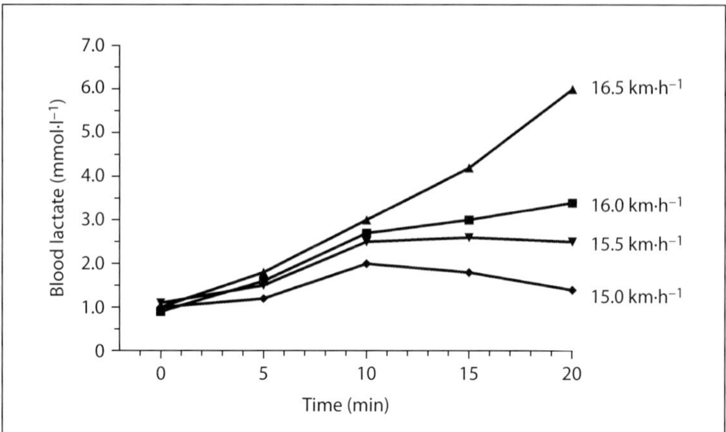

Fig. 4. Blood lactate profile in an adolescent runner during a series of 20 min treadmill runs to determine his MLSS. Capillary blood samples were obtained every 5 min and the MLSS occurred at a velocity of 15.5 km·h⁻¹. Adapted from Almarwaey et al. [29].

pre-pubertal runners, although their contributions appear to be less strong than the individual influence of $\dot{V}O_{2max}$ (r = 0.83) [46, 53].

Knowledge of the blood lactate threshold is important from training and monitoring perspectives, as this physiological marker represents the division between the moderate and heavy exercise intensity domains. The former represents exercise intensities where $\dot{V}O_2$ reaches a steady-state with blood lactate circa baseline concentrations (~1.0 mmol • l⁻¹), whereas the latter represents exercise intensities where $\dot{V}O_2$ reaches a delayed steady state and blood lactate stabilizes above baseline at ~2.0–5.0 mmol • l⁻¹. The upper limit of the heavy exercise domain is demarcated by the MLSS, which represents the highest velocity or power output that can be sustained where the accumulation and removal of blood lactate is at equilibrium [54]. Exercise above the MLSS, termed the very heavy intensity domain, is therefore characterised by a sustained rise in blood lactate and the projection of $\dot{V}O_2$ either towards, or to attain, $\dot{V}O_{2max}$ as fatigue ensures [55].

Middle and long-distance runners can use these exercise intensity domains to identify training zones termed 'easy' (moderate), 'steady' (heavy) and 'tempo' (very heavy) [30]. Training

at a velocity or power output corresponding to $\dot{V}O_{2max}$ or above (severe intensity exercise), is classified as the 'interval' training zone [30]. An improvement in aerobic fitness is characterised by a reduction in blood lactate, $\dot{V}O_2$ and heart rate when exercising at a given velocity or power output within an intensity domain (preferably close to competition pace). This method of fitness monitoring is commonly used by cyclists [28], and time-trial endurance performance tests have been demonstrated to have good reliability (~4% typical error) with trained adolescent cyclists [56].

Unlike the blood lactate threshold, the determination of the MLSS is time consuming and demanding. This could require up to six (possibly four with previous test data) separate visits to the laboratory with each visit consisting of a 20- to 30-min exercise bout at a constant velocity or power output, with blood lactate concentration determined every 5 min (fig. 4). The velocity or power output where the blood lactate concentration rises less than 0.5 or 1.0 mmol • l⁻¹ over the final 10 min of the test is deemed to represent the MLSS [29, 57].

The MLSS has been shown to occur at a mean blood lactate of ~2.0–3.0 mmol • l⁻¹ in trained adolescent runners [29]. Consequently, it has been proposed that the running velocity at the $2.5 \text{ mmol} \cdot l^{-1}$ blood lactate concentration, determined during a traditional discontinuous, incremental test to exhaustion, may be an appropriate method to estimate a young athlete's MLSS [29]. However, due to the considerable inter-individual variation in the blood lactate concentration at MLSS (typically $1.0–6.0 \text{ mmol} \cdot l^{-1}$), the fixed lactate concentration method clearly has its shortcomings and is inappropriate for use with young athletes.

Expressing the running velocity or the percentage of $\dot{V}O_{2max}$ at MLSS (or above) might be meaningful for training and monitoring purposes. The running velocity corresponding to a blood lactate concentration of $2.5 \text{ mmol} \cdot l^{-1}$ (presumably circa MLSS) has been shown to be the strongest physiological correlate, alongside $v–\dot{V}O_{2max}$, with 1,500 m race performance in adolescent runners [44]. Similarly, Fernhall et al. [53] noted a strong correlation ($r = 0.74–0.77$) between the $\dot{V}O_2$ at a fixed blood lactate concentration of $4.0 \text{ mmol} \cdot l^{-1}$ (presumably above MLSS in the very heavy intensity exercise domain) and 2 and 3 mile run performance in adolescent cross-country runners. To our knowledge, no study has directly measured MLSS in young athletes and examined its relationship with athletic performance.

Critical Power

In adults, it has been demonstrated that the critical power (CP) concept, which represents the asymptote of an individual's power-duration curve, demarcates the boundaries between the heavy and very heavy intensity domains [58], and is broadly considered analogous to MLSS. Theoretically, CP represents the maximal power output which can be sustained indefinitely [59], highlighting its importance as a parameter of aerobic function. According to the two component model, CP represents the maximal rate at which ATP turnover can be supplied aerobically, whereas the curvature constant of the hyperbolic curve, represents the

finite anaerobic energy stores (W', representing the work that can be performed above CP) within the muscle [59]. During exercise above the CP, exhaustion will occur when W' is depleted – the rate of which is determined by 'how far' an individual is exercising above their CP:

$$\text{Time to exhaustion} = W'/(P\text{-}CP) \qquad (2)$$

Given the physiological bases for CP and W', and the fact that the CP concept can be easily applied to running (termed critical velocity [CV] and D' [60]), knowledge of CP or CV may be useful for monitoring an young athlete's aerobic fitness, predicting performance, prescribing training intensities and/or assembling pacing decisions, when the velocity or power output is above an individual's CV or CP respectively [see 61, for review]. For example, based on equation 2, time to exhaustion (and therefore performance) for a given velocity or power output can be predicted during exercise above CP. Alternatively, if the objective is for an athlete to complete a given amount of work or distance in a training session within the 'tempo' zone, the (theoretical) time to achieve this feat can be calculated from the following equation [61]:

$$\text{Time to exhaustion} = (W\text{-}W')/CP \text{ or}$$
$$(D\text{-}D')/CV \qquad (3)$$

The coach will be able to manipulate time and/ or training intensity to ensure the athlete experiences the training stimuli desired.

The CV concept has also been applied to young swimmers and shown to correlate highly ($r > 0.86$) with swimming velocity over distances ranging from 183 to 2,286 m [62]. In young swimmers, it has been shown that CV occurs at a lower velocity than that measured at a blood lactate concentration of $4.0 \text{ mmol} \cdot l^{-1}$ [63].

The traditional method to determine CP requires the participant to complete 3–5 exhaustive bouts lasting 2–15 min on separate days in order to construct an individual's power-duration curve

Jumping Tests
The most common jump test is the vertical jump test, originally developed by Sargent [84] in 1921, which measures explosive leg power in the context of the jump height achieved. Energetically, this test therefore reflects the supply of ATP via the breakdown of muscle PCr. Typically, the best jump height out of three is taken as the performance measure (recorded in cm or m). Protocols should be standardised for the use of counter leg movement (i.e. rapid downward phase before jumping) and rapid arm swing, as jump performance can be increased significantly through using these movements [see 94]. We are unaware of any published report showing the test-retest reliability for the standing vertical jump test, although jump performance has been shown to correlate highly with the peak power achieved in a WAnT in adolescent boys [82]. Jump performance is routinely measured to monitor young athlete's short-term leg power in sports such as soccer, basketball and netball [39, 41, 70].

Sprint Running Tests
Sprint tests are commonly used to determine an individual's maximal running velocity or time taken to cover a set distance. The distance covered is usually between 30 and 50 m [83], although distances as low as 5–10 m have been used to monitor youth soccer players [70]. Docherty [85] has reported reliability coefficients ranging from 0.66 to 0.94 for the 50-m dash in untrained boys.

As successful participation in team sports requires the ability to perform multiple sprints, Oliver et al. [81] examined the reliability of repeated sprint ability during five trials of 7 × 30 m runs in untrained adolescent boys. The fastest and mean times to cover 10 and 30 m over the five trials had a coefficient of variation ranging from 1.6 to 1.7%. An indication of the fatigue over the repeated sprints was also calculated using either the percentage or time-based fall in running performance between the fastest and mean times. However, the reliability of fatigue during the sprints was poor (coefficient of variation 23–25%). Sport-specific adaptations of multiple-sprint ability are available in sports such as soccer, netball and basketball [39, 41, 70].

While not a sprint running test per se, the Yo-Yo intermittent recovery test has been used extensively to study young athletes' ability to perform repeated bouts of intense exercise, particularly in team sports [see 95]. Based on Leger and Lambert's [35] 20-metre shuttle test, the Yo-Yo intermittent recovery test consists of 2 × 20 m shuttle runs at increasing speeds, but with a 10-second active recovery between each run. When the athlete is no longer able to maintain the requisite speed, the total distance covered is recorded and used to reflect his/her ability to perform repeated maximal intensity exercise. It has been reported in junior basketball players that the Yo-Yo test produces reproducible results over three repeat tests (coefficient of variation 7.1%) [86], suggesting the development of an athlete's performance can be monitored with sufficient sensitivity. Unfortunately, there are few published studies of young athletes, although normative values for English premier league youth soccer players are available [70].

Sprint Swimming Tests
Due to the specific requirements of swimming (exercising in water in the prone position and whole-body muscle recruitment patterns), running and cycle tests lack the necessary specificity to monitor performance. Consequently, tethered swimming devices are available which allow swimmers to perform 'all-out' swims (typically over 30 s) in the pool whilst recording their peak and mean force [50]. Normative values are available for national level boys and girls aged between 10 and 15 years [50].

Considerations and Recommendations

Although there are few data concerning the young athlete in his/her sporting environment, in this section we will provide a summary of the key issues that should be considered when providing continued physiological assessment and support.

The physiologist or team of physiologists working with the young athlete must be aware of the unique ethical issues of working with minors. For example, in England and Wales, an individual under the age of 18 years cannot provide legal consent to partake in exercise tests. A common procedure to protect all parties, therefore, is to obtain consent from the athlete's parents/guardians and assent from the athlete [87], following an explanation appropriate to the athlete's level of comprehension of the purpose, procedures, and potential risk and benefits of the testing. In addition, a contract clearly outlining the role that the physiologist will play in providing support to the young athlete is recommended and should be signed by all parties (e.g. physiologist, athlete, parent, coach, sporting body) [4].

A unique consideration when providing physiological support to young athletes is the consequences of biological maturation on the athlete's development and performance [88, 89]. It is well documented that biological maturation does not change linearly with chronological age. Rather, an individual's stage of biological maturation can vary dramatically for a given chronological age, reflecting the inter-individual variation in the timing and tempo of the maturation process. Physiologists working with the young athlete must be aware of his/her maturity status as rapid physiological and performance-related improvements may be caused by advancing maturity, independent of training. Consequently, knowledge of the athlete's maturity status is likely to be useful from a talent identification perspective and for understanding changes in performance and fitness status. The delayed onset or slow progression of biological maturity may also identify athletes at risk [2], which if of concern, should be discussed with the coach and athlete in the context of modifying the athlete's training programme, and potentially a referral to a medical professional.

Assessing maturation is notoriously problematic. In youth soccer there has been great interest in using skeletal age to monitor maturity status in order to inform an athlete's training load or with the assignment of competitive groups [90]. This procedure, however, is not without criticism, especially in terms of the benefit (injury reduction) to risk (annual X-ray exposure) ratio [91]. In contrast, Tanner's secondary sex characteristics (e.g. pubic hair and genital development for boys, and pubic hair and breast development for girls) have been found to be accurately self-assessed in young athletes between 12 and 17 years of age [92]. However, some young athletes may view the Tanner method as intrusive. An alternative method is to use sex-specific prediction equations based on easy to administer anthropometrical measures (stature, body mass and sitting height) to estimate an individual's 'offset' age from peak height velocity as a marker of (somatic) maturity [93].

The key objectives of providing physiological support to the young athlete are to identify strengths and weaknesses, and through discussions with the coach and athlete, inform and evaluate training methods. It has recently been recommended that for most athletes physiological support should be provided every 3 months, allowing sufficient time for the adaptations from training (and owing to growth and maturation) to manifest [4]. However, the testing frequency should be discussed with the coach and focus around key periods in the athlete's training cycle and competition schedule, allowing a timely assessment of the last training cycle and new physiological data to inform the direction of the following cycle. To achieve this objective, the physiologist must be able to provide feedback on the athlete's performance in a manner which is easy for the coach and athlete to understand and where possible, delivered in the context of previous test scores. The physiologist should be prepared to provide an overview of the athlete's performance on the day, but follow this up with a written report such that the coach and athlete can use the test data to further develop the training programme.

The overall effectiveness of the physiological support will depend on the physiologist's knowledge of the physiological determinants of the athlete's event or sport, ability to select a valid test and interpret the data correctly, and provide evidence-based training recommendations. This requires a comprehensive understanding of the laboratory- and field-based measures that are available to the physiologist, and the art of selecting a battery of tests which is most relevant to the athlete's needs and environment. The physiologist may also have to consider the cost and practicalities when providing physiological support, as for large groups of athletes, for example in team-based sports, a low cost battery of tests to be implemented within a single training session, may be more appropriate. Field-based and sport-specific measures will inevitably increase the ecological validity of the test protocol, and where possible, this should be sought in the laboratory setting by matching the exercise ergometer and test protocol to the characteristics of the athlete's competitive environment. This may require, through communications with the coach and/or athlete, the modification of existing test protocols. However, whilst this is a reasonable approach, the physiologist must be aware of the reproducibility of the main outcome variables, to be certain of a 'true' improvement in fitness or performance.

Conclusions

Given the increasing number of young people engaging in competitive sport and seeking performance-related improvements, the demand to provide continual and high-level physiological support and monitoring to the young athlete has never been greater. In this chapter, we have provided a current overview of field- and laboratory-based methods to measure the key aspects of aerobic fitness and performance of maximal intensity exercise by young people, and, where possible, highlighted their relationship with athletic performance. It is clear that the availability of data concerning the physiological assessment of young athletes in their sporting environment is limited. Consequently, based on their understanding of the athletic event/sport and specific requirements of the young athlete, the challenge for exercise scientists is to: (1) select, in communication with the coach and athlete, the most appropriate physiological measure(s); (2) understand the different child-specific protocols at their disposal; (3) be aware of the validity and reliability of the testing procedures, and (4) consider how to communicate the test results in a context that is both athlete and coach friendly, and performance-related.

References

1 Mountjoy M, Armstrong N, Bizzini L, Blimkie C, Evans J, Gerrard D, Hangen J, Knoll K, Micheli L, Sangenis P, Van Mechelen W: IOC consensus statement: 'training the elite child athlete'. Br J Sports Med 2008;42:163–164.
2 Intensive training and sports specialization in young athletes. American Academy of Pediatrics. Committee on Sports Medicine and Fitness. Pediatrics 2000;106:154–157.
3 Winter EM, Bromley PD, Davison RC, Jones AM, Mercer TH: Rationale; in Winter EM, Bromley PD, Davison RC, Jones AM, Mercer TH (eds): Sport and Exercise Physiology Testing Guidelines. The British Association of Sport and Exercise Sciences Guide. London, Routledge, 2007, pp 7–10.
4 Davison RR, Van Someren KA, Jones AM: Physiological monitoring of the Olympic athlete. J Sports Sci 2009;27:1–10.
5 Winlove MA, Jones AM, Welsman JR: Influence of training status and exercise modality on pulmonary O_2 uptake kinetics in pre-pubertal girls. Eur J Appl Physiol 2010;108:1169–1179.
6 Barker A, Welsman J, Welford D, Fulford J, Williams C, Armstrong N: Reliability of ^{31}P-magnetic resonance spectroscopy during an exhaustive incremental exercise test in children. Eur J Appl Physiol 2006;98:556–565.

7 Barker AR, Welsman JR, Fulford J, Welford D, Armstrong N: Quadriceps muscle energetics during incremental exercise in children and adults. Med Sci Sports Exerc 2010;42:1303–1313.

8 Thomas JR, Nelson JK: Research Methods in Physical Activity. Champaign, Human Kinetics, 2001.

9 Hopkins WG: Measures of reliability in sports medicine and science. Sports Med 2000;30:1–15.

10 Atkinson G, Nevill AM: Statistical methods for assessing measurement error (reliability) in variables relevant to sports medicine. Sports Med 1998;26:217–238.

11 Helgerud J, Engen LC, Wisloff U, Hoff J: Aerobic endurance training improves soccer performance. Med Sci Sports Exerc 2001;33:1925–1931.

12 Wasserman K, Hansen J, Sue D, Stringer W, Whipp B: Principles of Exercise Testing and Interpretation. Including Pathophysiology and Clinical Application, ed 4. Philiadelphia, Lippincott Williams & Wilkins, 2005.

13 Bassett DR, Howley ET: Maximal oxygen uptake: 'classical' versus 'contemporary' viewpoints. Med Sci Sports Exerc 1997;29:591–603.

14 Taylor HL, Buskirk E, Henschel A: Maximal oxygen uptake as an objective measure of cardio-respiratory performance. J Appl Physiol 1955;8:73–80.

15 Barker AR, Williams CA, Jones AM, Armstrong N: Establishing maximal oxygen uptake in young people during a ramp cycle test to exhaustion. Br J Sports Med 2009;DOI:10.1136/bjsm.2009.063180.

16 Armstrong N, Welsman JR: Assessment and interpretation of aerobic fitness in children and adolescents. Exerc Sport Sci Rev 1994;22:435–476.

17 Rivera-Brown AM, Frontera WR: Achievement of plateau and reliability of VO₂ max in trained adolescents tested with different protocols. Pediatr Exerc Sci 1998;10:164–175.

18 Rivera-Brown AM, Rivera MA, Frontera WR: Achievement of VO₂ max criteria in adolescent runners: effects of testing protocol. Pediatr Exerc Sci 1994;6:236–245.

19 Armstrong N, Welsman J, Winsley R: Is peak VO₂ a maximal index of children's aerobic fitness? Int J Sports Med 1996;17:356–359.

20 Paterson DH, McLellan TM, Stella RS, Cunningham DA: Longitudinal study of ventilation threshold and maximal O₂ uptake in athletic boys. J Appl Physiol 1987;62:2051–2057.

21 Leger L: Aerobic performance; in Docherty D (eds): Measurement in Pediatric Exercise Science. Champaign, Human Kinetics, 1996, pp 183–224.

22 Armstrong N, Welsman JR: Aerobic Performance; in Armstrong N, Van Mechelen W (eds): Paediatric Exercise Science and Medicine. Oxford, Oxford University Press, 2008, pp 97–108.

23 Rivera-Brown AM, Rivera MA, Frontera WR: Applicability of criteria for VO₂ max in active adolescents. Pediatr Exerc Sci 1992;4:331–339.

24 Hebestreit H, Beneke R: Testing for aerobic capacity; in Hebestreit H, Bar-Or O (eds): The Young Athlete. Oxford, Blackwell, 2008, pp 443–452.

25 Sheehan JM, Rowland TW, Burke EJ: A comparison of four treadmill protocols for determination of maximum oxygen uptake in 10- to 12-year-old boys. Int J Sports Med 1987;8:31–34.

26 DiBella II JA, Johnson EM, Cabrera ME: Ramped vs. standard Bruce protocol in children: a comparison of exercise responses. Pediatr Exerc Sci 2002;14:391–400.

27 Armstrong N, Davies B: An ergometric analysis of age group swimmers. Br J Sports Med 1981;15:20–26.

28 Davison RR, Wooles AL: Cycling; in Winter EM, Jones AM, Davison RR, Bromley PD, Mercer TH (eds): Sport and Exercise Physiology Testing Guidelines. The British Association of Sport and Exercise Sciences Guide. Abingdon, Routledge, 2007, pp 160–164.

29 Almarwaey OA, Jones AM, Tolfrey K: Maximal lactate steady state in trained adolescent runners. J Sports Sci 2004;22:215–225.

30 Jones AM: Middle- and long-distance running; in Winter EM, Jones AM, Davison RR, Bromley PD, Mercer TH (eds): Sport and Exercise Physiology Testing Guidelines. The British Association of Sport and Exercise Sciences Guide. Abingdon, Routledge, 2007, pp 147–154.

31 Welsman JR, Armstrong N: Statistical techniques for interpreting body size-related exercise performance during growth. Pediatr Exerc Sci 2000;12:112–127.

32 Chamari K, Hachana Y, Kaouech F, Jeddi R, Moussa-Chamari I, Wisloff U: Endurance training and testing with the ball in young elite soccer players. Br J Sports Med 2005;39:24–28.

33 Pettersen SA, Fredriksen PM, Ingjer E: The correlation between peak oxygen uptake (VO₂ peak) and running performance in children and adolescents. aspects of different units. Scand J Med Sci Sports 2001;11:223–228.

34 Nevill A, Rowland T, Goff D, Martel L, Ferrone L: Scaling or normalising maximum oxygen uptake to predict 1-mile run time in boys. Eur J Appl Physiol 2004;92:285–288.

35 Leger LA, Lambert J: A maximal multistage 20-m shuttle run test to predict VO₂ max. Eur J Appl Physiol Occup Physiol 1982;49:1–12.

36 Tomkinson GR, Olds TS: Field tests of fitness; in Armstrong N, Van Mechelen W (eds): Paediatric Exercise Science and Medicine. Oxford, Oxford University Press, 2008, pp 109–128.

37 Voss C, Sandercock G: Does the twenty meter shuttle-run test elicit maximal effort in 11- to 16-year-olds? Pediatr Exerc Sci 2009;21:55–62.

38 Tomkinson GR, Olds TS: Secular changes in pediatric aerobic fitness test performance: the global picture. Med Sport Sci 2007;50:46–66.

39 Harley RA, Doust J, Mills SH: Basketball; in Winter EM, Jones AM, Davison RR, Bromley PD, Mercer TH (eds): Sport and Exercise Physiology Testing Guidelines. The British Association of Sport and Exercise Sciences Guide. Abingdon, Routledge, 2007, pp 232–240.

40 Smith RG, Harley RA, Stockill NP: Cricket; in Winter EM, Jones AM, Davison RR, Bromley PD, Mercer TH (eds): Sport and Exercise Physiology Testing Guidelines. The British Association of Sport and Exercise Sciences Guide. Abingdon, Routledge, 2007, pp 225–231.

41 Grantham N: Netball; in Winter EM, Jones AM, Davison RR, Bromley PD, Mercer TH (eds): Sport and Exercise Physiology Testing Guidelines. The British Association of Sport and Exercise Sciences Guide. Abingdon, Routledge, 2007, pp 249–255.

42 Bangsbo J, Lindquist F: Comparison of various exercise tests with endurance performance during soccer in professional players. Int J Sports Med 1992;13:125–132.

43 Chamari K, Hachana Y, Ahmed YB, Galy O, Sghaier F, Chatard JC, Hue O, Wisloff U: Field and laboratory testing in young elite soccer players. Br J Sports Med 2004;38:191–196.

44 Almarwaey OA, Jones AM, Tolfrey K: Physiological correlates with endurance running performance in trained adolescents. Med Sci Sports Exerc 2003;35:480–487.

45 Cole AS, Woodruff ME, Horn MP, Mahon AD: Strength, power, and aerobic exercise correlates of 5-km cross-country running performance in adolescent runners. Pediatr Exerc Sci 2006;18:374–384.

46 Unnithan VB, Timmons JA, Paton JY, Rowland TW: Physiologic correlates to running performance in pre-pubertal distance runners. Int J Sports Med 1995;16:528–533.

47 Krahenbuhl GS, Morgan DW, Pangrazi RP: Longitudinal changes in distance-running performance of young males. Int J Sports Med 1989;10:92–96.

48 Daniels J, Oldridge N, Nagle F, White B: Differences and changes in VO_2 among young runners 10 to 18 years of age. Med Sci Sports 1978;10:200–203.

49 Unnithan V, Holohan J, Fernhall B, Wylegala J, Rowland T, Pendergast DR: Aerobic cost in elite female adolescent swimmers. Int J Sports Med 2009;30:194–199.

50 Thompson KG, Taylor SR: Swimming; in Winter EM, Jones AM, Davison RR, Bromley PD, Mercer TH (eds): Sport and Exercise Physiology Testing Guidelines. The British Association of Sport and Exercise Sciences Guide. Abingdon, Routledge, 2007, pp 184–190.

51 Anderson CS, Mahon AD: The relationship between ventilatory and lactate thresholds in boys and men. Res Sports Med 2007;15:189–200.

52 Fawkner SG, Armstrong N, Childs DJ, Welsman JR: Reliability of the visually identified ventilatory threshold and v-slope in children. Pediatr Exerc Sci 2002;14:181–192.

53 Fernhall B, Kohrt W, Burkett LN, Walters S: Relationship between the lactate threshold and cross-country run performance in high school male and female runners. Pediatr Exerc Sci 1996;8:37–47.

54 Mader A, Heck H: A theory of the metabolic origin of 'anaerobic threshold'. Int J Sports Med 1986;7:45–65.

55 Whipp BJ, Rossiter HB: The kinetics of oxygen uptake: physiological inferences from the parameters; in Jones AM, Poole DC (eds): Oxygen Uptake Kinetics in Sport, Exercise and Medicine. London, Routledge, 2005, pp 62–94.

56 Montfort-Steiger V, Williams CA, Armstrong N: The reproducibility of an endurance performance test in adolescent cyclists. Eur J Appl Physiol 2005;94:618–625.

57 Beneke R, Heck H, Hebestreit H, Leithauser RM: Predicting maximal lactate steady state in children and adults. Pediatr Exerc Sci 2009;21:493–505.

58 Poole DC, Ward SA, Gardner GW, Whipp BJ: Metabolic and respiratory profile of the upper limit for prolonged exercise in man. Ergonomics 1988;31:1265–1279.

59 Hill DW: The critical power concept: a review. Sports Med 1993;16:237–254.

60 Berthoin S, Baquet G, Dupont G, Blondel N, Mucci P: Critical velocity and anaerobic distance capacity in prepubertal children. Can J Appl Physiol 2003;28:561–575.

61 Jones AM, Vanhatalo A, Burnley M, Morton RH, Poole DC: Critical power: implications for the determination of VO_2 max and exercise tolerance. Med Sci Sports Exerc DOI:10.1249/MSS.0b013e3181d9cf7f.

62 Hill DW, Steward Jr. RP, Lane CJ: Application of the critical power concept to young swimmers. Pediatr Exerc Sci 1995;7:281–293.

63 Denadai BS, Greco CC, Teixeira M: Blood lactate response and critical speed in swimmers aged 10–12 years of different standards. J Sports Sci 2000;18:779–784.

64 Fawkner SG, Armstrong N: Assessment of critical power with children. Pediatr Exerc Sci 2002;14:259–268.

65 Toubekis AG, Tsami AP, Tokmakidis SP: Critical velocity and lactate threshold in young swimmers. Int J Sports Med 2006;27:117–123.

66 Dekerle J, Williams C, McGawley K, Carter H: Critical power is not attained at the end of an isokinetic 90-second all-out test in children. J Sports Sci 2009;27:379–385.

67 Vanhatalo A, Doust JH, Burnley M: Determination of critical power using a 3-min all-out cycling test. Med Sci Sports Exerc 2007;39:548–555.

68 le Gall F, Carling C, Williams M, Reilly T: Anthropometric and fitness characteristics of international, professional and amateur male graduate soccer players from an elite youth academy. J Sci Med Sport 13:90–95.

69 Reilly T, Williams AM, Nevill A, Franks A: A multidisciplinary approach to talent identification in soccer. J Sports Sci 2000;18:695–702.

70 Barnes C: Soccer; in Winter EM, Jones AM, Davison RR, Bromley PD, Mercer TH (eds): Sport and Exercise Physiology Testing Guidelines. The British Association of Sport and Exercise Sciences Guide. Abingdon, Routledge, 2007, pp 241–248.

71 Williams CA: Children's and adolescents' anaerobic performance during cycle ergometry. Sports Med 1997;24:227–240.

72 Beneke R, Hutler M, Leithauser RM: Anaerobic performance and metabolism in boys and male adolescents. Eur J Appl Physiol 2007;101:671–677.

73 Williams CA, Ratel S, Armstrong N: Achievement of peak VO_2 during a 90-s maximal intensity cycle sprint in adolescents. Can J Appl Physiol 2005;30:157–171.

74 Bar-Or O: Anaerobic Performance; in Docherty D (ed): Measurement in Pediatric Exercise Science. Champaign, Human Kinetics, 1996, pp 161–182.

75 Cumming GR: Correlation of athletic performance and aerobic power in 12 17-year-old children with bone age, calf muscle, total body potassium, heart volume and two indices of anaerobic power; in Bar-Or O (ed): Paediatric Work Physiology. Netanya, Wingate Institute, 1973, pp 109–134.

76 Sutton NC, Childs DJ, Bar-Or O, Armstrong N: A nonmotorized treadmill test to assess children's short-term power output. Pediatr Exerc Sci 2000;12:91–100.

77 Santos AMC, Welsman JR, De Ste Croix MB, Armstrong N: Age and sex-related differences in optimal peak power. Pediatr Exerc Sci 2002;14:202–212.

78 Dore E, Duche P, Rouffet D, Ratel S, Bedu M, Van Praagh E: Measurement error in short-term power testing in young people. J Sports Sci 2003;21:135–142.

79 Mikulic P, Ruzic L, Markovic G: Evaluation of specific anaerobic power in 12–14-year-old male rowers. J Sci Med Sport 2009;12:662–666.

80 Meckel Y, Machnai O, Eliakim A: Relationship among repeated sprint tests, aerobic fitness, and anaerobic fitness in elite adolescent soccer players. J Strength Cond Res 2009;23:163–169.

81 Oliver JL, Williams CA, Armstrong N: Reliability of a field and laboratory test of repeated sprint ability. Pediatr Exerc Sci 2006;18:339–350.

82 Oliver JL, Armstrong N, Williams CA: Reliability and validity of a soccer-specific test of prolonged repeated-sprint ability. Int J Sports Physiol Perform 2007;2:137–149.

83 Rowland TW: Children's Exercise Physiology, ed 2. Champaign, Human Kinetics; 2005.

84 Sargent DA: The physical test of a man. Am Phys Ed Rev 1921;26:188–194.

85 Docherty D: Field tests and test batteries; in Docherty D (ed): Measurement in Pediatric Exercise Science. Champaign, Human Kinetics, 1996, pp 285–334.

86 Bangsbo J, Iaia FM, Krustrup P: The Yo-Yo intermittent recovery test: a useful tool for evaluation of physical performance in intermittent sports. Sports Med 2008;38:37–51.

87 Oliver S: Ethics and physiological testing; in Winter EM, Bromley PD, Davison RC, Jones AM, Mercer TH (eds): Sport and Exercise Physiology Testing Guidelines. The British Association of Sport and Exercise Sciences Guide. London, Routledge, 2007, pp 30–37.

88 Armstrong N, McManus AM: Physiology of elite young male athletes; in Armstrong N, McManus AM (eds): The Elite Young Athlete. Med Sport Sci. Basel, Karger, 2011, pp 1–22.

89 McManus AM, Armstrong N: Physiology of elite young female athletes; in Armstrong N, McManus AM (eds.), The Elite Young Athlete. Med Sport Sci. Basel, Karger, 2011, pp 23–46.

90 Johnson A, Doherty PJ, Freemont A: Investigation of growth, development, and factors associated with injury in elite schoolboy footballers: prospective study. BMJ 2009;338:b490.

91 Anand JK, Myles JW: Elitism and X-rays in child footballers: rapid responses to: Investigation of growth, development, and factors associated with injury in elite schoolboy footballers: prospective study. BMJ 2009. http://www.bmj.com/cgi/eletters/338/feb26_1/b490#211037.

92 Leone M, Comtois AS: Validity and reliability of self-assessment of sexual maturity in elite adolescent athletes. J Sports Med Phys Fitness 2007;47:361–365.

93 Mirwald RL, Baxter-Jones AD, Bailey DA, Beunen GP: An assessment of maturity from anthropometric measurements. Med Sci Sports Exerc 2002;34:689–694.

94 Krahenbuhl GS, Pangrazi RP: Characteristics associated with running performance in young boys. Med Sci Sports Exerc 1983;15:486–490.

95 Armstrong N, Welsman JR, Williams CA: Maximal Intensity Exercise; in Armstrong N, Van Mechelen W (eds): Paediatric Exercise Science and Medicine. Oxford, Oxford University Press, 2008, pp 55–66.

Dr. Alan R. Barker
Children's Health and Exercise Research Centre
University of Exeter
Exeter EX1 2LU (UK)
Tel. +44 0 1392 722766, Fax +44 0 1392 264726, E-Mail A.R.Barker@exeter.ac.uk

Armstrong N, McManus AM (eds): The Elite Young Athlete.
Med Sport Sci. Basel, Karger, 2011, vol 56, pp 126–149

Temperature Regulation and Elite Young Athletes

Bareket Falk · Raffy Dotan

Faculty of Applied Health Sciences, Brock University, St. Catharines, Ont., Canada

Abstract

Children and adults employ different thermoregulatory strategies, particularly in dealing with heat stress. Children rely more on 'dry' heat exchange, while evaporative heat loss is adults' foremost heat-dissipation venue. Several anatomical, physiological, and psychological factors can affect differential risk of thermal injury in the child vs. the adult athlete, in some situations. Children have greater surface-area-to-mass ratio, lower sweating rate, higher peripheral blood flow in the heat, and a greater extent of vasoconstriction in the cold. They can acclimatise to a similar extent but do so at a lower rate than adults. Differences in perceived exertion and thermal strain, cumulative experience, cognitive development, and decision-making capacity may negatively affect the young athlete's behaviour under competitive and other situations, possibly subjecting him/her to sub-par performance or to greater risk of thermal injury. However, except for very limited environmental conditions, children in general, and young athletes in particular, are physiologically as capable as adults to handle environmental challenges.

Youth sports participation in general, and elite sports in particular, are on an increasing trend [1]. Physical activity, exercise and sport participation have been shown to impart children with considerable health advantages such as cardiovascular and skeletal strength [2, 3], as well as social and scholastic benefits [4, 5]. Such activities, however,

also involve the risk of injury, particularly in competitive athletics. This chapter aims to provide an overview of the physiological challenges presented by environmental extremes and the differences in the thermoregulatory strategies employed by children and young athletes compared with adults (for detailed reviews, see [6, 9]). The chapter also attempts to elucidate the question of whether child athletes stand greater risks of thermal injury and, if so, under what situations; and recommend intervention and prevention strategies to minimise risks to the elite young athlete.

Environmental Conditions and Thermoregulatory Responses

Humans live, thrive, and athletically compete in a broad range of environmental conditions, having a remarkable ability to deal with and tolerate environmental extremes. These include the likes of hot-dry desert conditions, warm-humid tropical climate, and the bitter cold of the Arctic, extremes which can span more than 100°C. Nevertheless, humans are able to maintain body core temperature to within a relatively narrow range (35–41°C).

Human ability to regulate body temperature and successfully cope with metabolic and environmental extremes involves a host of physiological and behavioural responses, as well as the use of technological means. Physiological means may involve changes in blood flow distribution, increased cardiac output and sweating, or re-setting of thermoregulatory set points. Behavioural means may involve the selection of a better environment (e.g. shelter), selection of the micro-environment (e.g. clothing), or the adjustment of exertion level. Technological means can involve sheltering, the use of chilled or hot drinks, heating or air conditioning, special technical clothing, etc.

Metabolic heat production during sustained exercise may be 15–20 times higher than that produced at rest. In a hot (or warm-humid) environment, the need to dissipate this heat places particularly high demands on the thermoregulatory system. An inability to effectively meet the combined challenges of heat dissipation will invariably result in deterioration in athletic performance and, if not detected and responded to, may culminate in heat illness, organ failure, and eventually, death.

The excessive metabolic heat produced during exercise must be dissipated to the environment by means of dry heat exchange (radiation, conduction, convection), facilitated by augmented skin blood flow, or via evaporation, facilitated by sweating. The effectiveness of each of these two main venues depends on the environmental conditions. Evaporative heat loss is dependent on the evaporated sweat volume which, in turn, depends on the ambient relative humidity and level of convection (air movement, wind). As humidity rises, evaporative heat loss becomes progressively less effective. On the other hand, in hot and dry conditions, sweat evaporation becomes the main venue of heat dissipation. Effective dry heat loss is dependent on the exposed body surface area, as well as on the skin-to-environment temperature gradient. Therefore, the greater the temperature gradient between the skin and the surrounding medium (air, water), the greater the dry heat loss. As the ambient temperature rises, dry heat dissipation becomes less effective and when ambient temperature rises above skin temperature, heat is absorbed from, rather than dissipated to the environment.

For a given environmental heat stress, children's relative reliance on dry vs. evaporative heat dissipation is greater compared with adults [6, 8, 9]. This is due to children's relatively larger skin surface area which predisposes them to greater dry heat transfer. Consequently, children's thermoregulation manifests various physiological responses that are different from those of adults, as will be discussed later in this chapter.

Compared with heat stress, cold exposure lends itself better to behavioural responses – mainly in the form of appropriate clothing and shelter use. However, there is often a trade-off between athletic performance and thermal protection (i.e. added weight of clothing, restricted movement) and athletes often sacrifice the latter for the former, which puts them in a more vulnerable state. The increased heat production associated with exercise might not, by itself, suffice to offset heat loss and a heat-conservation response may still be necessary in the form of peripheral vasoconstriction.

Thermoregulation is affected by environmental conditions other than just temperature. These include humidity, relative air velocity (typically wind or movement through the air), and solar or other radiation. High humidity greatly reduces sweat evaporation in the heat. In the cold, typically low humidity mainly affects respiratory heat and water losses. Respiratory heat loss, while minor at rest, can become significant during high intensity exercise and can comprise as much as 15–20% of metabolic heat loss during exercise in the cold [10]. This may be more accentuated in children, who are characterized by a higher $\dot{V}_E/\dot{V}O_2$ ratio [11] and could, therefore, have greater respiratory heat loss. This is of practical significance only when heat production does not match heat loss in the cold, thus increasing the risk of hypothermia. Children's higher ventilatory heat loss also means greater water loss. While dehydration is typically inconsequential for thermoregulation in the cold, it may attain cardiovascular significance in endurance events where progressive, cumulative water loss may affect plasma and blood volume and consequently compromise cardiac output and work capacity. This risk can be compounded by the fact that, in the cold, thirst sensation may be considerably attenuated during physiological and psychological stresses typical of exercise in general [12], and athletic competition, in particular.

Windy conditions can enhance heat dissipation (increased convection and evaporation) and may be beneficial in the heat. In the cold, however, especially after competition is completed and heat production has dramatically subsided but the body is still sweaty and under-protected by clothing, wind can become a serious threat for hypothermia. With their greater body-surface-area-to-mass ratio, children stand a greater risk under such conditions, compared with adults (see next section).

Finally, radiation involves a combination of direct solar radiation, along with the indirect radiation reflected from the ground, bodies of water, and various structures and objects. Direct solar radiation is intuitively understood to be very high under exposure to sunny conditions and, depending on the time of day, can seriously contribute to thermal stress during long-duration outdoor events such as ball games, tournaments, long-distance running, etc. Indirect radiation from snow and ice is not always as intuitive but can add to the thermal stress in winter sports. Again, the impact of radiation on heat stress in children may be higher due to their higher surface-area-to-mass ratio (see next section). However, this is of secondary significance because heat stress under cold conditions can only be due to superfluous clothing, not to radiative heat gain.

For any given environmental condition, physical factors, such as body dimensions, composition, and proportions (e.g. surface-area-to-mass ratio), and physiological factors, such as level of acclimatization, aerobic fitness, and hydration state, can also affect the thermoregulatory effectiveness. The following section discusses physical and physiological differences between children and adults which may differentially affect their thermoregulatory effectiveness. Subsequently, some of the physiological factors (e.g. fitness, acclimation, hydration), as well as administrative means (e.g. scheduling) which can serve to prevent heat or cold injuries are also presented.

Child-Adult Differences Affecting Thermoregulation

Table 1 describes the anatomical, physiological, cognitive and behavioural factors which may differentially affect child and adult athletes in hot and cold environments. These factors are discussed in more detail in this section.

Body Surface Area-to-Mass Ratio

Children's smaller body- and muscle-mass can affect both heat production and heat dissipation or conservation. Children have a considerably greater surface area relative to their body mass (~20% for a 12-year-old). An implication of this difference is that in moderately warm environmental conditions, when skin temperature is higher than that of the environment, the flux of non-evaporative ('dry') heat is from the body outwards. Under these conditions, children can dissipate a greater proportion of body heat via dry means and, consequently, depend less on evaporative heat dissipation, as described above [8]. This thermoregulatory strategy can be advantageous in mild to moderate conditions. In fact, Dennis and Noakes [13] contend that small adult runners, because of their higher surface-area-to-mass ratio, actually have an advantage in

Table 1. Thermoregulatory factors in young vs. adult athletes

Category	Factor	Characteristics in children (compared with adults)	Effect in children and young athletes (compared with adults)		Comments
			heat stress	cold stress	
Anatomical	Body surface area-to-mass ratio	Considerably larger (relatively larger skin area)	– Higher capacity for 'dry' heat transfer – Greater risk of thermal injury at both temperature extremes		While other factors may be affected by training, pre-selection, or behaviour, this is the only inherently consistent difference between young and adult athletes
Physiological	Sweating and dehydration	– Lower sweating rate – Higher $\dot{V}_E/\dot{V}O_2$ ratio – More limited dehydration, but can approach adult levels in elite young athletes	Greater reliance on dry, non-evaporative, heat dissipation	The higher $\dot{V}_E/\dot{V}O_2$ may cause greater water loss, particularly during intense, prolonged exercise	– Lower sweating rate means lower evaporative cooling but also more fluid retention – Young athletes appear to have higher sweating capacity, near that of adults
	Cardiac output	– Slightly lower at similar absolute power outputs* – Similar response to similar change in power output			* – Likely, only a reflection of adults' larger resting cardiac output –Similar cardiac output when expressed per body surface area
	Cutaneous blood flow	– ~10% higher than in adults (depending on metabolic and environmental loads) – Greater vasoconstriction in the cold	Supports greater reliance on 'dry', non-evaporative, heat dissipation	The greater extent of vasoconstriction conserves heat and imparts partial cold protection**	** The protection is insufficient to counteract the larger, surface-area-related heat loss, compared with adults – particularly in extreme cold exposure
	Core temperature response	Faster rise in exercise- or environmentally induced heat stress	May bring the young athlete faster to critically-high core temperature in high heat stress		At least under moderate heat loads this may reflect children's greater reliance on dry heat-dissipation strategy, favouring higher skin-to-ambient temperature gradient

Category	Factor	Characteristics in children (compared with adults)	Effect in children and young athletes (compared with adults)		Comments
			heat stress	cold stress	
	Locomotive economy	– Lower in children – Improves with training	– May increase heat production at similar absolute workloads – Smaller, possibly negligible difference in elite athletes	May be beneficial in raising heat production under hypothermic threat	The lower economy does not affect relative thermal-injury risk, as each individual competes at an intensity relative to his/her own capacity
	Acclimatization	– Similar extent of heat acclimatization Passive heat exposure and exercise in thermo-neutral environment may suffice (adults need exercise in the heat for best acclimatization) – Cold acclimatization is much more limited; it is not clear how much of it is physiological or habitual and whether its nature is distinct from that of adults	In all but the extreme environments, proper acclimatization can be expected to provide the young athletes with protection or performance boost similar to that in adults	Children remain more susceptible to cold, particularly extreme cold, or any condition in which they cannot metabolically offset heat loss	– Children's lower tolerance to extreme heat stems from their larger relative surface-area and cannot be overcome by acclimatization – While they can heat-acclimatize to a similar extent as adults, children take longer to attain comparable acclimatization
Cognitive	Perceived exertion	– Tendency to underestimate, particularly in intermittent, variable- intensity exercise – Possible over-estimation in prolonged, monotonous exercise	Likelihood of faulty exertion management (e.g. pacing) and higher risk of thermal injury or premature fatigue	Hypothermia can ensue when failure to properly pace oneself results in premature fatigue and decreased metabolic heat production	

Category	Factor	Characteristics in children (compared with adults)	Effect in children and young athletes (compared with adults)		Comments
			heat stress	cold stress	
	Perceived thermal stress	– Apparently similar in heat exposure – Not known whether children have different cold-stress perception than adults	No known difference from adults	No known difference from adults	
Behavioural	Decision-making	Limited experience and lesser capacity to objectively assess hostile situations and make appropriate, informed decisions	Possible failure to sufficiently drink, properly pace, or employ other defensive measures	Possible failure to properly dress or use appropriate sheltering	

moderate heat conditions and can run at a higher pace before reaching uncompensable heat stress. However, in extremely hot conditions, when ambient temperatures are higher than skin temperature, or when radiative heat is very high, children's greater surface-area-to-mass ratio becomes a liability, resulting in greater heat absorption. This is also the case when training or competing outdoors, where weather conditions can make heat radiation a highly significant factor. Depending on ambient humidity, evaporative cooling may not suffice under such conditions, resulting in uncompensable heat stress.

Sweating Response

The most striking child-adult difference in the physiological response, to both resting and exercising in the heat, is the sweating response. Considerably lower sweating rates have been shown in children compared with adults, particularly in boys *vs.* men, and less so in girls compared with women [14]. Children's lower sweating rate has been observed under all metabolic loads in various heat-stress conditions [for reviews see 6, 14–18]. These sweating-rate differences are consistent, not only in absolute terms, but in normalized comparisons as well – per unit body surface area, per sweat gland, or when related to core temperature rise [19]. This difference in sweating rates grows larger with increasing exercise intensity or heat stress [18].

Sweating is central to thermoregulatory capacity due to the high heat-dissipation capacity of water vaporization. Therefore, the consistently lower sweating rates observed in children have traditionally been interpreted as a major liability and a potential cause for children's presumed relative heat intolerance. However, as suggested recently, the lower sweating rate may simply be a manifestation of children's different thermoregulatory strategy [8, 19]. That is, due to their larger surface-area-to-mass ratio and their greater reliance on 'dry' heat dissipation, children may simply not need to sweat as much as adults in order to thermoregulate effectively. Also, as a side effect, this strategy enables children to conserve body fluids, an important advantage in prolonged training or competition in the heat.

Comparative physiology shows that in warm-blooded animals, metabolic rate is better related to the body's surface area than to its mass [20]. From this perspective, and the fact that sweat dissipates heat by evaporating off the skin, it has made intuitive sense to relate sweating rate to body surface area. However, since exercise workloads are typically determined and normalized to body or lean-muscle mass (e.g. a given percentage of mass-relative $\dot{V}O_2$), sweating rate as a means for heat-loss should be evaluated in relation to mass or to the metabolic load ($\dot{V}O_2$), which is directly related to heat production. When sweat-induced dehydration was compared in this way between children and adults across several studies (as % body mass, calculated from [21]), adults' percentage loss was ~60% larger than that of the children. Thus, relative to actual heat production, this difference in sweating rate highlights children's lower reliance on evaporative heat loss and different thermoregulatory strategy.

While the maximal sweating rate of children or young athletes has not been determined, Rivera-Brown et al. [22] measured twice the normal reported peak sweating rates in trained, heat-acclimatized children (~500 vs. 200–300 ml $\bullet$ m^{-2} $\bullet$ h^{-1}). However, in many thermally-stressing environments, simple child-adult sweating-rate comparisons may be inconsequential due to sweat dripping. This has not been quantitatively reported but experience and anecdotal evidence suggests that sweat dripping is commonplace in adults (particularly males) but hardly, if ever, occurs in children. Dripped sweat is lost to both the evaporative cooling potential and the body's fluid balance. It is possible that under the severe conditions that lead to sweat dripping, adults' effective sweating rate (the amount actually evaporating off the skin) is significantly smaller than their raw sweating rate,

thereby lending added credence to the claim that children can be regarded as more efficient sweaters [19].

As children's thermoregulation is more dependent on peripheral (cutaneous) blood flow, a decrease in the latter would compromise their heat-dissipation capacity more than in adults and result in a greater core temperature rise for a given percentage of fluid loss. Children, therefore, seem to have an inherently greater need to conserve fluids. Thus, children's lower sweating rate should not be regarded as a liability that has to be compensated for by other means. Rather, the lower sweating rate is part of a thermoregulatory strategy that takes advantage of the unique characteristic of a high surface-to-mass ratio and minimizes the susceptibility to the pitfall of the heightened ill-effects of fluid loss.

Cardiac Output

At similar absolute metabolic loads ($\dot{V}O_2$), children produce somewhat lower cardiac outputs than adults [23]. Superficially, this appears to denote a paediatric cardiovascular deficiency. However, the apparent difference likely stems from the basal differences in cardiac output (e.g. ~5 vs. 2.5 litres $\bullet$ min^{-1} for adults vs. children, respectively). Indeed, when the cardiac index (cardiac output per unit surface area) is considered, at similar relative exercise intensity (60–65% $\dot{V}O_{2max}$), age-related differences have not been observed [24] or were statistically insignificant [25, 26]. This cardiac index similarity has been observed under different environmental conditions [24, 27], as well as in acclimated and non-acclimated subjects [24, 25].

In thermoregulatory terms, the similar cardiac index suggests that comparable proportions of cardiac output are available to children and adults for peripheral perfusion and hence, for heat convection. However, as children rely more heavily on peripheral perfusion for heat dissipation, their cardiovascular and thermoregulatory capacities can be expected to be more stressed under the conflicting demands of the working muscles and peripheral circulation under extreme heat stress.

Skin Blood Flow

Under similar heat-stress conditions, children have higher skin blood-flows per unit volume or mass, compared with adults [26, 28]. Likewise, Falk et al. [29] demonstrated a progressive decrease in forearm blood-flow with increasing maturity level in pre-, mid- and late-pubertal boys cycling in hot-dry conditions. Higher skin blood-flows in children have also been reported at similar rectal temperature values [28]. This is consistent with children's higher maximal skin vascular conductance at rest [30] and the lower peripheral vascular resistance recently demonstrated in children exercising in the heat [estimated from ref. 24]. Thus, children's higher cutaneous perfusion facilitates their greater reliance on 'dry' heat dissipation, compared with evaporative cooling.

Nonetheless, higher skin blood flow also suggests that a higher proportion of children's cardiac output is diverted to the periphery under heat stress. Higher skin blood flow and presumably a higher proportion of cardiac output diverted to the periphery, has not been observed to affect children's heat tolerance during moderate exercise-induced heat loads up to 30 min [24]. Due to the scarcity of direct evidence, it can only be speculated that as long as children have sufficient cardiac reserve and their thermoregulatory system can maintain stable core temperatures, they can continue their activity with no detriment. If the thermal load increases (due to increasing exercise intensity or duration, or with rising environmental stress), the ensuing increase in peripheral (cutaneous) vasodilation would compromise venous return and, consequently, cardiac output as well.

Under such conditions either performance (intensity, duration) or thermoregulation, or both, would be negatively impacted.

In cool or cold environments, children have been shown to have lower skin temperature of the extremities during rest [31, 32], as well as during exercise [33]. This lower skin temperature has been interpreted as reflecting greater peripheral vasoconstriction. However, more recently, Inoue et al. [34] demonstrated that cutaneous vascular conductance was not necessarily different between boys and men sitting in a cool environment and that differences in skin temperature may simply reflect differences in anthropometric characteristics. Thus, while greater peripheral vasoconstriction in children may be advantageous in cool and cold weather exposure, it is likely insufficient to counteract the disadvantage posed by their greater surface-area-to-mass ratio, at least under moderate to extreme cold conditions.

Locomotive Economy

Children in general, have lower locomotive economy compared with adults [11, 35–37]. That is, children expend more energy per unit mass at any given walking/running velocity. This subjects children to higher heat strain when matched with adults at similar velocities, as has been the case in several studies. While this is important for the interpretation of relative heat tolerance in those studies (see later in this chapter) and is worth mentioning here, it likely does not expose young athletes to a greater risk in competition for the following two reasons: (1) children, and particularly properly coached and guided young athletes, compete relative to their own capacities (e.g. at 80% max $\dot{V}O_2$), regardless of how economical they are – locomotive economy, therefore should not affect their relative heat tolerance, and (2) elite young athletes may have already reached or approached adult levels of locomotive economy.

Running economy has been shown to increase significantly more in 10-year-old runners over a 2-year period [38] than it did in their untrained counterparts [39]. Thus, age-related differences in economy may well be much smaller among trained athletes than in the untrained, general population.

Exertion and Heat-Stress Perception

The perception of physical exertion is a complex psycho-physiological process. Noble and Robertson [40] defined it as 'the act of detecting and interpreting sensations arising from the body during physical exercise'. With environmentally rather than just exercise-induced stress, the definition may be expanded to include the detection and subjective perception of thermal stress.

Very little is known about the subjective judgement of thermal sensation in children compared with adults. Among well-trained acclimated girls, thermal sensation was comparable to that of similarly trained women during the first 30 min of cycling at 60% $\dot{V}O_{2max}$ in hot and humid conditions [25]. However, after 40 min of cycling and until exhaustion (at ~1 h), thermal sensation was higher in the girls. On the other hand, during ~90 min of intermittent cycling at 50% $\dot{V}O_{2max}$ in hot, dry conditions, no differences in thermal comfort were observed between pre-, mid- and late-pubertal boys [41].

Exercise intensity appears to be perceived differently by children compared with adults. For example, over an 8- to 10-min progressive exercise bout Bar-Or [42] demonstrated that among 10- to 46-year-olds exercising at comparable exercise intensities, the ratio between the rating of perceived exertion (RPE) and the corresponding heart rate (HR), expressed as a percentage of maximal HR, increased with rising age. He argued that at a given cardiovascular strain (reflected by %HR$_{max}$), children perceive exercise intensity to be lower than do adolescents, who in turn, perceive it to be lower compared with adults. He suggested that children's lower perceived exertion may also partly explain why children are inherently more active (less exercise-reluctant) than adults. A probable implication to the athletic realm is that young athletes may perceive a given strain as lighter than would older athletes and would therefore be less likely to adjust their exercise intensity to the environmental conditions in an appropriate and timely fashion.

On the other hand, Timmons and Bar-Or [43] found that during prolonged cycling (60 min at 70% $\dot{V}O_{2max}$), 10- to 11-year-old boys perceived exercise as more intense than did adults. Compared with the earlier study with 8–10 min of progressive exercise, exertion in this study was characterized by both longer duration and uniform intensity. Although children have been shown to possess a shorter attention span [44], it is not directly known how their perception might be affected by task duration or monotony. It is possible that children's higher RPE in the 60-min effort reflected a relative difficulty to cope with prolonged, monotonous efforts rather than an elevated physical strain.

In their recent review, Groslambert and Mahon [45] conclude that children (not necessarily athletes) are able to reliably reproduce a cycling intensity based on their perceived effort. However, the reproduced intensities are often significantly lower than the intensity during the reference trial [46]. If this is indeed the case, it would mean that although children's perceptions may be consistent, they are not necessarily a true reflection of the objective strain the children are subjected to. Indeed, this statement conforms with the findings of the RPE-HR relationship varying with age [47] and increasing from childhood to adolescence [42].

Thus, while dependence on perception may be a valid strategy for adjusting exertion to environmental stress among adult athletes, this may not be the case among children and young athletes. It appears that during training or competition of short to medium duration at high or variable intensity (e.g. track and field, a tennis set, an interval-training set), children may underestimate their objective physiological strain, possibly putting them at increased risk of heat illness or sub-optimal performance in subsequent exposure and efforts. During exertions of long duration, particularly of constant intensity and monotonous nature (e.g. distance running), this may cause the young athlete to overestimate the objective physiological strain, possibly resulting in some heat-illness protection but also in sub-optimal athletic performance. It is less clear how prolonged, intensity-variable and emotionally charged exertion (e.g. a soccer match) would affect RPE. At present, it seems wise and safer to presume that this type of exertion would result in RPE underestimation similar to that shown for shorter efforts but with potentially higher risk.

It should be pointed out that the body of experimental data on the perception of exertional and thermal stress in children is small and that specific data on highly trained or athletically elite children are considerably more limited. It stands to reason that high-level training in general, and in thermally adverse conditions in particular, can only improve the acuteness of this perceptual capacity and bring it closer to adult levels.

Behaviour and Decision Making

Children and adolescents, including highly trained young athletes, possess less life- and sports-specific experience and are less capable of informed, objective decision-making than their adult counterparts [48]. Children's athletic behaviour may, to a large extent, be adult-guided. Nevertheless, when faced with the conflicting demands of maximising performance vs. heat-stress management (e.g. pacing, proper hydration), young athletes' ability to make the most appropriate decisions may not be on par with that of adults.

As was postulated for exertional and thermal perception, high-level training and competition can be expected to significantly augment experience, knowledge, and understanding of both the woes of athletic endeavour in a wide range of situations and the means available to counter or minimize them. Thus, while young elite athletes are likely still to be inferior to their adult counterparts in their relevant experience and decision-making capacity, they could nevertheless be expected to be closer, in this respect, to adult athletes than would be expected of their age.

Dehydration Effects on Cognition

Previous studies have found compromised cognitive functions at hypohydration of $\geq 2\%$ body mass, in adults [49–51]. However, among 10- to 13-year-old boys, who exercised in the heat at 40–45% $\dot{V}O_{2max}$, a 2% hypohydration could not be shown to affect cognitive and perceptual-motor functions [52]. This may suggest that children are more resistant to the deleterious effects of excessive dehydration on cognition or perceptual motor functions. However, the limited nature of the available data calls for caution in drawing this conclusion.

Children's Heat Tolerance

It is not clear whether or to what extent do the above-mentioned physiological and cognitive child-adult differences jeopardize elite young athletes more than their adult counterparts. Despite children's employment of a different thermoregulatory strategy and the notion that children's thermoregulation could be disadvantaged in some environments (e.g. extremely hot), we know of no epidemiological data, not even from extreme conditions such as heat waves, that can support the contention of children's greater susceptibility to heat exhaustion or illness. Brun and Mitchell

[53] recently reported that in Australia's tropical region, over a 10-year period, the prevalence of heat injury in children was not different than that in adults, and no heat-related incidents were reported in child athletes.

For ethical considerations, it is difficult to experimentally examine children's absolute tolerance to environmental extremes that may lead to heat injuries. Yet, numerous studies suggest reduced heat tolerance in children, especially in very hot conditions, i.e. when air is considerably hotter than skin [26, 54–56]. That is, children reach high core temperatures faster than adults [56–58] and appear to accumulate relatively more heat [26, 54]. This seemingly lower tolerance has been attributed to children's lower sweating rate [54, 56, 58, 59], which may result in insufficient evaporative cooling in very hot conditions. More recently, on the contrary, Inbar et al. [19] demonstrated that in extreme environmental heat (41°C), children thermoregulated their core temperature as efficiently or, arguably, even better than did adults. Similar findings were later reported by others as well [24, 25].

The apparent contradictory findings in the above studies are likely related to the different exercise modalities. Most studies determine and match work load intensities as given percentages of maximal or peak $\dot{V}O_2$, whilst those who have studied children and adults at similar treadmill velocities [54, 56] inadvertently compound the comparison with children's lower locomotive economy. As peak cycling $\dot{V}O_2$ is typically 10–15% lower than the peak or maximum attained in treadmill walking or running [60, 61], due to the smaller active muscle mass, blood flow to the working muscles would also be correspondingly lower in cycling tasks. This means that at any given percentage of peak cycling $\dot{V}O_2$, a greater proportion of the cardiac reserve is available for cutaneous blood flow compared with the same percentage of treadmill-determined peak $\dot{V}O_2$. This, in turn, differentially affects thermoregulatory capacity, putting children at a relative disadvantage in treadmill compared with cycling tasks. It appears that the typical 60–70% peak $\dot{V}O_2$ exercise intensity, employed in many heat tolerance studies, is the tipping point between cardiac sufficiency and insufficiency for children's thermoregulation in hot environments. Due to its dependence on body proportions, this relative disadvantage is not expected to be different in young athletes compared with untrained children. Better heat tolerance, expected of highly trained athletes, would be due to their superior heat acclimatisation and/or higher maximal cardiac outputs.

More fundamentally, in considering differential heat-dissipation strategies, it appears that reports of child-adult differences in heat gain/storage have thus far been misinterpreted as reflecting children's thermoregulatory deficiency or predisposing to it. Relying more heavily on dry heat dissipation, an earlier rise in core temperature may be advantageous to children because it raises cutaneous temperature and thus widens the skin-to-environment temperature gradient. The question of whether this predisposes children to earlier over-heating and reduced heat tolerance cannot be answered directly, at present. However, the extent of data suggesting that children thermoregulate on par with adults under most conditions, suggests that an early core temperature rise is inconsequential to subsequent heat tolerance unless the conditions are beyond the individual's thermoregulatory capacity to begin with, be it a child or an adult. Adults, relying more on sweating and its evaporation, do not gain from an earlier rise in core temperature, which would mainly serve to limit their heat storage capacity.

It should be noted, however, that such extreme ambient conditions, as examined in many of the studies cited above, are not typically encountered in sports events and competitions, in general, and those involving children, in particular. According to current guidelines and recommendations [62, 63], sports events are generally cancelled or postponed in such adverse conditions. In milder conditions, when air temperature is similar or lower than skin temperature, children's heat tolerance appears to be comparable to that of adults [9]. Indeed, under conditions of high relative humidity, children may actually have an advantage over adults. That is, the high humidity could nullify the effectiveness of the sweating mechanism, favouring those with a better 'dry' heat-dissipating mechanism, namely children. Thus, under humid conditions, where 'dry' heat dissipation is critical, children are possibly more efficient thermoregulators than adults.

It is unclear at present to what extent, if any, young athletes' performances are affected by the smaller proportion of cardiac output available to their working muscles. It should be emphasized, however, that if children's performance is indeed more adversely affected by high ambient temperatures, then this very fact would serve as a self-regulating safety mechanism. That is, while not eliminating their risk of heat injury, having a more limited muscular work capacity in extreme heat exposure also limits the amount of metabolic heat that children generate and must dissipate.

Intervention and Prevention Strategies

Heat stress is the only condition (other than trauma) that is potentially fatal in healthy individuals. Among North American high school athletes, it was estimated that the third leading cause of death was heat illness [64]. Yet, such deaths are preventable. Overall, strategies for the prevention of heat injuries in elite young athletes are very similar to those applicable for adult athletes. They involve an acclimation process and the attainment of reasonable fitness level before any high-intensity training or competition. Maintenance of proper hydration status before, during, and following exertion is a major means in preventing heat injuries. In fact, hypohydration can promptly nullify all the thermoregulatory benefits of acclimation and fitness.

Clothing should match environmental conditions. Light-coloured, sweat-wicking, and loose-fitting garments should normally be preferred in the heat. In the cold, layered, dark-coloured, light-weight, insulating, wind protective, and snug but unrestrictive clothing should be the norm [65].

Experimental active-cooling garments are presently available or being developed for military, fire-fighting, or other occupational uses (see reference [66] for details). They are absolutely impractical for athletic competition and would be sports-illegal if used. However, they could be considered, in special circumstances, as a means for pre-cooling, along with other less exotic means. The latter could include consumption of cold water or other beverages, cold showers or cool-water immersion, use of fans or air-conditioned quarters, etc. Lee et al. [67] showed, in adults, that drinking 900 ml of water at 4°C before exercise, lowered core temperature by 0.5°C. This, in turn, resulted in reduced cardiovascular and thermal strain during exercise in heat and increased exercise tolerance by >20%.

Other means of minimizing some of the ill-effects of pre-competition heat exposure could be the curtailment of unessential heat exposure and the minimization of warm-up exercise intensity and duration to reflect the faster heat gains under these conditions and the need to avoid excessive heat build up prior to the onset of competition.

Several reviews and position statements are currently available, regarding the prevention of heat injuries in young athletes [6, 9, 62, 68–71]. Table 2 provides recommendations for reducing or preventing thermal injuries among young athletes. The recommendations are directed toward athletes and coaches, as well as event organizers. This section will highlight only those aspects of heat injury prevention which are unique to young athletes. These aspects include hydration practices, acclimatization, training and competition scheduling (time of day, breaks), and general education of athletes, coaches, and parents.

Table 2. Conditions and situations of particular risk of thermal injury

Category	Condition/situation	Suggested strategy	Comments
Environmental	Extreme dry heat ($\geq$~35°C at <~30% RH)	– Consider forgoing the competition or training session – Have plenty of cool water or other beverages – Seek shade, shelter, air-conditioning, cold showers, etc., prior to and between actual competitive events – Be alert for signs or symptoms of heat disorders	Environmental heat stress that poses particular risk for children is likely too extreme for any sensible athletic competition
	Extreme heat-humidity combination (high WBGT index)	– As above for dry heat – The American Academy of Pediatrics WBGT guidelines (2000): >29°C – cancel all events; 26-29°C – exclude high-risk individuals (e.g. unacclimatised, over-weight), curtail long-duration activities (e.g. most ball games, distance running); 24--26°C – allow longer rest periods and hydration breaks every 15 min	– While children could be at risk, it is no higher in this type of heat stress than for adults – It is recommended that a child-specific WBGT index be developed to reflect children's different reliance on dry vs. evaporative heat dissipation routes – A more appropriate, proposed tentative index would be: $WBGT_{child} = 0.5T_{wet} + 0.3T_{globe} + 0.2T_{dry}$
	Extreme cold	– Consider forgoing the competition or training session – Consider extra protective clothing/gear – Seek wind shelter, heated indoor shelter, etc., prior to and between actual competitive events – Have hot beverages – Be alert for signs of hypothermia	– Take wind-chill factor into account – Lean athletes stand higher risk than overweight ones – Extreme cold, that poses particular risk for children wearing sport-appropriate protective gear, is likely too extreme for any sensible athletic competition
	Warm-water swimming/activity (from ~30°C up)	If possible, have frequent out-of-water breaks and implement cooling strategies	Risk may be higher than in hot air exposure because: – There is no evaporative heat dissipation – Skin-to-water temperature gradient is small

Category	Condition/situation	Suggested strategy	Comments
	Cold-water swimming/activity (at ~15–20°C and below)	– Use protective clothing (e.g. wet suit), if and when permitted – In cold weather, use water-protective clothing in above-water sports, such as rowing and kayaking, to avoid getting wet from splash and spray	– Higher risk compared with cold air exposure. The high specific-heat of water makes for greatly accelerated conductive and convective heat losses – Lean athletes stand higher risk than overweight ones – Risk threshold is difficult to determine due to the complex interactions between environmental conditions, metabolic intensity, and clothing
Nature of activity	Intensity-duration interaction	– High-intensity/short-duration events (e.g. sprint and field events) may be minimally affected by heat (sprint, power events often benefit from it), but could be negatively affected by cold; risk of heat injury is very small – Low-intensity events (e.g. archery, golf) may be little affected by heat but stand higher risk of thermal injury in the cold – Long-duration/medium-to-high intensity events (e.g. distance running, many ball games) will be greatly affected by heat and stand an elevated risk of heat injury; performance may benefit from moderate cold; risk of hypothermia is high for exhausted athletes who fail to maintain essential metabolic heat production	
Administrative, organizational	Repetitive exertions (tournaments, qualifying heats, multiple entries)	*In the heat* – Optimize time-of-day scheduling – Extend breaks between events – Consider timed finals rather than numerous qualifying heats – Make water and other beverages available and urge athletes to consume them – Provide shade, air-conditioned shelter, cold showers, etc. *In the cold* – Provide wind shelter, heated indoor shelter, etc. – Provide hot beverages and urge athletes to consume them	– In the cold, take wind-chill factor into account – Have appropriate medical support available – Consider cancelling/postponing the event in extreme conditions – See above WBGT recommendations of the American Academy of Pediatrics – Deliberate thermal risk should be permitted, if at all, only to informed consenting adults
	Endurance events (distance running, walking, cycling)	– Optimize time-of-day scheduling	

Category	Condition/situation	Suggested strategy	Comments
		In the heat – Make cool water/other beverages available at start/finish areas and along the course and urge athletes to consume them *In the cold* – Have hot beverages available – Have officials scattered along the course or patrol it to detect early signs of heat injury (or hypothermia, in the cold)	

Hydration

Exercise in the heat can result in significant fluid losses, mainly via sweating, and the resultant dehydration and hypohydration. Sweating rate, and hence sweat loss, is generally lower in children compared with adults, suggesting that hypohydration might not be as great a concern in young athletes as it is in adults. However, as mentioned earlier [22], sweating rates of acclimatized highly trained boys, while still lower than those of adults, have been shown to greatly exceed previously measured rates in untrained, non-acclimatized boys. Wilk et al. [72] demonstrated that during a triathlon competition in hot conditions (Costa Rica), nearly 50% of the young athletes reached a hypohydration level of 2–3%, while 7% of participants exceeded 3%. Thus, coaches and event organizers should keep in mind that, in spite of the typically lower sweating rates, elite young athletes can extensively dehydrate during exercise in the heat.

The most prominent result of dehydration is a decrease in plasma volume [73]. Therefore, dehydration can potentially lead to cardiovascular insufficiency (decreased cardiac output and blood pressure), an increase in body temperature [74, 75], and a remarkable increase in the risk of heat injury [76, 77]. Naturally, it can also lead to a reduction in athletic performance. This decline in performance has been demonstrated consistently in adults, especially in endurance performance [74, 78], and to a limited extent also in short-duration, high-intensity intermittent exercise [79, 80]. While there are limited comparable data on the effect of dehydration on endurance performance in children [26, 52], Dougherty et al. [76] recently demonstrated a reduction in basketball-related skills among 12- to 15-year-old boys, following dehydration induced by exercise in the heat. The maintenance of hydration status can prevent the decrements in cardiovascular function, as copiously demonstrated in adults [81–85], and recently in boys [7]. In adults, maintenance of euhydration has also been shown to prevent the decline in performance [81, 86], while in children this is also presumed to be the case [69].

Non-athletes, both children and adults, have been shown to consume insufficient amounts of liquids during exercise in the heat [86, 87]. This phenomenon has been labelled 'involuntary dehydration' [88]. This has also been shown to occur among junior athletes [89]. When drinking water ad libitum during exercise in the heat, Bar-

Or et al. [87] demonstrated that children involuntarily dehydrate to a similar extent as adults. While the extent of dehydration may be similar in children and adults, its effect on body temperature is apparently greater in children. Children's core temperature rise for a given percentage of body-weight loss is roughly twice that of adults [87]. As proposed earlier, this is likely due to children's greater reliance on dry heat dissipation, mediated by enhanced peripheral blood flow. Fluid loss can directly diminish cardiac output and cutaneous blood flow, thus precipitating an accelerated rise in core temperature. Therefore, while children are the better body-water conservers via lower sweating, their higher core-temperature sensitivity to dehydration calls for extra caution.

Many young athletes may begin their training session or competitive event in a hypo-hydrated state. For example, during a summer training camp, over 50% of 10- to 14-year-old soccer players and 14- to 16-year old football players were hypo-hydrated at the beginning of each day's training session [90, 91]. In some sports, where competitive division is determined by weight categories (e.g. wrestling, martial arts), athletes often intentionally dehydrate pre-competition in order to 'make weight'. While such practices are officially discouraged [92], many athletes continue to engage in dangerous weight management practices [93]. For example, a 5-year-old wrestler was reportedly pressured to compete at a weight category requiring him to lose 10% of his body weight pre-competition [94]. Beginning exercise in a hypo-hydrated state can independently affect exercise performance, whether full rehydration during exercise is attained or not [78].

Flavouring of water, with or without the addition of electrolytes or carbohydrates, can increase fluid intake and even completely prevent the involuntary dehydration associated with exercise in the heat [22, 95, 96]. That is, the palatability of the available beverage can make a significant impact on the magnitude of voluntary rehydration during exercise. Taste preferences can vary between individuals and in different environmental conditions. For example, while exercising in the heat many individuals prefer beverages that are less heavily sweetened [97]. Also, taste preferences may vary between children and adults. For example, while exercising in the heat children were shown to prefer grape-flavoured beverages over orange or apple flavour [98]. There are no data to suggest universal flavour preferences and these should be verified for each athlete.

Beverage temperature may also impact the amount of fluid consumed during exercise. Boulze et al. [99] demonstrated that, after dehydrating to variable degrees, adult men consumed water at 15°C to a greater extent than at higher or lower temperatures. While similar data are not available for children or adolescents, the preference of water at 15°C suggests that event organizers need not provide iced water.

It is unclear what 'adequate' hydration entails. Intuitively, ideal re-hydration would appear to aim to encourage athletes to drink as much as tolerable and to replace all fluid losses through sweat. For adults, this was indeed the American College of Sports Medicine (ACSM) recommendation in 1996 [100]. However, during moderate exertion of long duration (>4 h), this approach can lead to 'water intoxication' or hyponatremia [101]. That is, in events such as a marathon, slow runners, who are probably working at a lower intensity and producing lower sweating rates, spend more time on the course and can therefore consume more fluids. This is also true for young athletes who may participate in long endurance events. Thus, the current consensus for adults is that fluid replacement during exercise should aim to limit dehydration to <2% of body weight [102].

The optimal hydration strategy for young athletes depends on many factors. These include, age and body size, fitness level, typical sweat and urine losses, and the degree of acclimatization and beverage palatability. The recent ACSM position statement on exercise and fluid replacement suggests a range of 0.4–0.8 litres $\cdot$ h^{-1} of fluid ingestion for adult athletes depending on individual variability and exercise intensity [102]. Expressed relative to body mass, this recommendation can be translated to approximately 5–11 ml $\cdot$ kg^{-1} $\cdot$ h^{-1}. Higher hydration rates may be needed, although practically unattainable in severe situations such as marathon running in the heat. Holding this kind of event under such conditions should be avoided, in general, and particularly when children are involved. Although children sweat less than adults, they may be more prone to dehydration's ill-effects [87]. Thus, the adoption of the size-modified adult guidelines seems reasonable for young athletes. However, in view of the large individual variability in fluid preferences, both adult and child athletes should experiment with different beverages and hydration strategies to develop a plan which best suits their needs and preferences [103].

Hydration in the cold deserves a special note. As mentioned earlier, dehydration can occur in the cold due to ventilatory water loss and the general desensitization of thirst perception under stressful conditions. In sub-freezing conditions there is the risk of water/beverage freezing and unless measures are taken to avoid that, it might become difficult or impossible to fend off dehydration.

Acclimatisation

The physiological adaptations to heat acclimatization, via repeated exposures to heat, include lower heart rate, lower body temperature and higher sweating rate, along with lower sweat electrolyte levels during exercise in the heat [104]. These adaptations are similar in children and adults [105]. Acclimatization improves not only thermoregulation, but also exercise capacity and thermal comfort [104]. The main child-adult difference is in the rate, rather than the overall extent of acclimatization. In a 2 week, seven exposure acclimatization study, men attained most of their thermoregulatory adaptations in the first week, while boys attained them mostly in the second week [106].

It has been suggested that in adults, reasonable acclimatization may be attained by 4–7 exposures to exercise in the heat, while 8–14 exposures may be needed for maximal acclimatization [104]. There are no comparable data in children, but in view of their apparent slower response it is recommended that at least six acclimatization sessions be administered for incomplete but reasonable acclimatization. Indeed, specific acclimatization recommendations have been delineated for youths participating in some sports (e.g. American football), progressively increasing the number and duration of training sessions per day, as well as the amount and type of clothing and equipment [71].

The optimal nature of the acclimatization regimen appears to differ between children and adults. Physical conditioning alone (in a thermo-neutral environment) can induce many of the adaptations associated with heat acclimatization. While in adults this has been found insufficient for full acclimatization, children have been shown to attain similar acclimatization by simple conditioning as through exercise in the heat [105]. This difference may stem from children's greater dependence on peripheral circulation and elevated cardiac output, which can be attained by cardiovascular conditioning. Improved sweating response, upon which adult acclimatization more heavily depends, apparently needs heat stress greater than what can be achieved by cardiovascular exertion alone. The child-adult difference in the rate of acclimatization may therefore be ascribed to different adaptation kinetics of the cardiovascular system vs. the sweating response. It is possible that cardiovascular changes take longer than sweating changes and since children rely more heavily on the former they are slower in making comparable adaptations to those of adults.

The perceived stress of a given exercise-in-the-heat was shown to decrease faster during acclimatization in boys compared with men [107]. Although intuitively, this appears to be advantageous, it is not known whether children's reduction in perceived stress ends in appropriate or rather under-estimation of stress. The latter, of course, could be potentially dangerous.

Training and Competition Scheduling

Time of Day
To minimize thermal stress in hot weather, competition or intense training should be scheduled for the early or late parts of the day, while in exceptionally cold weather, mid-day should be preferred [100, 108]. These recommendations are similarly appropriate for both young and mature athletes.

Breaks and Recovery Periods
Exertion can have a residual effect on a subsequent, same-day exercise session, even in a thermo-neutral environment. This residual effect has been demonstrated consistently in adults, in which an initial exercise bout of 30–80 min resulted in higher heart rate, core temperature and RPE in a subsequent bout [109–111], even when the recovery period between bouts was as long as 6 h [112]. The residual effect seen in these studies was due to incomplete recovery of core temperature, heart rate, and hydration status.

Comparable data in children are scarce. Repeated exercise bouts in the heat (up to 30 min) have been shown to result in progressively higher heart rate and core temperature in subsequent bouts [19, 41, 113]. However, rest periods were typically short (10–25 min) and did not result in full recovery. In a recent study, Bergeron et al. [114] demonstrated in 12- to 13-year-old children and 16- to 17-year-old adolescents that when core temperature and hydration status were allowed to return to baseline levels (following a 60-min period of thermo-neutral recovery), a repeated 80-min session of intermittent cycling and running in the heat elicited a similar response of core temperature, heart rate, and thermal perception. The authors concluded that 60 min of 'optimal' recovery was sufficient for most young athletes, although it should be noted that 4 subjects still demonstrated elevated cardiovascular and thermal strain [114].

Typically, optimal recovery is not achievable in competitive situations. Bergeron et al. [115] observed that although given the opportunity, junior tennis players tended to only partially rehydrate from an earlier, same-day match, by the time they started their second match. To that effect, Coyle [116] examined a 7-year period of junior (14-year-old) US tennis national championships and showed that cumulative heat stress can affect the outcome of the second match of the day. After removing the effect of seeding, the winner of an afternoon singles match could be predicted based on the accumulated stress (product of WBGT index and duration) from morning matches, although players were all heat acclimatised. Thus, insufficient recovery, especially in hostile environments, can affect performance and increase the risk of heat injury, especially in highly motivated young athletes. While this has been consistently demonstrated in adults, the data are scarce and less consistent in youth. However, although children typically recover faster than adults [117], it is notable that even when their recovery appears to be complete, some young athletes still demonstrate increased cardiovascular and thermal responses in repeated performances [114].

Formal breaks are common in organized sports (e.g. soccer, baseball, tennis, track and field). Rules of some organised sports stipulate special limitations for young athletes (e.g. pitching limitations in baseball, number of games per day or per tournament), but, typically, minimum time between same-day contests is not defined. In North America, public school systems and sports associations governing bodies, typically have specific, although not uniform, guidelines for scheduling sports events. However, the sports associations guidelines are applicable only to the higher calibre competitions (e.g. regional, national competitions), not to local events. Most organized youth sports leagues do not have specific restrictions or guidelines [68].

Children recover from intense exercise faster than adults in terms of cardiovascular function, metabolic processes and performance capacity [117], suggesting that the necessary rest periods in competitions could be shorter for youth than for adults. However, the recovery from thermal stress and hypo-hydration has not been shown to differ between children and adults. Thus, the prudent approach should allow for at least 60 min of recovery in thermo-neutral conditions, allowing for fluid and nutrient replenishment and the return of cardiovascular responses and body temperature to resting values.

Drug Use

Although not common in children, drug use is becoming troublesome in adolescents [118]. Aside from being, for the most part, ethically objectionable and sports-illegal, many drugs could be physiologically or behaviourally detrimental to the athlete's thermoregulatory capacity. Amphetamines, ephedrine, alkaloids, and other stimulants increase exertional drive and consequently heat production and core temperature, while lowering pain sensation and perceived stress [119]. Pharmaceutical diuretics, but also sports-legal caffeine and alcohol, can predispose to hypohydration and electrolyte imbalance. Atropine and β-blockers can adversely affect cardiovascular capacity and the sweating response [120, 121]. It is unknown how anabolic steroids may affect the thermoregulatory response to exercise in the heat.

Creatine is considered a legal supplement in sports and many young athletes use it [122], often unaware of the amount they consume [123].

A recent meta-analysis found that among adults, there is no evidence that creatine hampers the body's thermoregulatory response or hydration status [124]. However, in view of the scant available knowledge about its potentially deleterious effects in the paediatric population, its use by young athletes is not recommended.

Finally, there is heightened awareness of attention deficit/hyperactivity disorder (ADHD) in children [125] and increased use of medications, mainly stimulants (e.g. Ritalin and Adderall), to manage the condition. While these stimulants are not permitted for use during competition by the International Olympic Committee, young athletes with ADHD competing in regional level competition may still be on these medications. ADHD medications have been shown to increase heart rate and blood pressure in children during exercise, while not affecting RPE [126, 127]. These effects, with presumably higher peripheral resistance, could result in elevated myocardial oxygen demand. Additionally, while stimulants often increase metabolic rate and heat production, it has recently been demonstrated that ADHD medication does not increase children's whole body oxygen uptake during exercise [126]. Thus, the thermoregulatory-related consequences of ADHD medication use are yet unclear.

Education

The fact that it is now commonplace for both athletes and non-athletes to go about with water or beverage bottle in hand attests to the effectiveness of educational/marketing campaigns, emphasizing the importance of hydration.

Recent hydration studies in children show little or no dehydration during exercise in the heat, even when only water is available. Heat-acclimatized girl athletes, exercising intermittently in hot, humid conditions (3 × 20 min cycling at 60% $\dot{V}O_{2max}$ with 25-min rest intervals, for a total exposure of >3 h) and drinking ad libitum, developed no dehydration [113]. Also, elite boy athletes, who exercised in similar, hot and humid conditions, but had considerably less time for drinking (5×15 min exercise at 65% $\dot{V}O_{2max}$ with 5 min rest intervals, 110 min exposure) did not develop any hypohydration (Wilk et al. personal communications). These findings contrast with the early findings of Bar-Or et al. [87], who found that 10- to 12-year-old non-athletes lost 1.2% of body weight during ~3.5 h exposure to heat, in which they had five 20-min cycling sessions at 40–45% peak $\dot{V}O_2$. These seemingly contradictory findings, may be suggesting that growing public and coach awareness, via directed education and advertising in the elapsed 30-year period, has affected children's hydration behaviour.

Special Safety Recommendation

In general, most adult oriented safety recommendations [63] for training and competition in adverse thermal conditions should be adhered to by young athletes, as well. It is proposed, however, that the Wet Bulb Globe Temperature (WBGT) index be modified for children.

The WBGT is considered a 'gold standard' index, universally used to assess environmental heat stress. It is a weighted composite of the humidity (wet bulb), absolute ambient temperature (dry bulb), and the incident radiation (black globe) contributions to the overall thermal stress (WBGT = 0.7 T_{wet} + 0.2 T_{globe} + 0.1 T_{dry}). This weighted scheme is based on adult data and thus reflects the typical relative effect of its three components on adults. Since, compared with adults, children have larger relative skin surface area and rely more on dry heat dissipation, a child-appropriate WBGT index should be more heavily weighted in the globe and dry temperature and less in the wet one. As a child-appropriate weighting scale has not yet been worked out (and is also expected to change with growth), it is suggested that critical scrutiny of meteorological data be used to re-assess heat-stress, at least in the more extreme conditions. Tentatively, a more appropriate index for pre- and early-pubertal children is proposed as:

$$\text{WBGT}_{child} = 0.5\, T_{wet} + 0.3\, T_{globe} + 0.2\, T_{dry}.$$

Conclusions

Revisiting existing data and re-evaluating long-held concepts has shed new light on the understanding of the young athlete's thermoregulatory capacity. Primarily due to their larger surface-area-to-mass ratio, children and young athletes must employ differing thermoregulatory strategies compared with adults. The different strategies, however, do not constitute an inferior thermoregulatory response. Children may be at a thermoregulatory disadvantage only in the most extreme conditions, in which training and competition are typically not held. Under some conditions (e.g. high humidity) children may even have an advantage over adults. Nevertheless, compared with adults, children and young athletes cannot be expected to benefit from the same level of experience and maturity of judgement regarding their athletic conduct and environmental-stress management. Thus, while any athlete should preferably be properly acclimatized and well-trained, the main emphasis when preventing heat illness in young athletes should be behavioural. Therefore, proper guidance and instruction (e.g. concerning proper pacing and hydration practices) is where the young athlete needs the most attention.

References

1 Zahner L, Muehlbauer T, Schmid M, Meyer U, Puder JJ, Kriemler S: Association of sports club participation with fitness and fatness in children. Med Sci Sports Exerc 2009;41:344–350.

2 Rowland TW, Boyajian A: Aerobic response to endurance exercise training in children. Pediatrics 1995;96:654–658.

3 Hind K, Burrows M: Weight-bearing exercise and bone mineral accrual in children and adolescents: a review of controlled trials. Bone 2007;40:14–27.

4 Hillman CH, Pontifex MB, Raine LB, Castelli DM, Hall EE, Kramer AF: The effect of acute treadmill walking on cognitive control and academic achievement in preadolescent children. Neuroscience 2009;159:1044–1054.

5 Melnyk BM, Jacobson D, Kelly S, O'Haver J, Small L, Mays MZ: Improving the mental health, healthy lifestyle choices, and physical health of Hispanic adolescents: a randomized controlled pilot study. J Sch Health 2009;79:575–584.

6 Falk B, Dotan R: Temperature regulation in children; in Armstrong N, Van Mechelen W (eds): Paediatric Exercise Science and Medicine. New York, Oxford University Press, 2008, pp 309–324.

7 Rowland T, Pober D, Garrison A: Cardiovascular drift in euhydrated prepubertal boys. Appl Physiol Nutr Metab 2008;33:690–695.

8 Davies CT: Thermal responses to exercise in children. Ergonomics 1981;24:55–61.

9 Falk B, Dotan R: Children's thermoregulation during exercise in the heat: a revisit. Appl Physiol Nutr Metab 2008;33:420–427.

10 Cain JB, Livingstone SD, Nolan RW, Keefe AA: Respiratory heat loss during work at various ambient temperatures. Respir Physiol 1990;79:145–150.

11 Astrand PO: Experimental Studies of Physical Work Capacity in Relation to Sex and Age. Copenhagen, Mundsgaard, 1952.

12 Kenefick RW, Hazzard MP, Mahood NV, Castellani JW: Thirst sensations and AVP responses at rest and during exercise-cold exposure. Med Sci Sports Exerc 2004;36:1528–1534.

13 Dennis SC, Noakes TD: Advantages of a smaller bodymass in humans when distance-running in warm, humid conditions. Eur J Appl Physiol Occup Physiol 1999;79:280–284.

14 Bar-Or O: Thermoregulation in females from a life span perspective; in Bar-Or O, Lamb DR, Clarkson PM (eds): Exercise and the Female – A Life Span Approach. Traverse City, Cooper Publishing Group, 1996, pp 250–283.

15 Bar-Or O: Climate and the exercising child – a review. Int J Sports Med 1980;1:53–65.

16 Bar-Or O: Temperature regulation during exercise in children and adolescents; in Gisolfi CV, Lamb DR (eds): Youth, Exercise and Sports. Indianapolis, Benchmark Press, 1989, pp 335–362.

17 Falk B: Effects of thermal stress during rest and exercise in the paediatric population. Sports Med 1998;25:221–240.

18 Inoue Y, Kuwahara T, Araki T: Maturation- and aging-related changes in heat loss effector function. J Physiol Anthropol Appl Human Sci 2004;23:289–294.

19 Inbar O, Morris N, Epstein Y, Gass G: Comparison of thermoregulatory responses to exercise in dry heat among prepubertal boys, young adults and older males. Exp Physiol 2004;89:691–700.

20 Kleiber M: Body size and metabolic rate. Physiol Rev 1947;27:511–541.

21 Meyer F, Bar-Or O: Fluid and electrolyte loss during exercise: the paediatric angle. Sports Med 1994;18:4–9.

22 Rivera-Brown AM, Gutierrez R, Gutierrez JC, Frontera WR, Bar-Or O: Drink composition, voluntary drinking, and fluid balance in exercising, trained, heat-acclimatized boys. J Appl Physiol 1999;86:78–84.

23 Turley KR, Wilmore JH: Cardiovascular responses to treadmill and cycle ergometer exercise in children and adults. J Appl Physiol 1997;83:948–957.

24 Rowland T, Hagenbuch S, Pober D, Garrison A: Exercise tolerance and thermoregulatory responses during cycling in boys and men. Med Sci Sports Exerc 2008;40:282–287.

25 Rivera-Brown AM, Rowland TW, Ramirez-Marrero FA, Santacana G, Vann A: Exercise tolerance in a hot and humid climate in heat-acclimatized girls and women. Int J Sports Med 2006;27:943–950.

26 Drinkwater BL, Kupprat IC, Denton JE, Crist JL, Horvath SM: Response of prepubertal girls and college women to work in the heat. J Appl Physiol 1977;43:1046–1053.

27 Rowland T, Popowski B, Ferrone L: Cardiac responses to maximal upright cycle exercise in healthy boys and men. Med Sci Sports Exerc 1997;29:1146–1151.

28 Shibasaki M, Inoue Y, Kondo N, Iwata A: Thermoregulatory responses of prepubertal boys and young men during moderate exercise. Eur J Appl Physiol Occup Physiol 1997;75:212–218.

29 Falk B, Bar-Or O, MacDougall JD: Thermoregulatory responses of pre-, mid-, and late-pubertal boys to exercise in dry heat. Med Sci Sports Exerc 1992;24:688–694.

30 Martin HL, Loomis JL, Kenney WL: Maximal skin vascular conductance in subjects aged 5–85 yr. J Appl Physiol 1995;79:297–301.

31 Araki T, Tsujita J, Matsushita K, Hori S: Thermoregulatroy responses of prepubertal boys to heat and cold in relation to physical training. Human Ergonomics 1980;9:69–80.

32 Wagner JA, Robinson S, Marino RP: Age and temperature regulation of humans in neutral and cold environments. J Appl Physiol 1974;37:562–565.

33 Smolander J, Bar-Or O, Korhonen O, Ilmarinen J: Thermoregulation during rest and exercise in the cold in pre- and early pubescent boys and in young men. J Appl Physiol 1992;72:1589–1594.

34 Inoue Y, Nakamura S, Yonehiro K, Kuwahara T, Ueda H, Araki T: Regional differences in peripheral vasoconstriction of prepubertal boys. Eur J Appl Physiol 2006;96:397–403.

35 Allor KM, Pivarnik JM, Sam LJ, Perkins CD: Treadmill economy in girls and women matched for height and weight. J Appl Physiol 2000;89:512–516.

36 Robinson S: Experimental studies of physical fitness in relation to age. Int Z Angetv Physiol Einschl Arbeitsphysiol 1938;10:251–323.

37 Unnithan VB, Eston RG: Stride frequency and submaximal treadmill running economy in adults and children. Pediatr Exerc Sci 1990;2:149–155.

38 Daniels J, Oldridge N, Nagle F, White B: Differences and changes in VO$_2$ among young runners 10 to 18 years of age. Med Sci Sports 1978;10:200–203.

39 Daniels J, Oldridge N: Changes in oxygen consumption of young boys during growth and running training. Med Sci Sports 1971;3:161–165.

40 Noble BJ, Robertson JR: Perceived Exertion. Champaign, Human Kinetics, 1996.

41 Falk B: The Thermoregulatory Response of Pre-, Mid- and Late-pubertal Boys Exercising in the Heat. Hamilton, McMaster University, 1991.

42 Bar-Or O: Age-related changes in exercise perception; in Borg GI (ed): Physical Work and Effort. Oxford, Pegamon Press, 1977, pp 255–266.

43 Timmons BW, Bar-Or O: RPE during prolonged cycling with and without carbohydrate ingestion in boys and men. Med Sci Sports Exerc 2003;35:1901–1907.

44 Elliott R: Simple reaction time in children: effects of incentive, incentive shift, and other training variables. J Exp Child Psychol 1972;13:540–557.

45 Groslambert A, Mahon AD: Perceived exertion: influence of age and cognitive development. Sports Med 2006;36:911–928.

46 Eston RG, Lamb KL, Bain A, Williams AM, Williams JG: Validity of a perceived exertion scale for children: a pilot study. Percept Mot Skills 1994;78:691–697.

47 Tenenbaum G, Falk B, Bar-Or O: The measurement and the accumulation of perceived exertion in a progressive cycling maximal power test in children and adolescents. Int J Sport Psych 2002;33:337–348.

48 Jacobs JE, Klaczynski PA: The development of judgement and decision making during childhood and adolescence. Curr Dir Psychol Sci 2002;11:145–149.

49 Cian C, Koulmann N, Barraud PA, Raphel C, Melin B: Influence of variation in body hydration on cognitive function: effect of hyperhydration, heat stress, and exercise-induced dehydration. J Psychophysiol 2000;14:29–36.

50 Epstein Y, Keren G, Moisseiev J, Gasko O, Yachin S: Psychomotor deterioration during exposure to heat. Aviat Space Environ Med 1980;51:607–610.

51 Gopinathan PM, Pichan G, Sharma VM: Role of dehydration in heat stress-induced variations in mental performance. Arch Environ Health 1988;43:15–17.

52 Wilk B, Yuxiu H, Bar-Or O: Effect of body hypohydration on aerobic performance of boys who exercise in the heat. Med Sci Sports Exerc 2002;34:S48.

53 Brun S, Mitchell G: The incidence of heat related illness in the child athlete in Cairns Far North Queensland Australia and the associated environmental variables. Med Sci Sports Exerc 2006;38:S111.

54 Haymes EM, Buskirk ER, Hodgson JL, Lundegren HM, Nicholas WC: Heat tolerance of exercising lean and heavy prepubertal girls. J Appl Physiol 1974;36:566–571.

55 Bar-Or O, Magnusson LI, Buskirk ER: Distribution of heat-activated sweat glands in obese and lean men and women. Hum Biol 1968;40:235–248.

56 Wagner JA, Robinson S, Tzankoff SP, Marino RP: Heat tolerance and acclimatization to work in the heat in relation to age. J Appl Physiol 1972;33:616–622.

57 Leppaluoto J: Human thermoregulation in sauna. Ann Clin Res 1988;20:240–243.

58 Sohar E, Shapiro Y: The physiological reactions of women and children marching during heat, in Israel Physiology and Pharmacology Society, Israel 1965, p 50.

59 Meyer F, Bar-Or O, MacDougall D, Heigenhauser GJ: Sweat electrolyte loss during exercise in the heat: effects of gender and maturation. Med Sci Sports Exerc 1992;24:776–781.

60 Hill DW, Davey KM, Stevens EC: Maximal accumulated O$_2$ deficit in running and cycling. Can J Appl Physiol 2002;27:463–478.

61 Basset FA, Boulay MR: Specificity of treadmill and cycle ergometer tests in triathletes, runners and cyclists. Eur J Appl Physiol 2000;81:214–221.

62 American Academy of Pediatrics Committee on Sports Medicine and Fitness: Climatic heat stress and the exercising child and adolescent. Pediatrics 2000;106:158–159.

63 Armstrong LE, Casa DJ, Millard-Stafford M, Moran DS, Pyne SW, Roberts WO: American College of Sports Medicine position stand: exertional heat illness during training and competition. Med Sci Sports Exerc 2007;39:556–572.

64 Lee-Chiong TL Jr, Stitt JT: Heatstroke and other heat-related illnesses: the maladies of summer. Postgrad Med 1995;98:26–36.

65 Pascoe DD, Bellingar TA, McCluskey BS: Clothing and exercise. II. Influence of clothing during exercise/work in environmental extremes. Sports Med 1994;18:94–108.

66 Cheung SS: Advanced Environmental Exercise Physiology. Campaign, Human Kinetics, 2010.

67 Lee JK, Shirreffs SM, Maughan RJ: Cold drink ingestion improves exercise endurance capacity in the heat. Med Sci Sports Exerc 2008;40:1637–1644.

68 Bergeron MF: Youth sports in the heat: recovery and scheduling considerations for tournament play. Sports Med 2009;39:513–522.

69 Rowland T: Thermoregulation during exercise in the heat in children: old concepts revisited. J Appl Physiol 2008;105:718–724.

70 Naughton GA, Carlson JS: Reducing the risk of heat-related decrements to physical activity in young people. J Sci Med Sport 2008;11:58–65.

71 Bergeron MF, McKeag DB, Casa DJ, Clarkson PM, Dick RW, Eichner ER, Horswill CA, Luke AC, Mueller F, Munce TA, Roberts WO, Rowland TW: Youth football: heat stress and injury risk. Med Sci Sports Exerc 2005;37:1421–1430.

72 Wilk B, Aragon-Vargas L, Bar-Or O: Involuntary dehydration in children and adolescents following a triathlon race in a hot climate. Med Sci Sports Exerc 2001;33:S137.

73 Costill DL, Cote R, Fink W: Muscle water and electrolytes following varied levels of dehydration in man. J Appl Physiol 1976;40:6–11.

74 Gonzalez-Alonso J, Mora-Rodriguez R, Below PR, Coyle EF: Dehydration reduces cardiac output and increases systemic and cutaneous vascular resistance during exercise. J Appl Physiol 1995;79:1487–1496.

75 Montain SJ, Coyle EF: Influence of graded dehydration on hyperthermia and cardiovascular drift during exercise. J Appl Physiol 1992;73:1340–1350.

76 Dougherty KA, Baker LB, Chow M, Kenney WL: Two percent dehydration impairs and six percent carbohydrate drink improves boys basketball skills. Med Sci Sports Exerc 2006;38:1650–1658.

77 Coris EE, Ramirez AM, Van Durme DJ: Heat illness in athletes: the dangerous combination of heat, humidity and exercise. Sports Med 2004;34:9–16.

78 Cheung SS, McLellan TM: Influence of hydration status and fluid replacement on heat tolerance while wearing NBC protective clothing. Eur J Appl Physiol Occup Physiol 1998;77:139–148.

79 Burge CM, Carey MF, Payne WR: Rowing performance, fluid balance, and metabolic function following dehydration and rehydration. Med Sci Sports Exerc 1993;25:1358–1364.

80 McGregor SJ, Nicholas CW, Lakomy HK, Williams C: The influence of intermittent high-intensity shuttle running and fluid ingestion on the performance of a soccer skill. J Sports Sci 1999;17:895–903.

81 Sawka MN, Montain SJ, Latzka WA: Hydration effects on thermoregulation and performance in the heat. Comp Biochem Physiol A Mol Integr Physiol 2001;128:679–690.

82 Murray R: Rehydration strategies – balancing substrate, fluid, and electrolyte provision. Int J Sports Med 1998;19(suppl 2):S133–S135.

83 Noakes TD: Fluid replacement during exercise. Exerc Sport Sci Rev 1993;21:297–330.

84 Maughan RJ, Noakes TD: Fluid replacement and exercise stress: a brief review of studies on fluid replacement and some guidelines for the athlete. Sports Med 1991;12:16–31.

85 Maughan RJ, Leiper JB, Shirreffs SM: Factors influencing the restoration of fluid and electrolyte balance after exercise in the heat. Br J Sports Med 1997;31:175–182.

86 Bar-Or O, Harris D, Bergstein V, Buskirk ER: Progressive hypohydration in subjects who vary in adiposity. Isr J Med Sci 1976;12:800–803.

87 Bar-Or O, Dotan R, Inbar O, Rotshtein A, Zonder H: Voluntary hypohydration in 10- to 12-year-old boys. J Appl Physiol 1980;48:104–108.

88 Bar-Or O, Rowland TW: Pediatric Exercise Medicine. Champaign, Human Kinetics, 2004.

89 Iuliano S, Naughton G, Collier G, Carlson J: Examination of the self-selected fluid intake practices by junior athletes during a simulated duathlon event. Int J Sport Nutr 1998;8:10–23.

90 Casa DJ, Yeargin SW, Decher NR, McCaffrey M, James CT: Incidence and degree of dehydration and attitudes regarding hydration in adolescents at summer football camp. Med Sci Sports Exerc 2005;37:S463.

91 Decher NR, Casa DJ, Yeargin SW, Levrealt ML, Cross CL, McCaffrey M, Psathas E: Attitudes towards hydration and incidence of dehydration in youths at summer soccer camp. Med Sci Sports Exerc 2005;37:S463.

92 National Federation of State High School Associations: Wrestling 2002–2003 Rules Book. Indianapolis, National Federation of State High School Associations, 2002.

93 Oppliger RA, Steen SA, Scott JR: Weight loss practices of college wrestlers. Int J Sport Nutr Exerc Metab 2003;13:29–46.

94 Sansone RA, Sawyer R: Weight loss pressure on a 5 year old wrestler. Br J Sports Med 2005;39:e2.

95 Meyer F, Bar-Or O, Salsberg A, Passe D: Hypohydration during exercise in children: effect on thirst, drink preferences, and rehydration. Int J Sport Nutr 1994;4:22–35.

96 Wilk B, Kriemler S, Keller H, Bar-Or O: Consistency in preventing voluntary dehydration in boys who drink a flavored carbohydrate-NaCl beverage during exercise in the heat. Int J Sport Nutr 1998;8:1–9.

97 Talavera K, Yasumatsu K, Voets T, Droogmans G, Shigemura N, Ninomiya Y, Margolskee RF, Nilius B: Heat activation of TRPM5 underlies thermal sensitivity of sweet taste. Nature 2005;438:1022–1025.

98 Wilk B, Bar-Or O: Effect of drink flavor and NaCl on voluntary drinking and hydration in boys exercising in the heat. J Appl Physiol 1996;80:1112–1117.

99 Boulze D, Montastruc P, Cabanac M: Water intake, pleasure and water temperature in humans. Physiol Behav 1983;30:97–102.

100 Convertino VA, Armstrong LE, Coyle EF, Mack GW, Sawka MN, Senay LC Jr, Sherman WM: American College of Sports Medicine position stand: exercise and fluid replacement. Med Sci Sports Exerc 1996;28:i–vii.

101 Noakes T: Fluid replacement during marathon running. Clin J Sport Med 2003;13:309–318.

102 Sawka MN, Burke LM, Eichner ER, Maughan RJ, Montain SJ, Stachenfeld NS: American College of Sports Medicine position stand: exercise and fluid replacement. Med Sci Sports Exerc 2007;39:377–390.

103 Maughan RJ, Shirreffs SM: Development of individual hydration strategies for athletes. Int J Sport Nutr Exerc Metab 2008;18:457–472.

104 Armstrong LE, Maresh CM: The induction and decay of heat acclimatisation in trained athletes. Sports Med 1991;12:302–312.

105 Inbar O, Bar-Or O, Dotan R, Gutin B: Conditioning versus exercise in heat as methods for acclimatizing 8- to 10-yr-old boys to dry heat. J Appl Physiol 1981;50:406–411.

106 Inbar O: Acclimatization to dry and hot environments in young adults and children 8–10 years old; Doctor of Education thesis, Columbia University, New York, 1978.

107 Bar-Or O, Inbar O: Relationship between perceptual and physiological changes during heat acclimatization in 8–10 year-old boys; in Lavalee H, Shephard RJ (eds): Frontiers of Activity and Child Health. Quebec, Pelican Press, 1977, pp 205–214.

108 Armstrong LE, Epstein Y, Greenleaf JE, Haymes EM, Hubbard RW, Roberts WO, Thompson PD: American College of Sports Medicine position stand: heat and cold illnesses during distance running. Med Sci Sports Exerc 1996;28:i-x.

109 Sawka MN, Knowlton RG, Critz JB: Thermal and circulatory responses to repeated bouts of prolonged running. Med Sci Sports 1979;11:177–180.

110 Kruk B, Szczypaczewska M, Opaszowski B, Kaciuba-Uscilko H, Nazar K: Thermoregulatory and metabolic responses to repeated bouts of prolonged cycle-ergometer exercise in man. Acta Physiol Pol 1990;41:22–31.

111 Brenner IK, Zamecnik J, Shek PN, Shephard RJ: The impact of heat exposure and repeated exercise on circulating stress hormones. Eur J Appl Physiol Occup Physiol 1997;76:445–454.

112 Ronsen O, Haugen O, Hallen J, Bahr R: Residual effects of prior exercise and recovery on subsequent exercise-induced metabolic responses. Eur J Appl Physiol 2004;92:498–507.

113 Rivera-Brown AM, Ramirez-Marrero FA, Wilk B, Bar-Or O: Voluntary drinking and hydration in trained, heat-acclimatized girls exercising in a hot and humid climate. Eur J Appl Physiol 2008;103:109–116.

114 Bergeron MF, Laird MD, Marinik EL, Brenner JS, Waller JL: Repeated-bout exercise in the heat in young athletes: physiological strain and perceptual responses. J Appl Physiol 2009;106:476–485.

115 Bergeron MF, McLeod KS, Coyle JF: Core body temperature during competition in the heat: National Boys' 14s Junior Championships. Br J Sports Med 2007;41:779–783.

116 Coyle E: Cumulative heat stress appears to affect match outcome in a junior tennis championship. Med Sci Sports Exerc 2006;38:S110.

117 Falk B, Dotan R: Child-adult differences in the recovery from high-intensity exercise. Exerc Sport Sci Rev 2006;34:107–112.

118 Hindmarsh KW, Opheim EE: Drug abuse prevalence in western Canada and the North West Territories: a survey of students in grades 6–12. Int J Addict 1990;25:301–305.

119 Gill ND, Shield A, Blazevich AJ, Zhou S, Weatherby RP: Muscular and cardiorespiratory effects of pseudoephedrine in human athletes. Br J Clin Pharmacol 2000;50:205–213.

120 Kolka MA, Stephenson LA, Bruttig SP, Cadarette BS, Gonzalez RR: Human thermoregulation after atropine and/or pralidoxime administration. Aviat Space Environ Med 1987;58:545–549.

121 Gordon NF, Kruger PE, van Rensburg JP, van der Linde A, Kielbloack AJ, Cilliers JF: Effect of beta-adrenoreceptor blockade on thermoregulation during prolonged exercise in the heat. Med Sci Sports Exerc 1984;16:S138.

122 Metzl JD, Small E, Levine SR, Gershel JC: Creatine use among young athletes. Pediatrics 2001;108:421–425.

123 Nemet D, Eliakim A: Pediatric sports nutrition: an update. Curr Opin Clin Nutr Metab Care 2009;12:304–309.

124 Lopez RM, Casa DJ, McDermott BP, Ganio MS, Armstrong LE, Maresh CM: Does creatine supplementation hinder exercise heat tolerance or hydration status? A systematic review with meta-analyses. J Athl Train 2009;44:215–223.

125 Scahill L, Schwab-Stone M: Epidemiology of ADHD in school-age children. Child Adolesc Psychiatr Clin N Am 2000;9:541–555,vii.

126 Mahon AD, Stephens BR, Cole AS: Exercise responses in boys with attention deficit/hyperactivity disorder: effects of stimulant medication. J Atten Disord 2008;12:170–176.

127 Boileau RA, Ballard JE, Sprague RL, Sleator EK, Massey BH: Effect of methylphenidate on cardiorespiratory responses in hyperactive children. Res Q 1976;47:590–596.

Prof. Bareket Falk
Faculty of Applied Health Sciences, Brock University
St. Catharines, ON, L2S 3A1 (Canada)
Tel. +1 905 688 5550, Ext. 4979, Fax +1 905 688 8364, E-Mail bfalk@brocku.ca

Armstrong N, McManus AM (eds): The Elite Young Athlete.
Med Sport Sci. Basel, Karger, 2011, vol 56, pp 150–170

Environmental Factors Affecting Elite Young Athletes

Craig Williams

Children's Health and Exercise Research Centre, University of Exeter, Exeter, UK

Abstract

To date, much of the research concerning the performance of elite young athletes has focused on physical and physiological factors and how these relate to age and maturation. Little attention has been paid to other factors which might limit performance such as nutrition or environmental stressors. The paucity of research on the environmental effects on performance in young athletes is unsurprising given the need for experimental studies, the ethics of which would generally be untenable. As an outcome, there is a reliance on observational and case study data, e.g. observing the stressors which occur during jet lag and effects on sleep patterns, altitude and pollution. The effects of environmental factors have been predominantly researched from a health context in youngsters rather than a performance context. However, the evidence of those few empirical studies combined with coach and/or sports science support teams' experience have provided professionals with some guidelines. These applied guidelines include sleep patterns, jet lag, pollution and altitude research, to aid those preparing young athletes for training and competition in environments that present potential challenges to performance. The limitations of data extrapolated from adults are acknowledged and in all cases it is emphasised that recommendations and implementing practice should be based on data collected from young people.

Elite young athletes are now more likely to face a greater variety of environmental stressors than competitors 30 years ago. The increasing professionalisation of youth competition has resulted in a greater emphasis on success at the youth level and more opportunity for travel, particularly international travel. This greater access to competition in different localities and other countries has introduced a range of stressors which the competitor might not have encountered if competition had been confined to their region. Travel increases the risk of jet lag and disrupted sleep patterns, competitions may take place at higher altitude or in locations with high levels of air pollution. All these factors can affect performance and if a young athlete is to develop into a successful adult athlete, these stressors must be overcome or minimised.

There are very few published data on environmental stressors in young elite athletes and much of what is known has been inferred from adult studies. Due to the expense and ethical concerns that studies on environmental stressors would generate, the scarcity of data is likely to remain so for the foreseeable future. Most sports organisations are more likely to use their own personal experience in an attempt to minimise the disruptive effect of environmental stressors. The most pertinent stressors which affect elite athletes are circadian rhythms, jet lag, sleep, altitude and pollution and these form the focus of this chapter. Other factors such as climate and seasonal change are beyond the scope of this review.

Circadian Rhythms

Circadian rhythms were first described in 1729 by De Marian [1] when he observed the rhythmic opening and closing of the mimosa pudica plant leaves, even when the plant remained in total darkness. It was not until 1959 that Franz Halberg coined the term circadian from the Latin, meaning circa or 'about' and dies or 'day'. Just over a decade later, the suprachiasmatic nucleus (SCN), a set of small paired nuclei in the hypothalamus, was identified as the internal clock or pacemaker in the circadian mammalian system.

The most commonly known circadian rhythm that relates to sport and exercise is core body temperature, but there are many other examples. These include the sleep/wake cycle, reproduction, blood pressure, hormonal secretion and airway resistance. These all follow coordinated sequential patterns which oscillate within a time period of ~24.5 h but, due to a process called entrainment, light synchronises the SCN to the 24-hour day. The variation in daylight and darkness is the prime stimulus for synchronising the circadian timing system. In particular, the light at dusk and dawn has the greatest effect on the circadian pacemaker and at midday the least effect.

One hormone which oscillates with the circadian rhythm is melatonin. Melatonin levels are virtually absent in the day time, rise in the evening near bedtime, remain relatively constant during the night and decline at the time at which waking approaches. Melatonin is suppressed by light and is often used as a marker of the circadian timing system, as is core body temperature. However, the onset of melatonin secretion is considered a more reliable measure than body temperature measures.

Sleep and Circadian Rhythms

The two most important factors for determining sleep are the sleep-wake homeostatic system and the circadian timing system. The homeostatic sleep-wake system accounts for both the accumulation of pressure for sleep whilst awake and the dissipation of this pressure whilst asleep [2]. The circadian system regulates the timing of sleep and waking across each cycle. According to one theoretical model, the homeostatic and circadian systems work interactively, whilst another model proposes the two systems work in opposition to one another, such that a circadian timing system promotes wakefulness whilst opposing the homeostatic force which promotes sleep. In addition, the times of falling asleep and waking up are closely related to core temperature, so that when the body clock is desynchronised (e.g. after a time-zone transition), the changes in sleep habits that are observed can be accounted for by this relationship between sleep and circadian rhythmicity.

Irrespective of whichever model researchers in this field favour, what has been found is that these systems undergo developmental change through childhood, adolescence and into adulthood. Table 1 provides a chronological sequence of the maturation of the circadian system as applied to sleep patterns. One striking feature often observed by many parents and coaches is the adolescent tendency towards later bedtime and consequently an increase in daytime sleepiness. Studies by Carskadon and colleagues have found that the intrinsic circadian period is prolonged in adolescence, often >25 h, compared to the adult population circadian period of 24.5 h. This prolonged period was at first attributed to psychosocial factors, e.g. increasing burden of school work, greater independence and activities in the evening with peers, part-time employment and increased participation in sport. However, although the above factors are important they have now been superseded by evidence

Table 1. Age and maturation effects of the circadian system as applied to sleep patterns

Age	Observations
18 weeks' gestation	suprachiasmatic nucleus evident in developing foetal brain
First weeks postnatal	almost no obvious circadian rhythm
From ~4 weeks	circadian rhythms becoming noticeable
From ~12 weeks	majority of babies sleeping at east 5 h per night
From ~12–24 weeks	babies sleep pattern organised into morning and afternoon naps and night time sleep
From ~1.5 years old	toddler moves to just ~mid-day nap and night time sleep
By 6 years	for the majority of children, day time napping ceased
Adolescence	tendency to sleep later, an increased total amount of sleep required plus increases in day time sleepiness; effects of puberty and gonadal hormonal influence
Adulthood	attenuation of sleep patterns shown in adolescence
Older adults	propensity for earlier bedtimes and wake up times, frequent awakenings during sleep, consequently increased evening napping also a possibility

that indicates it is a biological process which accounts for the changes in sleep-wake cycles.

Evidence supporting a biological mechanism underlying the changes in sleep during adolescence includes the observation that girls appear to experience a delay in the onset of sleep about 1 year before boys, mirroring, to a degree, their earlier onset of puberty. The maximum delay in sleep onset also occurs earlier in girls at ~19.5 years compared to boys 20.9 years [3]. However, given the limited amount of data and evidence of cultural/racial differences, which have found the peak delay to occur earlier in youngsters of differing races [4–7], these averages should be treated with some caution.

The coupling of sleep onset to pubertal development has been observed using animal models and although there are some weaknesses related to methodological protocols and the lack of established longitudinal data, there are strong associations between the delay in the circadian phase related to sleep and the onset of puberty. Developmental changes according to a theoretical model in the homeostatic drive and circadian timing have been proposed by Carskadon [8]. It has been suggested that adolescents have a resistance to sleep pressure thus permitting them to stay up later compared to pre-pubertal children. Concomitantly, their circadian phase is delayed thus providing an urge to stay awake later in the evening and to sleep later in the morning. Cross-sectional studies have found that more mature adolescents are slower to fall asleep (after being awake for 14.5 and 16.5 h) and are able to stay awake compared to younger adolescents [9]. One suggestion is that the build up of sleep pressure (detected using electroencephalographic wave activity) was slower in post-pubertal compared to pre-pubertal youngsters [10].

Changes in the circadian regulation of sleep during adolescence have also been related to changes in light sensitivity. Although the circadian pacemaker is set internally by the SCN and its rhythm is ~24 h, it is also influenced by external factors such as time cues brought about by light. Adolescents have been found to have a blunted response to light in the morning (affecting waking up time) and an exaggerated phase delay response to light exposure in the evening (affecting sleep pressure and staying awake) [11].

Currently researchers are investigating whether the homeostatic and circadian regulation of sleep is influenced by gonadal hormones. Oestrogen, testosterone and progesterone ingestion in rodents are known to effect sleep via modulation of the pacemaker in the SCN. There are also anatomical growth changes in the SCN at mid-puberty in rats linking gonadal hormones to the delay phase in adolescence. It should also be noted that the hormone melatonin may be linked to the timing of puberty. This key circadian hormone, which is secreted maximally during the night and least during daylight, is thought to inhibit gonadotropin-releasing hormone secretion. It is proposed that although the concentration of melatonin release remains constant, its effectiveness is reduced on account of increases in body size, such that when melatonin falls below a threshold point, gonadotropin-releasing hormone is then released and the pubertal process is initiated [12]. How these changes are associated with or affected by training and performance are yet to be determined.

Application of Sleep Research for Elite Young Athletes

There are no published sleep-wake data on elite young athletes, although some data are available for healthy school-age children. Sleep need is defined as 'when a child wakes spontaneously in the morning and does not sleep more on weekends than weekdays' [2, p. 321]. On average children aged 9–10 years require ~10 h of sleep per night, although with any mean figure there is considerable variation between individuals. The consequences of daily training for the elite athlete on sleep-wake patterns are unclear. Whilst the physical exertion from training will make young athletes more tired than their untrained peers, whether there is any compensatory response in sleep pressure in children or adolescents is not known.

It has been established that when bedtimes are clearly set and adhered to that children will not experience deficits in sleep. Training either early in the morning or late at night will certainly impose challenges to the needs of sleep in some athletic youngsters. In our laboratory, self-reported disturbances to sleep were found in 20% of 365 young athletes [unpubl. data] and data have shown that a lack of sleep may augment pressure at school, interfere with the ability to socialise and affect mood, e.g. depression [13, 14]. Sleep disturbance is an indicator of over-reaching/overtraining, and the importance of appropriate amounts of sleep therefore cannot be underestimated. Coaches must be attentive to issues related to tiredness, either as a consequence of training and/or lack of sleep. Chronic insufficient sleep is likely to be a causal factor of under-performance in young athletes whose training schedules involve early starts, multiple sessions in a day and/or high training volumes across a week.

Sleep research in youngsters has found that when sleep is optimal, pre-pubertal children are alert and awake throughout the day. In contrast, the pubertal adolescent experiences mid-afternoon declines both in alertness and performance, which occur approximately 8 h after waking. If sleep is deficient, then pre-pubertal children will be most tired in the afternoon and evening, whilst the pubertal adolescent experiences significant impairments in the morning. This morning impairment is related to the change in the biological timings for arousal to awake and alert signals to sleep if the youngster has not benefited from a good night's sleep. In contrast to the pre-pubertal child, an uplift of energy in the late afternoon is often experienced by adolescents as they benefit from the alert systems preparing for the evening [15]. The key educational message about the importance of sleep for coaches and their athletes is that although it is easier for adolescents to stay awake, the need for sufficient sleep is just as important as it was in childhood.

Despite a sound understanding of some of the key influential variables related to sleep, the timing of training is more likely to be based on pragmatism rather than physiological rationale. Training schedules for sports such as swimming, diving, ice-skating or ice-hockey are often dictated by the financial aspects of hiring the facilities, i.e. early morning or late evening starts, and not by consideration of when it is best to practise. However, if there are opportunities for dictating the timing of practices, e.g. in an Academy setting, it would make sense for the coaches to consider the amount of training being undertaken and its possible consequences on sleep patterns. A summary of studies on self-reported rise times noted that these were significantly later on weekend mornings in comparison to school mornings [16]. Additionally, the sleep/wake patterns tend to shift to later, particularly for adolescents during the summer holidays compared to the school year, but any impact this may have on performance has yet to be verified.

If early starts or late training are unavoidable, the practice of napping might be a strategy worthy of future consideration for young athletes. In one study on napping, Carsdakon and Dement [17] found that a 45-min midday nap, which occurred 6 h after waking, was found to enhance alertness and mood for up to 8 h later. Conversely, an afternoon nap did not provide benefit for alertness or mood the following day, in fact sleepiness worsened in the pre-nap morning hours with each passing day.

In summary, despite accumulated evidence related to sleep in the normal healthy child and adolescent, little is known about sleep deficit on performance in young athletes. It is common that factors beyond the control of coaches will dictate

sleep patterns, such as pre-arranged competition start times, international flight travel and crossing of time zones. All these will have an affect on sleep (see section on jet lag) and efforts to minimise these effects should be sought. In general, is it likely that the sleep needs of the healthy youngster apply equally to athletic youth and therefore some practical suggestions related to maximising optimal sleep are summarised in table 2.

Jet Lag

Jet lag is a term used to collectively describe a range of undesirable symptoms brought about by a rapid transition across time zones. These symptoms, commonly resulting in a malaise, include disrupted sleep patterns, fatigue, decreased motivation, loss of concentration, alterations in mood and irritability, loss of appetite, feeling 'bloated' after eating and bowel dysfunction. The number of symptoms, severity and duration are dependent on several factors including the length of the flight and number of time zones crossed, and altitude change. It should be noted though that there is considerable inter-individual variation [18].

Jet-lag symptoms are believed to emanate from the circadian rhythms being out of synchrony with the new local time. The most substantial circadian disruption affects the sleep/wake cycle. To date, most research has been conducted on adults often in a work setting such as pilots and flight attendants [19–21]. To the best of the author's knowledge there are no published data for children and adolescents. However, given what is known about sleep in youngsters, it is unlikely that the consequences of jet lag will be substantially different to those in adults.

The differential consequences of travel direction (westwards or eastwards) on the sleep/wake cycles are likely to be the same in children as adults. For example, travelling westwards across six time zones will mean that the fatigue in the evening will be high and the traveller is unlikely

Table 2. Summary of common factors related to youngsters' sleep patterns and recommendations to delimit the effect of their evolving sleep patterns

1	Although adolescents will have a tendency to go to bed later, this is not because they need less sleep In the case of elite young athletes experiencing high volumes of training (e.g. most days of the week and greater than 2 h per day), recovery through sleep is even more important
2	Activities at bed time such as TV watching, using the computer, phone or internet, acts which arouse children and adolescents, should be limited
3	Sleep times that are regularly set and adhered to are more likely to benefit performance
4	Pre-pubertal youngsters function better earlier in the day compared to late afternoon and evening Monitoring will help to evaluate the effects of sleep patterns on individual performance
5	Circumpubertal and post-pubescent adolescents' performance is worst in the morning, monitoring will help to evaluate the effects of sleep patterns on individual performance

to have difficulty going to sleep, partially as a result of a sleep delay due to travelling and partially due to the external cue of darkness. However, premature waking is likely to occur because the waking signals (rising plasma adrenaline and core temperature) are conditioned to an earlier rise. Conversely, a flight eastwards, crossing the same number of time zones results in a reversal of this pattern, with the initiation of sleep difficult, but no premature waking as the new waking time corresponds to the original destination night time.

Jet lag symptoms were assessed in 39 adults (some of them Olympian adult athletes), who crossed ten time zones eastwards, en route to the 2000 Sydney Olympics. Key findings showed that the perception of jet-lag was strongly related to ratings of fatigue. Early morning jet lag symptoms were predicted by earlier waking time and decreased alertness 30 min after waking. Whereas, jet lag symptoms during the day were predicted by feeling bloated after meals and by an increased inability to concentrate. Mood, mental performance and bowel function appeared to adjust more rapidly than did other symptoms of jet lag and as such Waterhouse et al. [22] rendered them poor markers of the process of body clock adjustment. One key practical point emphasised in this study was that the various jet lag symptoms do not all adjust in synchrony within an individual and there are likely to be considerable inter-individual variations in symptoms too. Nonetheless, the key symptoms of sleep and fatigue should be the target of attempts to adjust to local time as quickly as possible. Such a focus is supported by findings from Lowden and Akerstedt [23], who showed rating of jet lag symptoms for aircrew were most closely associated to sleepiness and the number of awakenings.

In order to extend sleep and reduce the effects of fatigue, a pharmacological approach has often been used. The effectiveness of using drugs such as those in the benzodiazepine group or melatonin, has been studied. Although it is claimed these medications have had some success, it is not clear whether they directly affect the body clock, have a hypnotic effect or both. In fact, the timing of administration of the drug is dependent on whether a soporific (sleep inducing) or chronobiotic (phase shifting) effect is required [24]; however, no studies investigating time-of-day effects upon the efficacy of such drugs are available. For further information on advice on air travel and children's health issues, the reader is directed to the Position statement of the Canadian Paediatric Society [25].

As the level of competition for the elite young athlete increases so too does the likelihood of international travel. For the first time traveller this is bound to be a time of great excitement, but also increased anxiety and stress. Therefore, coaches and support staff need to plan to limit the effects of sleep disruption as best as is practically possible.

For example, it is likely that teams travelling westwards and crossing time zones will have an advantage over the opposition when the performance is earlier rather than later in the day. But, on their return, school and training schedules are likely to be disrupted, particularly if the period away has been of several weeks duration. Therefore, coaches might have to alert schools of the possible effects on school work due to the significant sleep-phase delay.

Although melatonin has often been prescribed in an attempt to alter circadian rhythm, its use in young athletes is not justified. The timing of ingestion of melatonin is crucial to its effects on the circadian system. Melatonin ingestion, although having a sleep inducing effect has been found to have the opposite intended effect when mis-timed in adults and consequently might impair performance [26–28]. Using natural daylight or artificial lighting when timed appropriately is more effective in resetting the sleep-phase than use of melatonin.

Melatonin, as well as benzodiazepine, has been used for treatment of clinical sleep disorders in children, but utilization is controversial. The effects of these drugs on the brain and on the body of growing children are unknown. In the United States melatonin is not regulated by the Food and Drug Administration but in other countries is freely available as a certified medication. However, the use of such treatments is not warranted in young athletes and is best avoided unless authorised by suitably qualified medical staff.

In summary, although there appear to be no published data on the effects of jet lag on performance in children and adolescents, most findings in adults would likely be applicable, particularly with regards to sleep deprivation. Table 3 provides a summary of the key issues and applied recommendations to reduce the effects of jet lag.

Air Pollution

Concerns about the level of air pollutants during the Athens Olympics in 2004 and the Beijing Olympics in 2008 brought much attention to the issues of air pollution and sporting performance. It is interesting to note that during the 1996 Atlanta Olympics, traffic was limited in an attempt to restrict air pollution and there was a noticeable decrease in hospital admissions for asthma related exacerbations [29]. This provides some evidence of the positive effect of reducing air pollution by controlling traffic. Other pollutants, including those affecting water and sanitation, might also exert profound effects on children and adolescents, but for the purposes of this section, only air pollution will be considered.

Organisations such as the North American Commission for Environmental Cooperation, the United Nations, and the World Health Organisation (WHO) have begun systematic programmes to evaluate the consequences of children's exposure to air pollutants. The significance of these programmes is naturally concerned with health and well-being rather than sports performance and is specifically aimed at documenting the effects of chronic exposure. This work is particularly important because of children's immature and developing lungs, as well as the relative immaturity of their immune system. Equally as important is that children and adolescents tend to spend more time outdoors compared to adults, thus predisposing children and adolescents to increased air pollution exposure to pollutants. Air pollution research has been concerned with

Table 3. Summary of key issues and applied strategies to reduce the effects of jet lag in young athletes

1	Flying to the new country in plenty of time to adapt to the new local time is optimal in terms of delimiting the deleterious effects of jet lag on performance, but might incur greater expense Alternatively, preparing a training/competition schedule which factors in adjustment to the new time zone is recommended and this would include reducing training in the days immediately after the flight When training/competition schedules dictate otherwise, athletes and coaches might need to adopt a more pragmatic approach such as keeping busy during the new waking time, in spite of some compromise to performance, in an attempt to adjust quicker It is important that young athletes are made aware of the possible reduction in performance they may experience during the adjustment period
2	Travelling westwards will result in premature waking This is likely to be beneficial for training or performance if competitions are scheduled earlier in the day, but may be detrimental when scheduled later in the day or evening
3	Travelling eastwards will result in initial difficulties in sleeping and less likelihood of premature waking When training or competition times are scheduled in the early morning, this will require arrangements to ensure the athlete is awoken in plenty of time If training or competition is scheduled later in the afternoon or early evening this may be beneficial as feelings of fatigue should be lessened
4	Focus on monitoring sleep and fatigue to gauge the extent of jet lag and adjust training accordingly
5	Coaches and support staff should be aware of temporary changes in mood, concentration, motivation, appetite and bowel function which will vary considerably in magnitude and duration in their young athletes
6	Pharmacological intervention, notably through sleeping tablets (melatonin or benzodiazepine), is not recommended for healthy young athletes

exacerbating acute illnesses, with broader and encompassing studies associating pollution with foetal death, preterm delivery and low birth weight [30–34]. Although causality has yet to be established, possible mechanisms for these associations continued to be explored. For a brief synopsis of the research relating air pollution to children's health, see Schwartz [35].

Air pollution is usually classified according to acute effects (short-term fluctuations) or chronic effects (long-term exposure). The type of exposure therefore depends upon the athlete's home location, but for many young athletes in regions of low pollution, exposure is more likely to be acute and related to competitions held elsewhere. This of course does not diminish the importance of avoiding habitual sports practice near sites of pollutants, e.g. next to a road side. It is hoped that either due to the implementation of environmental laws or to a common sense approach, exposure to air pollutants in young athletes can be reduced to an absolute minimum. Although air quality has improved in many countries around the world, there are an equal number of countries which still suffer significant problems with air quality in major cities. Such cities, including Athens, Beijing, Hong Kong, Los Angeles and Mexico City, suffer not only because of their industrial landscape but also due to their topography, environmental climate and a lack of implementation of environmental law.

The most commonly measured air pollutants are sulphur dioxide (SO_2), carbon monoxide (CO), nitrogen dioxide (NO_2), particulate matter

(PM$_{10}$) and ozone (O$_3$). The first three pollutants are classified as primary pollutants as they either remain in their current form when emitted or are synthesised via a chemical reaction between the source and the target. The PM$_{10}$ is defined as particles less than 10 µm in diameter and this is used as a standard measure for establishing air quality around the world. Although the WHO has established acceptable standards for some pollutants such as O$_3$, others such as PM$_{10}$ may vary globally. Other sources of primary pollutants are dust and smoke. Ozone and related nitrates are formed from the reaction of ultraviolet radiation with a primary pollutant, e.g. NO$_2$, and are known as secondary pollutants.

Air pollution is most problematic in those with known respiratory disease and is most commonly associated with increased incidence of asthma or decreased pulmonary function, particularly when exposure concentrations are chronic and/ or high. Therefore, in young athletes with known respiratory problem, pollutants are a serious consideration when training or competing. For young athletes with no known respiratory deficit, it is generally considered that low-dose exposure to daily air pollution does not exert any significant effect on pulmonary function. Nevertheless, a recent review of studies in adults suggests that adverse health effects occur even when levels of air pollutants are low [36]. Despite noting substantial methodological weakness in both design and instrumentation in many of the available studies, the authors argue that the public health implications for children and adolescents cannot be ignored, even for low level air pollutant exposure.

The effects of the pollutants on the airways, and in particular the sensitive lining of the epithelial cells and alveoli, will be influenced by factors such as the individual's ventilatory rate, atmospheric temperature, pressure and rainfall. Ozone is a very reactive gas evoking oxidative stress and damage within the lungs, but because ozone is produced by chemical reactions within the atmosphere, its production and appearance is influenced by seasonal and diurnal patterns. It is higher in the summer and in the afternoon and lower in the winter, early morning and at night time.

Peak respiratory flow decrements have been noted during the summer months [37, 38], during the winter months in asthmatics [39], at residential schools [40] and during summer camps [41, 42]. Overall, declines in lung function were associated with incidences of high air pollution and symptoms were recorded and were worst for those on asthma medication than for non asthmatics. Animal models support the epidemiological evidence and point towards altered macrophage activity and epithelial damage as consequences of exposure to air pollutants [43–45].

Despite the majority of studies investigating air pollution in children being focused on health outcomes, it is logical to conclude that these results are equally applicable to child athletes. Compared to resting values, as exercise intensity increases, the rate of ventilation increases and with changes in water content of the inspired breath, any pollution effects are likely to be accentuated. Already, it is clear that children exposed to high levels of ambient air pollution have reduced lung development [46]. Part of this exposure occurs during outdoor play, either during or after school. In one cross-sectional study in primary school children in Taiwan, declining lung function coincided with increasing hourly exposure to O$_3$ [47]. Furthermore, in a group of 249 clinically healthy children from south west Mexico City, an area chronically exposed to O$_3$ levels which exceed the US air quality standards, over half the children exhibited bilateral hyperinflation and increased linear marking of the lungs. Spirometry data also confirmed acute decrements in lung functions tests that could be related to chronic exposure to the polluted environment [48].

Scant data are available for young athletes, but one study of 16 adolescent (mean age 14.9 ± 0.9 years) high school cross-country runners from Atlanta, USA, examined ozone, PM$_{2.5}$ and pH of exhaled breath condensate (EBC) before and after a daily run (4–5 p.m.) on 15 consecutive days [49]. The EBC contains a range of particles from the surfaces within the respiratory tract and is thought to indicate inflammation. More specifically, the pH of EBC has been used as an indicator of inflammation reflecting the acid-base balance of the airways. Spirometry measures, including forced expired volume in 1 s (FEV_1) were also collected. Despite the study taking place in August (smog season) and on 4 days when air quality warnings were issued, results surprisingly demonstrated that compared to resting values there was no acute effect of air pollution exposure during vigorous outdoor exercise on breath pH, contrary to the original hypothesis. Unfortunately, no information was provided on quantifying the intensity of the training runs or the quality of the training sessions. However, the authors did note very low and variable measures of EBC pH within the athletes, similar to values indicative of severe asthma or to those in sickle cell anaemia patients. Despite a robust defence against alternative explanations for the low values, the authors concluded that additional studies were needed to establish the validity of EBC as a useful biomarker and as to whether these low values were pathological or normal biological variants.

Air pollution is not just an outdoor problem. Although pollutants such as ozone are generally higher outdoors compared to indoors, air quality indoors is just as important. It has been observed that winter sport athletes have a higher prevalence of exercise-induced asthma than summer sport athletes [50, 51]. This fact has been ascribed to the high levels of ventilation under cold and dry ambient conditions, thus causing damage to the ventilatory airways [52]. However, indoor winter athletes (ice and speed skaters, ice hockey players, etc.) experience a greater prevalence of exercise induced bronchi-constriction compared to outdoor winter athletes, coupled with lower resting lung function and greater airway dysfunction. As these athletes compete in an environment that is not as extreme as the outdoor weather conditions, thermal damage via temperature and humidity cannot be the cause. One factor postulated is the high concentrations of fine and ultra-fine particulate matter less than 1 μm in diameter (PM_1) that are emitted from the ice resurfacing machines used in ice rinks. Rundell et al. [53] found in a comparison of 10 ice rinks pre- and post-resurfacing, high concentrations of ultra-fine and fine PM_1 emitted from gasoline or diesel ice resurfacing machines. Additionally, the ventilation and air circulation system of the rink also influenced the extent of the PM_1 dissipation. Unfortunately, Rundell and colleagues did not measure the airway characteristics of any athletes at the same time as measuring the air quality in the rink. They argue that there is enough indirect support of the association between the increased hyperreactivity and exercise induced asthma of indoor skaters and the poor air quality of ice rinks. They concluded that future studies were needed to define the relationship between PM_1 and the high prevalence and pathology of exercise-induced asthma in ice-skating athletes. Importantly, these future studies should also provide information on the effects on athletic performance.

Application of Pollution Research to the Elite Young Athlete

In the absence of specific empirical information related to young elite athletes, information obtained from healthy, but less active youth have been used to provide guidelines for reducing exposure to air pollution when training. The guidelines presented in table 4 offer a common sense approach to training in an environment where pollutants might be present. Although it is recognised that this might not always be under the control of the athlete and coach, e.g. for geographical reasons, it is logical to reduce the duration of exposure to such contaminates.

Table 4. Guidelines for reducing the effects of pollution during training

1	Avoid regular training near road sides and traffic If training on roads and amongst congested traffic has to take place, then avoid the rush hours
2	Try to locate open or rural park-land as a training venue to avoid more polluted districts
3	Train early in the morning or late in the evening to avoid the most concentrated effects of pollutants in the air
4	If the environment is cold and smoggy, avoid exercise in these conditions and train indoors instead Make use of the local meteorological office for advice and guidance on the quality of the air This would be particularly important when a training camp or competition is held abroad
5	If environmental conditions are less than favourable and training has to occur, ensure that the asthmatics in the squad take and use their inhalers
6	Consideration of possible pollution effects should be given not just for outdoor locations, but also for indoor facilities such as ice-rinks
7	Be aware of the symptoms of exposure to air pollution when training which include airway irritation, coughing, wheezing, pain upon inhalation and breathing difficulties

Altitude

There is a well-known relationship between altitude and pressure, such that the air becomes less dense with increasing altitude and each litre of air contains fewer molecules of gas. As the O_2, CO_2 and N_2 percentages are the same at altitude as they are at sea level, the change in the partial pressure of each gas is a result of the atmospheric pressure. The inverse relationship between altitude and partial pressure has a direct effect on the haemoglobin saturation and the amount of oxygen transport. This lowered partial pressure in O_2 (PO_2) is termed hypoxia. Thus, at an altitude of 3,500 m the atmospheric air has a PO_2 equivalent to 13% O_2 at sea level. The effect of the lowered partial pressure has both acute and chronic consequences on the respiratory, cardiovascular and neural systems, as well as important implications on sleep and nutritional habits [54–57].

Although there are increasing numbers of publications related to the effects of altitude on adults, the published literature related to athletic performance in the younger population is sparse. The scarcity of data for young athletes at natural altitude is likely due to a number of reasons. Firstly, altitude studies are often related to extreme environmental conditions and usually involve mountaineering type activities, thereby precluding young people's participation. When at a higher altitude the impact of decreases in humidity, increases in solar radiation and wind chill have to be considered, all of which add considerably to safety concerns. Physiological responses of adults at altitude have become a source of great interest because of the potential ergogenic advantage of altitude training in adult athletes, and because of the need for more information on acute mountain sickness with the advent of greater accessibility of adult adventure holidays [54]. Finally, the few altitude studies that have attempted to involve children and adolescents, often do so by studying those who reside at altitude, without consideration of other confounders such as nutritional and socioeconomic status.

Although it is possible to simulate altitude in laboratories, the known risk of hypoxic events

Table 5. The acute physiological responses of children to altitude

Reduction in	Increases in
Peak flow/FEV_1	Heart rate
Lung gas transfer	$\dot{Q}$
Arterial PO_2 and O_2 saturation	Erythropoietin red blood cell production
CO_2 production	Minute ventilation
RER	Vital capacity/residual volume
	Less active sleep
	Periodic breathing

See references [56, 59, 60, 63, 69].
FEV_1 = Forced expired volume in 1 s; RER = respiratory exchange ratio; $\dot{Q}$ = cardiac output.

delimits the extent of altitude exposure to moderate hypoxia only. Therefore, exercise events that are held in locations with natural altitude, such as Everest ascents or competitions held ≥2,000 m (e.g. Mexico City Olympics in 1968), have often served as 'natural experiments' in which the physiological effects of altitude are tested. The easiest methods to study the effects of altitude are to monitor travellers going to altitude or to compare residents based at sea level to those living at high altitude (<3,000 m). Most of this work has been conducted with adults but as more children and adolescents are undertaking travel opportunities in regions of high altitude, more data are becoming available. As it is likely that the young elite athlete will be travelling to a region to compete rather than to train or live for a substantial period of time, acute responses will be the focus of this section.

Data on children resident at altitude have been published and report the effects of long-term adaptations to residing at altitude, as well as genetic [58] and environmental [59, 60] influences. Therefore, the scenario facing the young athlete who is normally resident at low altitude and who

is competing in an event at high altitude is likely to be quite different to that of those resident at altitude athletes. Table 5 provides a summary of the acute physiological effects being at high altitude induces in children compared to sea level measurements. Studies have found increased ventilatory and respiratory responses such as higher minute ventilation, tidal volumes, vital capacity and oxygen extraction. Similarly, higher cardiovascular responses, such as higher heart rate, cardiac output and red blood cell production, have been observed.

These increased responses are an outcome of the lower arterial PO_2 and oxygen saturation. Most of the extant literature has focused on clinical questions, for example, administration of oxygen therapy [61], or investigating possible cellular hypoxia in critically ill patients [62]. One such study documented cardiovascular autonomic function after exposure to moderate altitude [63]. Eight healthy but untrained children (mean age 9.5, range 6–12 years) completed a battery of cardiovascular, blood pressure and oxygen saturation tests both at their home residence (200 m above sea level) and at 2,950 m. The cardiovascular and oxygen saturation measures were taken once at 200 m above sea level, and twice at altitude; first within 1 h of arrival and second 24 h later. The blood pressure, a 24-hour ambulatory measure, was taken once at 200 m and once at altitude commencing on arrival. It was observed that there was an immediate, small, but statistically significant, increase in heart rate and blood pressure, as well as a significant decrease in oxygen saturation on exposure to 2,950 m altitude in comparison to the basal (200 m) condition. Results from the 24 h exposure to altitude showed no significant differences in any cardiovascular values compared to the 1 h exposure values. Oxygen saturation values in the basal condition, on arrival and 24 h later were $95.1 \pm 1.3\%$, $88.5 \pm 1.7\%$ and $91.7 \pm 2.4\%$, respectively. Observations from a group of adults (age range 32–45 years) and elderly (range 60–83 years) that were also tested at the same time showed similar patterns. Four adults and one child complained of a headache and insomnia, but none were reported as displaying acute mountain sickness (AMS) as defined by the Lake Louise Consensus on Definition and Quantification of Altitude Illness questionnaire [64] (table 6).

Another study which involved children travelling to altitude assessed responses of 20 prepubertal children (16 boys and 4 girls, age range 9–12 years) and their fathers as they travelled from 490 m to 2,450 m and spent 2 nights at altitude [56]. Specifically, this study investigated the respiratory adaptation to hypoxia and in particular nocturnal breathing and quality of sleep, symptoms of AMS. Baseline measurements at 490 m included the use of nocturnal polygraphic measurements, including respiratory inductive plethysmography, pulse oximetry and capnography of expired air to estimate end-tidal CO_2 tension (PETCO$_2$) as a surrogate for arterial PCO$_2$. Clinical examinations for symptoms of AMS were also conducted using the environmental symptoms questionnaire [65]. The key findings from the 17 children and 19 adults who completed all measurements produced some interesting data. Similar to previous

findings [63], the mean O_2 saturation decreased by 11–13% during the first night for both children and adults compared to baseline. This was accompanied by significant increases, compared to baseline, for measures of minute ventilation, inspiratory flow and a decrease in PETCO$_2$. The increase in children's minute ventilation during the night was accomplished by increasing the breathing rate, whilst adults increased both breathing rate and tidal volume. Paralleling other studies, heart rates were also higher for children in comparison to baseline values. It was also found that rest time and sleep efficiency were significantly decreased in the first night at altitude in both children and adults. Most interestingly, differences in periodic breathing, a symptom found at altitude where breathing patterns alternate rapidly and often uncontrollably, were found between the children and adults.

Children demonstrated much less periodic breathing even though the effects of hypoxaemia and increased proportional minute ventilation were similar to adults. The children's greater stability of breathing was explained by a higher CO_2 reserve, a lower apnoea threshold for CO_2 and a shorter circulation time. These responses coupled with an increased heart rate and ventilatory response during the hypoxic environment is consistent with the proposition that children have a more dynamic cardiorespiratory adaptation to altitude than adults. However, it is important to note that this did not translate into any significant difference in sleep duration between adults and children, as measured by actigraphy. Nor was the occurrence of AMS symptoms lower in children than adults as a result of the children's more dynamic adaptation. In this regard, 50% of the children (n = 10), including one child who was withdrawn from the study due to severe AMS [66] and 30% of the adults (n = 6) experienced significant symptoms of AMS. Although breathing patterns in the children were more stable at night, they presented with a similar degree of nocturnal O_2 desaturation and hyperventilation as the adults,

Table 6. The Lake Louise Classification and Scoring of AMS

Symptom	Scoring	
Headache	0	none at all
	1	mild headache
	2	moderate headache
	3	severe headache, incapacitating
Gastrointestinal symptoms	0	good appetite
	1	poor appetite or nausea
	2	moderate nausea or vomiting
	3	severe, incapacitating nausea and vomiting
Fatigue and/or weakness	0	not tired or weak
	1	mild fatigue/weakness
	2	moderate fatigue/weakness
	3	severe fatigue/weakness
Dizziness/light-headedness	0	none
	1	light
	2	moderate
	3	severe headache, incapacitating
Difficulty in sleeping	0	slept as well as usual
	1	did not sleep as well as usual
	2	woke many times, poor night's sleep
	3	could not sleep at all

AMS is determined as a total score of 3 or more following recent ascent to altitude, but only if headache and at least one other symptom is present (i.e. did not sleep as well as usual, mild fatigue and poor appetite scores 3 but is not AMS; similarly, a severe headache alone scores 3 and is also not AMS).
Reproduced with permission from Scrase et al. [69].

leaving the authors to conclude that the enhanced breathing stability in children was likely related to a lower apnoea threshold for CO_2.

In a more recent study by Bloch et al. [67], 48 healthy but non-acclimatised children and adolescents were taken to the same altitude research centre as used in the study of Kohler et al. [56]. The 20 girls and 28 boys (mean ± age; 13.7 ± 0.3 years) were assessed for AMS at serial time-points, 6, 18 and 42 h after arrival at the altitude station (3,450 m). Ascension to the station was considered rapid via a 2.5 h train journey. Using the Lake Louise

AMS questionnaire outlined in table 6, the prevalence rate of AMS in the children was 37.5%, with similar rates for the boys (39% or 11 of 28) and girls (35% or 7 of 20). With increasing time at altitude, occurrence of symptoms decreased significantly, with the majority of cases reported upon arrival at the centre (within the first few hours) and reaching their maximal effect in the evening of the first day's arrival. Unlike the previously cited study [56], no evacuation of any adolescent was required and five participants were provided with a single tablet of paracetamol to reduce the effect of headaches. Bloch and colleagues concluded that the prevalence of AMS appears to be lower in adolescents compared to adults where rates as high as 84% have been recorded [68]. However, it should be noted that physical exertion was rigorously standardised (defined as mild effort on the first and moderate on the second day) and it is unknown whether the more random variation in exercise intensity in 'real life' competitive settings would alter these findings.

Observational data on 9 healthy children (5 boys and 4 girls) aged between 6 and 13 years and their parents were collected during a trek from 1,300 to 3,500 m in Nepal, with a period of 9 days of acclimatisation at 3,500 m [69]. The children and their parents were tested at sea level, 1,500 and 3,500 m and after the acclimation period for a range of physiological measures, plus the Lake Louise classification for AMS [70]. Table 7 represents the data for the children and shows a similar cardiorespiratory response to altitude as that noted for adults.

It can be seen from table 7 that with continued exposure to altitude, increases in ventilation coupled with decreases in end tidal CO_2 and some recovery of oxygenation occurred. However, Scrase et al. [69] recorded wide inter-individual variability and this aspect requires further study. For the Lake Louise scores of AMS, although the children coped well with the trek, there appeared to be under, as well as over reporting of symptoms (table 7). This is most probably due to the lack of

validation of this scale in children, confirmed by a lack of agreement with more objective physiological and subjective measures recorded during the trek. Although some authors have highlighted this as an important issue to be resolved [71], the ethics and practicalities of conducting the research to resolve the problem are very difficult. Interestingly, with regard to the quality of sleep the general guidance for children less than 10 years was not to allow them to sleep above 3,000 m. Although Scrase and colleagues questioned the utility of the Lake Louise questionnaire, it did appear that the children could cope at this altitude and sleep was not unduly compromised. Based on the results of this study, Scrase and co-authors concluded that with healthy children, vigilant parents and a slow ascent, children as young as 6 years could be taken to altitudes of 3,500 m. However, it should be remembered that this conclusion is drawn from a sample of just 9 children who were accompanied by experienced trekkers and appropriate medical supervision. For further guidance on children at high altitude (including case reports on incidences of altitude illness), the reader is directed to the International Consensus Statement by the International Society for Mountain Medicine [71].

Application of Altitude Research on Performance Measures

The information presented thus far has focused largely on the development of AMS symptoms and not performance. Aerobic fitness, as assessed by a peak oxygen uptake (peak $\dot{V}O_2$) test to volitional exhaustion has been investigated in children at altitude [73]. At high altitude values for peak $\dot{V}O_2$ were 10–20% lower (35–45 ml $\cdot$ kg^{-1} $\cdot$ min^{-1}) than those values found at low altitude. The values for these Bolivian boys were similar to those of Ethiopian boys aged 10–12 years living at 3,000 m, ~40 ml $\cdot$ kg^{-1} $\cdot$ min^{-1}. Apart from lower maximal heart rates at high altitude compared to low

Table 7. Effect of altitude on vital signs, lung function and symptoms in children

	Sea level	Katamandu day 1	Phakding day 2	Namche Bazaar day 5	Namche (repeat) day 14
Altitude					
Metres	30	1,300	2,600	3,500	3,500
Feet	98	4,265	8,530	11,483	11,483
Barometric pressure, mm Hg	760	652	560	503	503
PiO_2, mm Hg	150	127	108	96	96
Equivalent FiO_2	0.21	0.18	0.15	0.13	0.13
Respiratory rate/min	21 (4)	NA	NA	23 (5)	22 (5)
Heart rate/min	78 (13)	86 (12)	89 (14)	99 (14)	98 (14)
BP, mm Hg systolic/diastolic	100 (8)/ 61 (7)	96 (7)/55 (12)	NA	98 (96)/57 (16)	
$etCO_2$, mm Hg	42.5 (2.8)	NA	NA	35.8 (2.5)	32.7 (1.8)
SpO_2, %	98.5 (0.9)	95.9 (1.05)	93.2 (2.2)	88.9 (2.4)	91.8 (1.5)
Overnight SpO_2, %	96.8 (0.8)	94.1 (1.8)	NA	85.8 (3.3)	NA
Lake Louise*					
Total score	1 (0–4)	1 (0–2)	1 (0–3)	0 (0–5)	NA
Headache	0 (0–1)	0 (0–1)	0 (0–2)	0 (0–1)	NA
Gastrointestinal	0 (0)	0 (0–1)	0 (0)	0 (0–1)	NA
Sleep quality	0 (0–1)	0 (0–1)	0 (0–1)	0 (0–1)	NA
Fatigue	0 (0–1)	0 (0–1)	0 (0–1)	0 (0–2)	NA
Dizziness	0 (0–1)	0 (0–1)	0 (0–1)	0 (0–1)	NA

Results are expressed as mean (SD) except for *Lake Louise score expressed as median (range). BP = Blood pressure (results only presented for seven children due to missing data at 3,500 m); $etCO_2$ = end-tidal carbon dioxide; FiO_2 = fractional inspired oxygen; PiO_2 = partial pressure inspired oxygen; SpO_2 = peripheral oxygen saturation. Reproduced with permission from Scrase et al. [69].

altitude (mean difference of 10 beats · min^{-1}), no other explanatory variables were measured to explain the lower peak $\dot{V}O_2$ scores. Fellmann et al. [73] speculated that one limiting factor could be the lower O_2 diffusion in the muscle through a reduced O_2 differential pressure gradient between the capillaries and mitochondria.

Some observations related to anaerobic performance have been documented and have been laboratory based. Several studies by a French group in collaboration with a research group in Bolivia (La Paz, altitude 3,700 m) have been published [72–74]. The first study relates to measures of anaerobic performance. Anaerobic performance was assessed using force-velocity and Wingate tests of 8 and 30 s duration, respectively. Bedu et al. [72] studied 148 boys (age range 7–15 years) of which 47 were Bolivian boys living at altitude and 101 were French boys living at low altitude (330 m). Maximal anaerobic power as assessed by the force-velocity test was similar between the high and low altitude boys. This observation has also been replicated in adult studies [75]. However, mechanical power output as determined from the 30-second Wingate test was significantly different between high and low altitude boys. The lower mean power output sustained by the high altitude dwelling boys was explained by the lower lactate production at high altitude and a lower aerobic contribution under chronic hypoxic conditions [76–78]. Finally, it was concluded that the increase in anaerobic performance with growth was not affected by altitude and chronic hypoxia with the rate of increase similar in low and high altitude dwelling boys. Maximal anaerobic power standardised according to body mass increased over 70% from age 7 to 15 years for both groups, similar to previous findings [79, 80]. However, what could not be determined was if boys at low altitude cycling maximally at high altitude would experience a lower power output and vice versa.

This was the purpose of the next study by Blonc et al. [74]. They studied 10 boys living at low altitude (330 m) and 15 boys at high altitude (3,700 m) from Bolivia. Each participant performed two Wingate anaerobic tests in random order, one with ambient air and 3–4 days later, one either in acute hypoxia for the boys resident at low altitude and one in acute normoxia for the boys resident at high altitude. No significant differences were found in peak power, findings similar to those in adult studies [81, 82]. This finding is unsurprising given peak power is attained within the first 5 s of the test, with ATP turnover supported largely by the phosphagens, ATP and CP, which are generally unaffected by hypoxic conditions. Interestingly, there were no significant differences in mean power, oxygen consumption and blood lactate when the low altitude residents performed the tests in hypoxic conditions or when the high altitude residents performed the test in normoxic conditions. The only significant difference found was a lower delta change in blood lactate (before and after the Wingate anaerobic test) in those boys living in altitude than those boys living at low altitude. Further work is required to elucidate the so-called lactate paradox [83]. Therefore, in pre-pubertal boys when oxygen fractions were manipulated to simulate acute hypoxia conditions for boys normally resident at low altitude or normoxic conditions in those normally resident at high altitude, anaerobic performance and the aerobic contribution during a 30-second maximal Wingate test was unaffected.

Relevance of Altitude Research to the Elite Young Athlete

For many coaches and their athletes, travelling to competitions at altitude above 2,500 m is infrequent. However, with increased access to international flights, training camps and youth international competitions, as well as holidays, it is a possibility. There is a distinct lack of data on the child's responses to hypoxic conditions which provide direct guidance for ascent to altitude. Therefore, coaches and athletes must prepare assiduously for events which take place at altitude. If an event is being held at 2,500 m or above there is an increased risk of young athletes experiencing altitude sickness. The importance of having a sports medic available cannot be over estimated. Within a large national sports organisation this should not be a problem. However, for some athletes and their coaches who perhaps do not have

Table 8. Summary of key guidelines for youngsters ascending to altitude

1	Children and their carers should be fully briefed on the symptoms of altitude illness prior to travel above 2,500 m and should know how to manage the illness
2	Prior to travel a full medical history of the athlete should be conducted
3	Educational sessions should be held for both carers and athletes related to not only knowing the symptoms of altitude illness but other factors related to altitude, e.g. cold and sun exposure, changes in appetite, sleep, energy levels and fatigue
4	When ascending it is wise to treat any symptoms as a sign of potential altitude illness
5	Altitude illness for children 8 years and above will present in a similar manner to adults
6	There should be a clear plan in the event of an emergency including ensuring full medical insurance is sufficient to cover all eventualities

Based on recommendations presented by the International Society for Mountain Medicine, 2001.

regular medical support, it is advised that access to medical help is sought. Table 8 summarises the International Consensus Statement for children at altitude and provides critical recommendations [71].

In summary, whilst there are no data to determine a safe absolute altitude for ascent in children, ascending above 2,500 m and remaining overnight for short durations increases the risk of altitude illness. This risk will be increased further if the athlete is already suffering from a pre-existing illness and greater caution is then advised. In all scenarios, it is advised that the coach and the support team seek medical advice. Although these recommendations are considered to be cautious, until further evidence is presented, a safety first approach to the young athlete at altitude is warranted.

Conclusions

The continued professionalisation of youth sports will undoubtedly lead to increased research opportunities to gather data on topics such as sleep patterns, jet lag and altitude. Currently, the extant data are largely descriptive and observational, as opposed to experimental. This is largely an outcome of ethical constraints of the topics covered in this chapter. It is clear that there are different physiological responses to sleep patterns in adolescents compared to children and adults. Therefore, it is not appropriate to directly transfer adult recommendations to adolescents. The effects of jet lag appear to produce similar symptoms in children as in adults, as do the effects of altitude and there is perhaps more scope, in the absence of substantial paediatric data, to use results from adult studies to make recommendations. However, in all cases I propose that published paediatric data be sought when compiling recommendations and implementing practice. Finally, it is important for sports science teams and medical practitioners not to treat children and adolescents as 'mini-adults', but to acknowledge them as individuals, uniquely different to adults.

67 Bloch J, Duplain H, Rimoldi SF, Stuber T, Kriemler S, Allemann Y, Sartori C, Scherrer U: Prevalence and time course of acute mountain sickness in older children and adolescents after rapid ascent to 3450 meters. Pediatrics 2009;123:1–5.

68 Murdoch DR: Altitude illness among tourists flying to 3740 meters elevation in the Nepal Himalayas. J Travel Med 1995;2:255–256.

69 Scrase E, Laverty A, Gavlak JCD, Sonnappa S, Levett DZH, Martin D, Grocott MPW, Stocks J: The young Everest study: effects of hypoxia at high altitude on cardiorespiratory function and general well-being in healthy children. Arch Dis Child 2009;94:621–626.

70 Roach RC, Bartsch P, Oelz O, et al: The Lake Louise acute mountain sickness scoring system; in Sutton Jr, Houston CS, Coates G (eds): Hypoxia and Molecular Medicine. Burlington, Queen City Press, 2003, pp 272–274.

71 Pollard AJ, Niermeyer S, Barry P, et al: Children at high altitude: an international consensus by an ad hoc committee of the international society for mountain medicine, March 12, 2001. High Alt Med Biol 2001;2:389–403.

72 Bedu M, Fellmann N, Spielvogel H, Falgairette G, van Praagh E, Coudert J: Force-velocity and 30-s Wingate tests in boys at high and low altitudes. J Appl Physiol 1991;70:1031–1037.

73 Fellmann N, Coudert J, Spielvogel H, Bedu M, Obert P, Falgairette G, van Praagh E: Physical fitness of children resident at high altitude in Bolivia. Int J Sports Med 1992;13:S92-S95.

74 Blonc S, Falgairette G, Bedu M, Fellmann N, Spielvogel H, Coudert J: The effect of acute hypoxia at low altitude and acute normoxia at high altitude on performance during a 30-s Wingate test in children. Int J Sports Med 1994; 15:403–407.

75 Di Prampero PE, Mognoni P, Veicsteimas A: The effects of hypoxia on maximal alactic power in man; in Brendel W, Zink RA (eds): High Altitude Physiology and Medicine. Springer, New York, 1982, pp 88–93.

76 Macek M, Vavra J, Benesova H, Radvansky J: The adjustment of oxygen uptake at the onset of exercise: a comparison between prepubertal boys and young adults. Int J Sports Med 1980;1: 75–77.

77 Williams CA, Ratel S, Armstrong N: The achievement of peak $\dot{V}O_2$ during a 90 s maximal intensity cycle sprint in adolescent children. Can J Appl Physiol 2005; 30:157–171.

78 Chia M, Armstrong N, Childs D: The assessment of children's anaerobic performance using modifications of the Wingate anaerobic test. Pediatr Exerc Sci 1997;9:80–89.

79 Armstrong N, Welsman JR, Williams CA, Kirby BJ: Longitudinal changes in young people's short-term power output. Med Sci Sport Exerc 2000;32:1140–1145.

80 Dore E, Bedu M, Franca NM, Van Praagh E: Anaerobic cycling performance characteristics in prepubescent, adolescent and young adult females. Eur J Appl Physiol 2001;84:476–481.

81 McLellan TM, Kavanagh MF, Jacobs I: The effect of hypoxia on performance during 30- or 45 s of supramaximal exercise. Eur J Appl Physiol 1990;60: 155–161.

82 Richalet JP, Marchal M, Lamberto C, Le Tong JL, Antezana AM, Cauchy E: Alteration of aerobic and anaerobic performance after 3 weeks at 6542 m (Mt Sajama). Int J Sports Med 1992;13:86.

83 Green HJ, Sutton J, Young P, Cymerman A, Houston CS: Operation Everest. II. Muscle energetics during maximal exhaustive exercise. J Appl Physiol 1989;66:142–150.

Assoc. Prof. Craig Williams
Children's Health and Exercise Research Centre
University of Exeter
Exeter EX1 2LU (UK)
Tel. +44 1392 724890, Fax +44 1392 724726, E-Mail c.a.williams@exeter.ac.uk

Armstrong N, McManus AM (eds): The Elite Young Athlete.
Med Sport Sci. Basel, Karger, 2011, vol 56, pp 171–186

Prevention of Sudden Cardiac Death in Young Athletes: Controversies and Conundrums

Thomas Rowland

Department of Pediatrics, Baystate Medical Center, Springfield, Mass., USA

Abstract
Strategies for preventing sudden cardiac death in young athletes are predicated on the assumption that: (1) these events reflect pre-existing, clinically silent heart disease, and (2) means for detecting these abnormalities on the pre-participation evaluation are both feasible and accurate. Recent controversy has surrounded both of these presumptions. Some evidence suggests that the myocardial hypertrophy accompanying sports training itself might serve as a substrate for fatal arrhythmias. As well, vigorous debate has arisen over the optimal content of the pre-participation evaluation, particularly regarding the inclusion of routine screening electrocardiograms. As the rarity of these fatal events does not lend itself to an experimental approach, such disagreements are not easily resolved. Consequently, it is expected that decisions regarding approaches to prevention of sudden death in athletes will be dictated largely by region-specific financial, political, and cultural factors. This chapter examines the aetiologies of sudden cardiac death in young athletes as well as the controversies surrounding the prevention of these tragedies.

Identifying an effective and feasible means of preventing sudden unexpected cardiac death in young athletes continues to confound physicians, exercise scientists, and sports officials alike. From a public health standpoint the magnitude of the problem is not great, with an annual incidence of 0.5–3.0 per 100,000 athletes [1, 2]. In any given year in the United States the chance of an adolescent perishing in an automobile accident is approximately 500 times that of an athlete dying during sports play. Still, the poignancy and public visibility of these fatalities has commanded a great deal of attention toward understanding their causes and best means of prevention.

Traditionally, young athletes who suffer unexpected sudden death during play are considered to harbour an unsuspected cardiac anatomic or electrophysiologic abnormality which (a) is clinically silent, and (b) predisposes to sudden death during vigorous exercise from myocardial ischaemia or electrical instability as a consequence of sympathetic stimulation and/or increased demands for myocardial perfusion. In this aetiologic model, then, the athlete's demise reflects the existence of an occult pre-existing cardiac condition. Efforts to prevent such deaths have consequently focused on an optimal means of detecting would-be athletes with such abnormalities in the pre-participation medical screening and disqualifying them from sports play. In large populations, however, the feasibility of effectively identifying all such athletes at risk through such an evaluation is highly problematic.

Table 1. Frequency of different forms of heart disease (in %) in three autopsy series of youths <35 years of age dying suddenly during sports training or competition

	United States (n = 134)	United Kingdom (n = 89)	Italy (n = 47)
Hypertrophic cardiomyopathy	36	14	2
Left ventricular hypertrophy/fibrosis	10	34	0
Right ventricular cardiomyopathy	3	11	26
Congenital coronary artery anomaly	19	7	15
Atherosclerotic coronary artery disease	2	7	21
Mitral valve prolapse	2	0	13
Ruptured aortic aneurysm	5	0	2
Anatomically normal heart	2	32	11[1]

[1] Abnormalities of the conduction system identified at autopsy.

Recent information has challenged the precepts of this traditional model and may alter approaches to preventing sudden cardiac death in the young athlete population. In this chapter, I will review these controversies in respect to the causes of these tragedies, the fatal mechanisms involved, and the most effective means of decreasing their frequency. The discussion will be limited to sudden cardiac death in athletes below 35 years of age; sudden death in older individuals during sports play or vigorous exercise is most frequently a consequence of atherosclerotic coronary artery disease, which is generally not a consideration in the younger athlete. This review will not consider cases of commotio cordis, the arrhythmic death in athletes occurring when struck in the chest.

Aetiology and Mechanisms

The forms of heart disease which are responsible for sudden death in young athletes are uncommon in the general population. Defining the frequency that each contributes to these events is critical for formulating preventive strategies, yet the relative incidences of these abnormalities in autopsy series have varied considerably according to geographical area.

Table 1 outlines findings in three autopsy reports of causes of sudden unexpected cardiac death in athletes less than 35 years old in the United States [3], Great Britain [4], and Italy [1]. In the US series, hypertrophic cardiomyopathy (HCM) was the most common, followed by congenital coronary artery anomalies and idiopathic left ventricular hypertrophy. In the Italian report, on the other hand, there was only a single athlete with HCM. Instead, arrhythmogenic right ventricular cardiomyopathy (ARVC) was found to be the most frequent cause, a disease that was seen in only 3% of the American series. The British report describes idiopathic left ventricular hypertrophy/fibrosis as the most common cause of death, while HCM and ARVC were responsible for 14 and 11% of the cases, respectively. In that series one-third of the cases had no anatomic cardiac disease at all, suggesting a possible role of disorders of electrical activity.

While variation in factors such as pathologic disease definitions, genetic effects, racial and gender demographics, and type of sport might contribute to these differences, it is important to recognise that each of these reports gathered data by different means. The American series is an assemblage of cases identified by newspaper accounts, a national registry, and informal communications and school reports, which is based on autopsy diagnoses of multiple examiners. The United Kingdom series was derived from cases sent to a specialist tertiary centre for cardiac pathology by coroners and pathologists throughout the country. These, then, can be assumed to represent 'troublesome' difficult-to-diagnose cases. Those hearts with easily identified pathology, such as severe HCM or obvious coronary artery anomalies, would presumably not be referred and therefore not included in the series.

The Italian report represents a prospective study of cases referred from the Veneto region of north-eastern Italy, whose population of entirely white residents number over four million. The cases in this report represent, like the British series, cases sent by pathologists and medical examiners to an institute of pathology at the University of Padua. It was not known how many cases of sudden death occurred during this time that were not referred for post-mortem examination. The extent that these reports define a true profile of causes of death in young athletes is therefore problematic. The authors suggested that requisite pre-participation screening in Italy (see below) might have identified cases of hypertrophic cardiomyopathy and prevented their appearance on this mortality list.

Such uncertainties not withstanding, these data do identify specific disease entities that need to be targeted in efforts to prevent sudden death in young athletes. An awareness of utility and feasibility of particular diagnostic approaches needs to be considered in light of particular findings and mechanisms for sudden death in each.

Hypertrophic Cardiomyopathy

HCM is a genetic disease of the heart muscle characterized by dramatic ventricular hypertrophy, particularly involving the interventricular septum. In severe cases, septal thickness may exceed 3–4 times that of normal individuals, with virtual obliteration of the left ventricular cavity during systole and varying degrees of sub-aortic stenosis. Its prevalence in the general paediatric population over 1 year of age is approximately 2–3 cases per million [5]. Its occurrence among athletes is not known. In series numbering 501 and 3,500 athletes in the United States [6] and Great Britain [7], respectively, no cases of HCM were found after diagnostic cardiac evaluation. In Italy, routine screening that included electrocardiogram and limited stress test uncovered 22 cases among 33,735 would-be athletes [8].

Patients with recognized HCM carry a significant risk for sudden death. In studies from tertiary referral hospitals, sudden death in children and adolescents with HCM occurs at a rate of 1–3% per year [5, 9, 10]. In a general population, the risk is presumably significantly lower. Ischaemia-invoked ventricular dysrhythmias are likely responsible for these fatal outcomes. Exercise may act as a trigger via increased sympathetic activity and levels of circulating catecholamines as well as augmented myocardial oxygen demands [11]. Most deaths do not, in fact, occur with vigorous exercise, but a disproportionate percentage (approximately 40%) do [12]. Consequently, patients known to have HCM are generally restricted from vigorous sports play.

Patients with HCM may experience episodes of dizziness, syncope, or chest pain, often provoked by exercise, but most are asymptomatic. In approximately 20–40% of cases, a history of another family member with HCM can be obtained. The physical examination in those with HCM is often deceptively benign and can be, in fact, completely normal. When left ventricular outflow tract obstruction is present a systolic murmur can often be heard along the left sternal border.

The electrocardiogram is abnormal in 90% of cases, typically demonstrating left ventricular hypertrophy, abnormal Q waves, or ST-T wave changes. Transthoracic two-dimensional echocardiography provides the definitive diagnosis, revealing asymmetric left ventricular hypertrophy with a septal thickness usually greater than 15 mm, a septal:free wall thickness ratio of >1.3, systolic anterior motion of the mitral valve, a small left ventricular chamber, and evidence of ventricular diastolic dysfunction. In some patients, a degree of left ventricular outflow obstruction is observed, though seldom severe.

Patients with HCM are usually initially treated pharmacologically (beta blockers, calcium channel blockers). Those with drug-resistant ventricular tachyarrhthymias may undergo insertion of an implantable cardioverter-defibrillator (ICD). Surgical options include myectomy and cardiac transplantation.

Coronary Artery Anomalies

During foetal development the orifices of the coronary arteries appear early on as endothelial buds at the base of the truncus. A misdirection in the course of these events results in an abnormal origin of either the right or left main coronary artery with take off from the wrong sinus of Valsalva and a variable course to connect up with the normal distal coronary branches and distribution. Most of these anomalous coronary origins are benign, but certain forms are distinctly pathologic and have long been recognised to pose a risk for sudden death, particularly in the young athlete.

As indicated in table 1, such anomalies are found at autopsy in a high percentage of cases of sudden death in athletes, regardless of geographical location. The most common abnormality in these series is the left coronary artery (LCA) arising from the right sinus of Valsalva, with a much smaller number of cases of the right coronary (RCA) arising from the left sinus. In early autopsy studies, the specific type of abnormality which appeared to be related to sudden death was when the anomalous main artery coursed between the aorta and main pulmonary artery on its way to attach to its normal peripheral branches.

The mechanism of sudden death in these cases was not clear. The two most popular hypotheses suggested were (1) compression of the aberrant vessel as it passed between the great vessels, which expanded with exercise, and (2) relative stenosis of the take off of the artery from the wrong sinus because of its acute angle of origin. This, it was proposed, might create a limitation of coronary flow that fails to meet the demands of augmented myocardial metabolism with exercise [13].

More recent investigations using intravascular ultrasound have shed new insights on this question [14]. These findings have identified a specific mode of coronary insufficiency in patients with these anomalies and pinpointed more specifically particular anatomic forms of anomalous coronaries that pose risk for sudden death.

After the main LCA takes off from the right sinus of Valsalva, it can pass anteriorly or posteriorly to the pulmonary artery or, as noted above, between the great vessels. In the latter case, it can course around the base of the aorta within its wall (intramural) or through the myocardium of the ventricular septum. Of these, the only variety which poses risk for sudden death in athletes appears to be the intramural coronary artery.

When viewed by intravascular ultrasound techniques, the reasons are evident. The orifice of the portion of the anomalous coronary artery that traverses within the aortic wall is narrowed. Moreover, it is ovoid rather than circular in nature and is compressed during each systole by the pulsatile action of the aorta. Under pharmacologic stimulation (dopamine, atropine) to mimic the effects of exercise, the vessel lumen narrows further, to as little of 10% of its normal area.

The true incidence of this particularly fatal course of the LCA in the general population and the risk of death to the athlete is not entirely clear. An echocardiographic study in a paediatric population of over 14,000 subjects revealed 24 with RCA from the left sinus and 6 with LCA from the right [15]. Of the latter, four had a course between the aorta and pulmonary artery. This would suggest a population incidence of less than 1:3,600 for potentially fatal coronary anomalies. Another investigation of children and adolescents demonstrated a similar incidence of anomalous origin of LCA from the right sinus of 1:1,100 [16].

Among sudden deaths during military training, an incidence of 21 cases of abnormal coronary artery origin per 6.3 million recruits has been reported (1:300,000) [17]. The incidence of sudden death from these anomalies in young athletes in the United States has been estimated as 1:650,000. It is likely, then, that even in athletes with a coronary artery with predisposing anatomy the risk of sudden death is small.

Unfortunately, serious coronary artery anomalies are typically silent. Persons with these abnormalities can experience angina, palpitations, dizziness, and syncope – particularly with exercise – but in most cases they are asymptomatic, and the initial presentation is sudden collapse and death during sports play. Why athletes should suddenly and unexpectedly succumb from their coronary artery anomaly, often after many years of uneventful training and competition, remains a mystery. In retrospect their physical examinations had been normal, and those who had previous cardiac testing showed no abnormalities as well. Basso et al. [18] described the clinical profile of 27 young athletes who died with a coronary artery arising from the wrong aortic sinus, all during or immediately following vigorous exercise. The majority (21) were LCA from the right sinus. Premonitory symptoms were reported in only 37%. Of those who had undergone previous cardiac assessment, all had a normal electrocardiogram (9 of 9) and exercise stress test (6 of 6).

With current high resolution echocardiographic equipment, an abnormal origin of a main coronary artery from the aorta can usually be diagnosed in the short axis (cross-sectional) view. Identification of coronary anomalies, does, however, require a skilled ultrasonographer and greater attention than is afforded by a quick screening echocardiogram. Other tests (trans-oesophageal echocardiography, magnetic resonance imaging (MRI), radionuclide angiography) can be supportive for the diagnosis, but coronary angiography remains the most definitive technique for outlining the origin and course of the coronary vessels. Anomalous coronary arteries are amenable to surgical repair by several surgical options.

Arrhythmogenic Right Ventricle Cardiomyopathy

In patients with ARVC, the muscle walls of this chamber are replaced by fat and fibrous tissue. The disease is inherited, with a family history in approximately half of cases. Ventricular involvement varies in a spectrum of mild to severe. Fatal ventricular tachyarrhythmias, triggered by adrenergic stimulation, serve as the most serious complication. The left ventricle is usually spared, and there is often no cardiomegaly as viewed on chest X-ray. Premonitory symptoms of syncope and palpitations are not uncommon.

The diagnosis can be suspected from the electrocardiogram, which shows widened QRS complexes in the right precordial leads with undulation of the ST segments (epsilon waves) as well as T wave inversion (although the latter is common in healthy young subjects). During episodes of ventricular tachycardia, a left bundle branch block pattern is typical. On echocardiogram the diagnosis is indicated by right ventricular enlargement, focal right ventricular wall motion abnormalities, and an echodensity of the ventricular anterior wall. Magnetic resonance imaging (MRI) often provides better views of the right ventricle, however, and is the best means of establishing the diagnosis. Placement of an ICD is common in those with life-threatening arrhythmias.

Electrical Disorders

In all series of sudden athlete deaths a certain percentage is reported in which no abnormality – cardiac or otherwise – can be found at autopsy. As it has been considered that all such fatalities occur in the setting of underlying pathology, it has been presumed that these cases reflect fatal arrhythmias associated with cardiac electrical abnormalities. These include the 'channelopathies' (long QT syndrome), Brugada syndrome, and catecholamine-induced ventricular tachycardia [19].

The former is frequently associated with a positive family history and symptoms of syncope and palpitations. The diagnosis is suggested by a prolongation of the QT interval, indicating delayed ventricular repolarisation, on the electrocardiogram. Exercise is a recognized trigger for fatal ventricular tachyarrhythmias. Brugada syndrome is a genetic disease caused by abnormalities in transmembrane sodium transport. ST elevations in the right precordial leads on the electrocardiogram are characteristic. Most arrhythmic events occur during rest or sleep instead of during exercise. Patients with catecholamine-induced ventricular tachycardia have a normal electrocardiogram at rest but can develop fatal arrhythmias with exercise. The diagnosis is usually made with exercise stress testing.

The 'Athlete's Heart' and Sudden Cardiac Death

When Henschen first described heart enlargement in cross country skiers by chest percussion in 1898, he concluded that this characteristic reflected the beneficial effects of sports training [20]. That the cardiomegaly, ventricular hypertrophy, and electrocardiographic changes seen in the 'athlete's heart' mimicked that of patients with heart disease was not lost on clinicians, however, and many interpreted such responses as maladaptive, putting the highly trained athlete at risk. Over the past century, in what can be best described as a massive 'natural experiment', the well-being of the many millions of athletes who have participated in sports has revised this opinion to consider the athlete's heart as a benign physiologic training response. Those cases in which athletes collapse and die during sports play, it has been assumed, can always be accounted for by one of the underlying diseases outlined above. Recently, the debate has re-surfaced, with increasing evidence that the hypertrophy associated with athletic training may be arrhythmogenic and bears certain shared genetic and metabolic features with that of patients with heart disease. Specifically, some have considered that training-induced ventricular hypertrophy might serve as a substrate for sudden unexpected cardiac death in young athletes.

Ventricular hypertrophy – expansion of size and protein content of individual myocytes – is a response to increased heart stress. The form of this change depends on the type of work imposed. Among patients with heart disease, needs for generation of greater pressure, as in those with ventricular outflow obstruction (such as aortic valve stenosis), the ventricular response is an increase in wall thickness without increase in chamber size (concentric hypertrophy). If, on the other hand, pumping a larger volume of blood is required, as with aortic valve insufficiency, ventricular remodelling involves chamber dilatation. In this case, wall thickening is mild (eccentric hypertrophy), serving to maintain normal wall stress according to the dictates of LaPlace's Law.

Initially, these hypertrophic responses to heart disease are compensatory and adaptive. Given sufficient time or disease severity, however, the physiologic overwork eventuates in myocardial dysfunction, along with signs and symptoms of congestive heart failure. Ventricular hypertrophy in patients with heart disease is associated with an augmented risk for serious ventricular tachyarrhthymias. For example, in hypertensive adults Ghali et al. [21] found that for every 1-mm increase in thickness of the ventricular septum was accompanied by a 2- to 3-fold risk of serious ventricular arrhythmias. Indeed, mortality in patients with heart failure is typically a direct consequence of episodes of ventricular tachycardia or ventricular fibrillation.

The altered electrical properties of the hypertrophied myocardium reflect an increase in the surface area of the sarcolemma as the myocyte expands. The most common electrophysiologic features of this change which appear to predispose to arrhythmias are (1) a prolonged action potential duration, and (2) regional delays in cell repolarisation.

These features in patients with heart disease can be compared with those observed with the 'athlete's heart'. Some degree of ventricular hypertrophy is observed in virtually all competitive athletes [22]. The pattern of ventricular response appears, at least in a general fashion, to mimic that of pathologic hypertrophy. Athletes who engage in sports characterized by increases in systolic blood pressure (weight-lifting, wrestling) often exhibit concentric hypertrophy, while those participating in events requiring sustained increased cardiac output (distance running, swimming) show eccentric hypertrophy with chamber enlargement. In sports typified by both strength and endurance (combined ventricular pressure and volume work), such as cycling and rowing, a combination of remodelling is observed (increased chamber size and exaggerated hypertrophy).

These observations trigger the obvious question: is the nature of the cardiac hypertrophy of the athlete identical to that of patients with heart disease? And more specifically, does the thickened myocardium of the athlete possess the same adverse electrophysiologic properties predisposing to fatal ventricular tachyarrhythmias as that of pathologic hypertrophy? The question bears considerable importance and has been the recent focus of considerable research activity as well as expert opinion.

Such considerations usually begin with the obvious observation that pathologic hypertrophy deteriorates myocardial function, while physiologic hypertrophy of athletes is characterized by superior ventricular performance. It might be argued, though, that this is simply a reflection of the volume of overwork being performed. Athletes stress myocardial function a few hours a day, while the ventricular work of patients with heart diseases must be sustained continuously, 24 h a day, 7 days a week, without a rest. This explanation is supported by the observation that athletes, who do participate in extremely sustained heart work, such as during competition in ultra-marathons, demonstrate transient evidence of depressed myocardial function afterwards [23].

Many biochemical and metabolic features, as well as gene triggers, are shared by physiologic and pathologic hypertrophy, but each also possess certain separate distinctive characteristic features [24–26]. The relevance of such studies to human athletes versus cardiac patients is not clear, however. The evidence comparing the two has been derived from animal rather than human studies in which physiologic hypertrophy is created by an intermittent volume overload (rats swimming or training on a treadmill) while pathologic hypertrophy is stimulated by a constant pressure overload (such banding the aorta).

In athletes, the electrical properties of the heart are clearly altered, as witnessed by their high incidence of electrocardiographic abnormalities [27]. For the most part these are benign and reflect augmented parasympathetic tone or increased ventricular size which accompany sports training sinus (bradycardia, first-degree heart block, left ventricular hypertrophy). However, there is growing evidence that trained athletes, as a group, exhibit an increased incidence of ventricular ectopy, including ventricular tachycardia, which are the forms of electrical activity that predispose to death in heart disease patients.

For example, Biffi et al. [28] found that 77% of 175 elite-level Italian athletes demonstrated ventricular ectopy on 24 h electrocardiogram recordings. More than 1000 premature ventricular contractions per day were found in 12%, and among these, one third showed couplets (paired ectopic beats). In the entire group, eight of the athletes (5%) had periods of non-sustained ventricular tachycardia. When athletes experience a period of detraining, ventricular hypertrophy diminishes, and so does the frequency of ventricular arrhythmias [29, 30].

In an 8 year follow-up study by Biffi et al. [31] there was no evidence that ventricular arrhythmias in otherwise healthy athletes forecasted sudden death. Among the 93% of subjects with a structurally normal heart, no fatalities were observed. This information has led to the conclusion that 'in the absence of cardiovascular abnormalities, even frequent ventricular arrhythmias [in athletes] appear to be benign. . . . [these arrhythmias] are common in trained athletes and in the absence of heart disease they do not convey adverse clinical significance' [32]. In fact, the alterations in autonomic activity that accompany athletic training – increased parasympathetic, decreased sympathetic activity – should be expected to decrease rather than increase risk for fatal ventricular rhythms. Multiple studies in dogs, for example, have demonstrated a training-induced increase in threshold of ventricular fibrillation to ischemic stress [33].

The report by Heidbüchel et al. [34] of fatal arrhythmias among highly competitive cyclists, however, has raised concern. A total of 46 elite-level athletes were referred to a cardiac centre in Germany because of findings of ventricular tachycardia on routine screening. Thirty six had experienced episodes of syncope or pre-syncope. High-normal or mild increase in left ventricular chamber size and thickness was considered compatible with the 'athlete's heart'. Sustained ventricular tachycardia was found in 37%, usually with a left bundle branch morphology, indicating a right ventricular origin. Diagnostic criteria for ARVC were present in 59%, with borderline findings of this abnormality in another 30%.

Nine subjects, all cyclists, died suddenly during follow-up (median 2 years), all during light or moderate physical activity but not sports competition. While these may have represented cases of ARVC, the authors were not convinced. They noted that MRI evidence of wall fat infiltration was generally absent, there was familial ARVC in only one case, and ARVC is very rare in the German general population. Their conclusion: 'We speculate that endurance sport by itself may also lead to RV structural damage that might not have developed without the activity. Long-lasting volume overload could be the mechanism leading to or contributing to the development of RV structural changes'. Whyte et al. have noted that in its early stages the differentiation of ventricular tachycardia from ARVC, with its adverse outcome, can be difficult to distinguish from more benign forms of right ventricular outflow tract tachycardia [35]. They reported a case of the latter in a female sprinter with right ventricular dysfunction which disappeared after resolution of her tachyarrhythmia.

So, is the athlete's heart – with its arrhythmogenic hypertrophy – responsible for episodes of sudden unexpected death? In particular, does it explain those significant number of fatalities in which the autopsy reveals simply 'left ventricular hypertrophy'? The experimental evidence at hand is not sufficient to answer the question. As for expert opinion, it depends upon to whom one is listening. According to Maron and Pelliccia [36], 'There is no evidence at present showing that athlete's heart remodelling leads to long-term disease progression, cardiovascular disability, or sudden cardiac death'. On the other hand, Hart [37] has contended that 'intensive athletic training is associated with a small but finite risk of sudden death, which may be a consequence of the cellular electrical changes of mild-to-moderate cardiac hypertrophy'.

An additional perspective has been added by a recent suggestion that many of the cases of sudden death in athletes may have been falsely diagnosed as hypertrophic cardiomyopathy [38]. This conclusion was based on the observation that several of the demographic features of athletes dying in this category are not consistent with those typically seen in the clinical disease of HCM in the general population. Moreover, instead, these characteristics share in common a propensity for ventricular hypertrophy.

Almost all reported cases of sudden death in athletes from hypertrophic cardiomyopathy have occurred in males, which cannot be attributed to gender-related sports participation rates. In a 10-year review of sudden death in US athletes, 55 of the 56 cases of HCM or 'probable HCM' occurred in males [39]. In the general population of patients with HCM there is no sex predilection.

Compared to its reported high frequency among fatalities in athletes, hypertrophic cardiomyopathy is not a prominent cause of sudden unexpected cardiac death during exercise in nonathletic populations. For example, in a report of 17 deaths during exertion among 1,606,167 American military recruits that occurred over a 20-year period, only 2 cases of HCM were found [40].

Despite a very large number of participants, sudden death on the athletic field appears to be rare in pre-pubertal children. HCM is well recognized in the general nonathletic paediatric population, however, as a harbinger of sudden death [5].

Sudden death from HCM is disproportionately higher in African-American athletes. In one series of 158 deaths in American athletes, African-Americans actually suffered death from HCM more often than Caucasians [41]. At the same time, there is no racial bias for HCM in the general population.

These observations are consistent with the conclusion that at least some of the deaths attributed to HCM might instead be outcomes of well-recognized triggers for ventricular hypertrophy (sports training, androgenic hormonal effects, and African-American race).

Diagnostic Considerations

Table 2 summarizes the effectiveness of various diagnostic approaches in detecting the principal causes of sudden cardiac death in young athletes. It is clear that, at least hypothetically, the great majority of at-risk athletes would be identified if they were to undergo a complete battery of such evaluations and tests. Certain economic, statistical, and logistical barriers, however, have precluded a universal endorsement of such an approach. The controversies surrounding just what should be included in a pre-participation assessment will be addressed in the next section.

One particular dilemma in such an evaluation arises in distinguishing mild forms of HCM from those athletes with exaggerated hypertrophy as a physiologic response to training. A ventricular septal thickness >16 mm would be expected to indicate HCM, while a measurement of <13 mm could safely be considered normal. But between the two values rests a 'grey zone', an overlap between the two conditions. Certain criteria have been offered to identify HCM in this situation, including a positive family history, asymmetric ventricular hypertrophy without chamber enlargement, left-ventricular outflow obstruction, abnormalities in diastolic filling, normal or low maximal oxygen uptake, and failure of hypertrophy to resolve after a period of detraining [42]. Still, such criteria are not infallible, and play or no-play decisions in such cases can pose a particular challenge for clinicians [43].

Genetic testing is available for HCM. A high incidence of false negative tests, however, reflects the fact that many gene mutations are involved,

Table 2. Effectiveness in disease detection among diagnostic measures for the principal causes of sudden unexpected cardiac death in young athletes

Disease	Symptoms	Family history	Physical examination	EKG	Echocardiogram
Hypertrophic cardiomyopathy	+	+	0	++++	++++
Coronary artery anomalies	+	0	0	0	+++
Right ventricular cardiomyopathy	+	++	0	+++	+++
Non-HCM cardiomyopathy	0	+	0	++	++++
Aortic aneurysm	0	+	+++	0	++++
Prolonged QT syndrome	++	++	0	++++	0

Graded from 0 = none to ++++ = high.

and genetic screening of athletes is not currently recommended [43].

A different perspective on screening is created if, as some evidence suggests, the hypertrophy of the 'athlete's heart' can predispose to fatal arrhythmias and sudden death. Now the problem is not that of identifying a pre-existing cardiac condition but rather one that develops in the course of sports training. The specific issue would be to identify the one athlete among a half million (the number of such deaths associated with ventricular hypertrophy) who is predisposed to such electrical instability.

Unfortunately, little is known regarding the electrophysiological response to sports training in humans – normal or abnormal. There is reason to expect, however, that certain portentous markers of arrhythmia risk might exist. Measures such as heart rate variability, T wave alternans, and T wave variability on the electrocardiogram have been shown to be predictive of arrhythmic death in patients with heart disease. Following this lead,

Heinz et al. [44] analyzed variation of T wave vectors on 24-hour electrocardiograms in elite swimmers and untrained controls. While values were normal for both groups, variability was significantly greater in the athletes.

The question of whether arrhythmia-related death can be due to training-induced hypertrophy in athletes remains presently unresolved. The extraordinary infrequency of such events, if they happen at all, will make this possibility extremely difficult to address either experimentally or epidemiologically.

Controversies in Pre-Participation Strategies

The question of how this information should be best translated into screening strategies has become embroiled in vigorous controversy. Opinions have ranged from those who suggest no screening at all [45] to recommendations for mandatory state-funded evaluations for all athletes which include non-invasive testing [46]. In terms of national policy, the major point of debate is between statements of that of the American Heart Association (AHA) in the United States, which limits screening to history and physical examination, and that of the European Society of Cardiology (ESC), which recommends, based on the 25-year screening experience in Italy, universal electrocardiograms in the pre-participation assessment. Such differences reflect varying cultural settings, social structures, and legal climate in these countries as well as, to some extent, separate philosophical approaches in screening goals. In this section the essentials of this controversy will be outlined. The issue is complex, and a full review would exceed space allotment. The reader is thus referred to more comprehensive reviews for further discussion [46–53].

American Heart Association Statement

The recommendation of an expert panel of the AHA in 2007 was that 'a complete and targeted history and physical examination designed to identify or raise suspicion of those cardiovascular diseases known to cause sudden cardiac death in young athletes represent the most practical screening strategy for implementation in large populations of young competitive sports participants in the United States. . . . The AHA panel does not believe it to be either prudent or practical to recommend the routine use of tests such as the 12-lead ECG or echocardiography in the context of mass, universal screening' [52]. The 'history' includes not only that of the athlete's prior symptoms but, considering the hereditary nature of many causes of sudden cardiac death, those of heart disease or sudden demise in first-degree relatives as well.

The panel acknowledged that this approach limits the detection of athletes at risk and addition of additional testing by ECG or echocardiography may enhance the identification of cardiovascular diseases in athletes (in one study, for instance, which reviewed 134 athletes' deaths in Minnesota, only 3% had a cardiac abnormality previously suspected by the history and physical examination alone [3]). However, these tests were not recommended for large-scale screening based on the following considerations:

Cost
The number of athletes that would require yearly screening in the United States has been estimated to be approximately 10 million. It is expected that the expense involved in creating and sustaining a formal national screening programme that would include history, examination, and electrocardiogram, plus secondary cardiac evaluation for suspected abnormalities, would reach USD 2.0 billion per year.

False-Positives
'Abnormal' electrocardiograms are observed in as many as 30% of healthy, well-trained athletes, a physiologic training manifestation of the 'athlete's heart'. Borderline abnormal left ventricular hypertrophy on echocardiography in the athlete's heart is not rare, and needs to be distinguished from HCM. Based on the large pool of athletes, an unacceptably high number of healthy athletes with such findings would require further cardiac evaluation. This would prove not only costly but would generate unnecessary emotional stress on athletes and their families. Such an approach also poses a risk of unjustified disqualification of athletes from sports play.

Lack of Medical Resources
The United States lacks a sufficient number of trained professionals who are qualified to interpret testing findings in large-scale screening programmes. Currently, guidelines for screening vary widely from state to state, and pre-participation screening is often the responsibility of individuals with limited levels of cardiovascular training and expertise. Currently, two-thirds of the states allow non-physician examiners, and one-third

permit screening of athletes by chiropractors or naturopathic practitioners.

This statement indicates, then, that in large-scale screening programmes the 12-lead electrocardiogram, echocardiogram, and exercise stress test should be reserved for secondary evaluation of athletes with abnormal findings on the medical history and physical examination. In cases of individual pre-participation evaluations, however, the inclusion of these tests (or not) was considered to be at the discretion of the examining physician.

European Society of Cardiology Statement

A consensus statement from the ESC in 2005 recommended that, besides the medical history and physical examination, a standard 12-lead electrocardiogram be performed as part of routine screening of young athletes [46]. This recommendation reflected the point of view that this test carries an acceptable cost-benefit ratio and is capable of detecting, on a screening basis, the majority of diseases (at least 60%) responsible for sudden deaths. Most particularly, the ECG is abnormal in 90% of individuals with HCM, who typically have an unremarkable history and physical examination.

The document was based on a 25-year experience of mandatory pre-participation screening in Italy whereby, according to law, all wishing to compete in sports activities must first undergo such an evaluation. In this programme, referral is made for secondary cardiac evaluation (including echocardiography) when certain ECG criteria are recognized (such as rhythm and conduction disturbances, ST-T wave changes, prolonged QT interval, increased ventricular voltages, and ventricular conduction delays).

In a 17-year report from one of the Italian testing centres, the frequency of screened athletes referred for secondary evaluation was 9%, and 621 of 33,735 (2%) of screened athletes were disqualified from sports play because of detected cardiovascular abnormalities [8]. The most common conditions found for denying participation were rhythm and conduction abnormalities (38%), systemic hypertension (27%), valvular diseases (21%), and HCM (4%).

Assessment of sudden cardiac deaths in athletes in that country revealed a decline from 3.6:100,000 before onset of the mandatory programme (1979–1981) to 0.4:100,000 in the late screening period (1993–2004) [47]. This 9-fold reduction was considered due mainly to a decline in deaths from cardiomyopathies. It is not clear if this reduction would have been obtained through the personal or family history as well as the physical examination and electrocardiogram.

Cost

The Italian programme screens approximately 3 million young athletes yearly. The estimated cost is EUR 30 per person (not including infrastructure expenses, secondary testing, and training courses for personnel). Screening for athletes less than 18 years of age is paid for by the National Health System, while in older persons, the athletes themselves or sports teams cover the cost.

False-Positives

In the Italian experience, the rate of false-positive electrocardiograms (normal athletes with positive screening findings who required secondary evaluation) has been reported to be less than 10% [47].

Medical Resources

Screening and interpretation of testing results is conducted by full-time specialists who have undergone 4 years of postgraduate residency training in sports medicine and cardiology.

Other Considerations

The Italian population-wide screening model supported by the ESC, then, is mandated by law, financed by the government, staffed by trained physicians, and requires an electrocardiogram. None of these features has been considered by many American experts as feasible within the setting of the current non-structured screening of athletes in the U.S. [52]. The controversy over this issue has involved a number of considerations:

- Much of this debate between the two approaches has focused on the sensitivity and specificity of the electrocardiogram to detect heart disease in large scale screening programs [54, 55]. Abnormal ECGs are common in diseases that predispose to sudden death, but similar changes are often observed as a consequence of benign physiologic responses to sports training, particularly in endurance athletes. In the United States, the reported 10–30% of collegiate and high school athletes who have abnormal electrocardiograms (particularly excessive left ventricular voltages) would require costly secondary evaluation (that might amount to nearly a million athletes per year).

In the Italian experience, however, the rate of false positive electrocardiograms has been reported to be only about 7%. It has been suggested that the incidence of false positives would be lower in young, middle school and high school populations in which ECG manifestations of the 'athlete's heart' would be expected to be less than in older highly-trained elite athletes.

- The annual rate of sudden unexpected cardiac death in Italian athletes fell from 3.6 per 100,000 to 0.43 per 100,000 over a 25-year period, a trend attributed to institution of the mandatory national screening programme, which includes the ECG. In real numbers, this amounted to 8 sudden deaths per year in 1979–1980, 3 deaths per year between 1982 and 1992, and 1 per year between 1993 and 2004. It has been noted that at the end of this experience the incidence of sudden death was similar to that reported in the United States without such a screening programme (0.5–0.9 per 100,000) [48]. Douglas [50] commented that 'the diseases responsible for causing sudden cardiac death might differ in this region [of Italy] with its higher prevalence of right ventricular cardiomyopathy and higher death rate present before the beginning of the screening programmes, possibly affecting these results and their 'translatability' to other countries'.

- European guidelines are more restrictive for sports participation in those with recognized heart disease compared to those in the United States [50]. This reflects an overall more liberal approach to risk: benefit considerations in respect to athletic play in the US. In Italy, screening programmes have excluded 2% of athletes from sports play, although only 0.2% demonstrated potentially fatal conditions. This had led to concern that 'adoption of such a programme in the United States would lead to an unacceptable number of disqualifications in athletes who may be at low risk for sudden cardiac death' [49].

Or No Screening at All?

To gain a full perspective of this issue, it is valuable to consider the point of view that, based on the above information, mandatory screening of athletes prior to competitive sports participation is not justified at all. Viskin [45] argued that the cost of large-scale screening would be justified if (1) sudden cardiac death in athletes was sufficiently common, (2) tests were available to accurately detect athletes at risk, and (3) disqualification from sports would eliminate or at least substantially reduce the mortality associated with potentially fatal cardiac abnormalities. He concludes that 'none of these criteria are actually met'. To wit:

- Although such events are highly publicized, the occurrence of an asymptomatic, apparently healthy athlete dying suddenly during sports play is extraordinarily rare.
- Medical history and physical examination alone have been demonstrated to be ineffect-

ive in preventing these tragedies. The electro-cardiogram and echocardiogram should be expected to more accurately identify athletes at risk. However, because of the large number of false-positives and unknown significance of borderline findings, these tests, even in expert hands, have limited predictive value. 'The sensitivity and specificity of the tests available for identifying those at risk are so low that too many athletes would have to be disqualified to prevent all sport-related arrhythmias.'

- Restricting patients with potentially fatal diseases from sports play may reduce the risk of sudden death, but not to a large degree. The majority of patients who die suddenly with HCM, for example, do not do so during vigorous physical activity. Vishkin estimates that a reduction in risk by disqualification from sports would realistically amount to no more than 50%.

He concludes that 'mandatory screening of all competitive athletes would save too few lives at too large a cost. If one is willing to accept that endurance sports per se entail a very small risk for death while providing profound personal satisfaction for the athlete, then endurance sports become no different from mountain climbing or car racing, activities that entail a small – albeit inevitable – risk for fatal accidents.'

Conclusions

It is apparent from this brief review that a good number of difficult questions surrounding the prevention of sudden cardiac death in young athletes remain unanswered. Why do the reported causes of sudden cardiac death in youth athletes differ in various geographical locations? What is the true incidence of these tragedies? Do arrhythmias associated with the hypertrophic response to sports competitors mean that risk is created by athletic training? Can sudden cardiac death in athletes be prevented? If so, how might this best be accomplished? Will there be a role in the future for genetic testing?

The rarity of these fatal events coupled with ethical and procedural barriers do not easily permit an experimental approach to answering these important queries. Decisions regarding how screening should be performed in particular geographical regions will presumably continue to be dictated by financial, cultural, social, and experiential factors which define a certain approach as appropriate for that area or nation.

References

1 Corrado D, Basso C, Rizzoli G, Schiavon M, Thiene G: Does sports activity enhance the risk of sudden death in adolescents and young adults? J Am Coll Cardiol 2003;42:1959–1963.

2 Van Camp SP, Bloor CM, Mueller FO, Cantu RC, Olson HG: Non-traumatic sports death in high school and college athletes. Med Sci Sports Exerc 1995;27:641–647.

3 Maron BJ, Shirani J, Poliac L, Mathenge R, Roberts WC, Mueller FO: Sudden death in young competitive athletes: clinical, demographic, and pathological profiles. JAMA 1996;276:199–204.

4 De Noronha SV, Sharma S, Papadakis M, Desai S, Whyte G, Sheppard MN: Aetiology of sudden cardiac death in athletes in the United Kingdom: a pathological study. Heart 2009;95:1409–1414.

5 Colan SD, Lipshultz SE, Lowe AM, Sleeper LA, Messere J, Cox GF, Lurie PR, Orav EJ, Towbin JA: Epidemiology and cause-specific outcomes of hypertrophic cardiomyopathy in children. Circulation 2007;115:773–781.

6 Maron BJ, Bodison SA, Wesley YE, Tucker E, Green KJ: Results of screening a large group of intercollegiate competitive athletes for cardiovascular disease. J Am Coll Cardiol 1987;10:1214–1221.

7 Basavarajaiah S, Wilson M, Whyte G, Shah A, McKenna W, Sharma S: Prevalence of hypertrophic cardiomyopathy in highly trained athletes. J Am Coll Cardiol 2008;51:1033–1039.

8 Corrado D, Basso C, Sciavon M, Thiene G: Screening for hypertrophic cardiomyopathy in young athletes. N Engl J Med 1998;339:364–369.

9   Decker JA, Rossano JW, Smith EO, Cannon B, Clunie SK, Gates C, Jeffries JL, Kim JJ, Price JF, Dreyer WJ, Towbin JA, Denfield SW: Risk factors and mode of death in isolated hypertrophic cardiomyopathy in children. J Am Coll Cardiol 2009;54:250–254.

10 Yetman AT, Hamilton RM, Benson LN, McCrindle BW: Long-term outcome and prognostic determinants in children with hypertrophic cardiomyopathy. J Am Coll Cardiol 1998;32:1943–1950.

11 Seggewiss H, Blank C, Pfeiffer B, Rigopoulos A: Hypertrophic cardiomyopathy as a cause of sudden death. Herz 2009;34:305–314.

12 Maron BJ, Roberts WC, Epstein SE: Sudden death in hypertrophic cardiomyopathy: a profile of 78 patients. Circulation 1982;65:1388–1394.

13 Cheitlin MD, MacGregor J: Congenital anomalies of coronary arteries. Role in the pathogenesis of sudden cardiac death. Herz 2009;34:268–279.

14 Angelini P: Coronary artery anomalies: an entity in search of an identity. Circulation 2007;115:1296–1305.

15 Lytrivi ID, Wong AH, Ko HH: Echocardiographic diagnosis of clinically silent congenital coronary artery anomalies. Int J Cardiol 2008;126:386–393.

16 Davis JA, Cecchin F, Jones TK: Major coronary anomalies in a pediatric population: incidence and clinical importance. J Am Coll Cardiol 2001;37:593–597.

17 Eckart RE, Scoville SL, Campbell CL, Shry EA, Stajduhar KC, Potter RN, Pearse LA, Virmani R: Sudden death in young adults: a 25-year review of autopsies in military recruits. Ann Intern Med 2004;141:829–834.

18 Basso C, Maron BJ, Corrado D, Thiene G: Clinical profile of congenital coronary artery anomalies with origin from the wrong aortic sinus leading to sudden death in young competitive athletes. J Am Coll Cardiol 2000;35:1493–1501.

19 Kauferstein S, Kiehne N, Neumann T, Pitschner H-F, Bratzke H: Cardiac gene defects can cause sudden cardiac death in young people. Dtsch Arzbetl Int 2008;106:41–47.

20 Rost R: The athlete's heart: What did we learn from Henschen, what Henschen could have learned from us! J Sports Med Phys Fitness 1990;30:339–346.

21 Ghali JK, Kadakia S, Cooper RS, Liao Y: Impact of left ventricular hypertrophy on ventricular arrhythmias in the absence of coronary artery disease. J Am Coll Cardiol 1991;17:1277–1282.

22 Pelliccia A, Maron BJ: Outer limits of the athlete's heart, the effect of gender, and relevance to the differential diagnosis with primary cardiac diseases. Cardiol Clin. 1997;15:381–396.

23 Shave R, George K, Whyte G, Hart E, Middleton N: Postexercise changes in left ventricular function: the evidence so far. Med Sci Sports Exerc 2008;40:1393–1399.

24 Wikman-Coffelt J, Parmley WW, Mason DT: The cardiac hypertrophy process. Analyses of factors determining pathological vs. physiological development. Circ Res 1979;45:697–707.

25 Lips DJ, de Windt LJ, van Kraaij, Doevendans PA: Molecular determinants of myocardial hypertrophy and failure: alternative pathways for beneficial and maladaptive hypertrophy. Eur Heart J 2003;24:883–896.

26 Dorn GW: The fuzzy logic of physiological cardiac hypertrophy. Hypertension 2007;49:962–970.

27 Holly RG, Shaffrath JD, Amsterdam EA: Electrocardiographic alternations associated with the hearts of athletes. Sports Med 1998;25:139–148.

28 Biffi A, Maron BJ, Di Giacinto B, Porcacchia P, Verdile L, Fernando F, Spataro A, Culasso F, Casasco M, Pelliccia A: Relation between training-induced left ventricular hypertrophy and risk for ventricular tachyarrhythmias in elite athletes. Am J Cardiol 2008;101:1792–1795.

29 Maron BJ, Pelliccia A, Sparito A: Reduction in left ventricular wall thickness after deconditioning in highly trained Olympic athletes. J Am Coll Cardiol 1998;32:1881–1884.

30 Biffi A, Maron BJ, Verdile L: Impact of physical deconditioning on ventricular tachyarrhythmias in trained athletes. J Am Coll Cardiol 2004;44:1053–1058.

31 Biffi A, Pelliccia A, Verdile L, Fernando F, Spataro A, Caselli S, Santini M, Maron BJ: Long-term clinical significance of frequent and complex ventricular tachyarrhythmias in trained athletes. J Am Coll Cardiol 2002;40:446–452.

32 Giada F, Barold SS, Biffi A, et al: Sport and arrhythmias: a summary of an international symposium. Eur J Cardiovasc Prev Rehabil 2007;14:707–714.

33 Billman GE: Cardiac autonomic neural remodeling and susceptibility to sudden cardiac death: effect of endurance exercise training. Am J Physiol 2009;287:H1171-H1193.

34 Heidbüchel H, Hoogsteen J, Fagard R, Vanhees L, Ector H, Willems R, Van Lierde J: High prevalence of right ventricular involvement in endurance athletes with ventricular arrhythmias. Eur Heart J 2003;24:1473–1480.

35 Whyte GP, Stephens N, Senior R, Peters N, O'Hanlon R, Sharma S: Differentiation of RVOT-VT and ARVC. Med Sci Sports Exerc 2008;40:1357–1361.

36 Maron BJ, Pelliccia A: The heart of trained athletes: cardiac remodeling and the risks of sports, including sudden death. Circulation 2006;114:1633–1644.

37 Hart G: Exercise-induced cardiac hypertrophy: a substrate for sudden cardiac death in athletes? Exp Physiol 2003;88:639–644.

38 Rowland T: Sudden unexpected death in young athletes: reconsidering 'hypertrophic cardiomyopathy'. Pediatrics 2009;123:1217–1222.

39 Mueller FO, Cantu RC, Van Camp SP: Catastrophic Injuries in High School and College Sports. Champaign, Human Kinetics, 1996, pp 23–29.

40 Phillips M, Robinowitz M, Higgins JR, Boran KJ, Reed T, Virmani R: Sudden death in Air Force recruits. JAMA 1986;256:2696–2699.

41 Maron BJ, Carney KP, Lever HM: Relation of race to sudden cardiac death in competitive athletes with hypertrophic cardiomyopathy. J Am Coll Cardiol 2003;41:974–980.

42 Cheng TO: Hypertrophic cardiomyopathy vs. athlete's heart. Int J Cardiol 2009;131:151–155.

43 Scharag J, Kindermann W: Pitfalls in the differentiation between athlete's heart and hypertrophic cardiomyopathy. Clin Res Cardiol 2009;98:465–466.

44 Heinz L, Sax A, Robert F, Urhausen A, Balta O, Kreuz J, Nickenig, Ocklenburg R, Schwab JO: T-wave variability detects abnormalities in ventricular repolarization: a prospective study comparing healthy persons and Olympic athletes. Ann Noninvasive Electrocardiol 2009;14:276–279.

duration and frequency. It is important that the education of trainers and coaches is taken into account [13] and vital that coach education curricula include injury prevention. Information and education of the parents and the young athletes themselves should also be reinforced. Only an uninjured athlete is able to perform at his/her best.

The level of competition, type of sport, and standard of the injury surveillance system may have an effect on the incidence of injuries. At present, few studies are available to evaluate the long-term health outcomes of youth sports injury [14]. In this chapter, we begin with an overview of the musculoskeletal system of the elite child athlete, germane to injury; review types of sports injuries in the young and outline some sport injury prevention concepts which are applicable to young athletes.

Musculoskeletal System of the Young Athlete

An appropriate knowledge of the growing musculoskeletal system is needed to understand children's injuries. Indeed, the growing musculoskeletal system has typical peculiarities in comparison with the musculoskeletal system of the adult. Tendons and ligaments are relatively stronger than the epiphyseal plate, and considerably more elastic. Hence, in severe trauma, the epiphyseal plate, being weaker than the ligaments, gives way [15, 16]. Growth plate damage is more common than ligamentous injury [3]. Bones and muscles in children present increased elasticity and heal faster [17]. Around the period of peak linear growth, adolescents are prone to injuries because of imbalance in strength and flexibility and changes in the biomechanical properties of bone. As bone stiffness increases and resistance to impact diminishes, sudden overload may cause bones to bow or buckle. Physiological loading is beneficial for the skeleton, but excessive strains may produce serious injuries to joints [18]. High-intensity training can inhibit bone growth,

however, low-intensity training can stimulate it [19]. Up to puberty, muscle strength is similar in girls and boys, and adaptive changes to sport activity have been reported [20, 21]. Injuries in young athletes may result in progressive permanent effects as the skeleton is growing, affecting the bone and soft tissues [11]. Growth plate disturbances may result in limb length discrepancy, angular deformity or altered joint mechanics, and marked long term disability [22]. Also, as noted by Falk and Dotan [23], children produce more heat relative to body mass, have a low sweating capacity, and also tend not to drink enough compared with adults. This may produce heat exhaustion more promptly than in adults, especially if the sport activity is performed in hot climates. This may also result in an increased number of injuries [20].

Sports Injuries in Young Athletes

Physeal Injuries and Growth Disturbance

The epiphysis is located at the end of a long bone. The epiphyseal growth plate is usually called the physis in the long bones, and is a pressure growth plate. The apophysis, on the other hand, is a traction physis [22], and is located at the site of attachment of major muscle tendons to bone. The apophysis is subjected primarily to tensile forces. The apophyses contribute to bone shape but not to longitudinal growth. Although a sport injury may involve the apophyseal growth plates, it will not produce disruption of longitudinal bone growth [22].

Epiphyseal growth plates are mainly subjected to compressive and, at times, shearing forces. The process of endochondral ossification depends on the health of the growth plate [22, 24]. Growth disturbance can be a consequence of injuries to the epiphyses and their associated growth plates. These are weaker areas and are therefore predisposed to injury. Five types of injury of the epiphyseal plates have classically been described [25].

Type I injury is complete separation of the epiphysis from the metaphysic, without any bone fracture. In this type of injury, the germinal cells of the growth plate are separated in the epiphysis, and the calcified layer is located in the metaphysis. In type II injury, the most common, the line of separation is placed along the growth plate, then out through a portion of the metaphysis, producing a triangular-shaped metaphyseal fragment which has been described as the Thurston-Holland sign. Type III injury is intra-articular. It usually extends from the joint surface to the weak zone of the growth plate, and then along the plate to its periphery. Type IV injury extends from the joint surface through the epiphysis, across the full thickness of the growth plate and through a portion of the metaphysis, producing a complete split. In type V injury, the growth plate is compressed, and longitudinal growth is compromised.

Types I and II injuries have good prognoses because germinal cells usually remain with the epiphysis, and circulation is not impaired, even though there is an associated risk of growth impairment [26, 27]. In type III injuries, the prognosis is good if the blood supply in the separated portion of the epiphysis is not disturbed and there is no displacement of the fracture. If damage of the joint surface is present, surgery is necessary. Surgery is needed in type IV injuries. Anatomical reconstitution of the joint surface is necessary, and the growth plate must be perfectly aligned. Type IV injuries have a poor prognosis unless the articular surface and the growth plate are carefully realigned. At the time of injury, the diagnosis of Salter V injury can be difficult. Given the nature of the injury, growth can be disturbed, and this may become evident only later. The diagnosis by radiographs of physeal injuries can be challenging. However, if there is clinical suspicion of an injury, protection of the limb with a cast and repeat radiographs and examination after 2 weeks should be performed [28].

Unfortunately, case reports and case series data are the main source of knowledge about the frequency of acute sport-related physeal injuries. A systematic review of the frequency and characteristics of growth plate injuries affecting children and youth shows that 38.3% of 2,157 acute cases are sport related, and, among these, 14.9% are associated with growth disturbance [22]. These injuries occur in a variety of sports, although football is the sport most often reported. Berson et al. [29] reviewed 24 patients with distal tibial growth disturbance. The author classified disturbances as physeal bar (prior to deformity), angular, linear or combined deformities. Treatment consisted of osteotomy in 14 patients, epiphyseodesis in 7, excision of bony bar in 2, and observation in 1 patient.

Angular and linear deformities presented at an average 46 months (range 12–120 months) and physeal bars at an average 14 months (range 6–25 months) after injury. Patients with a delay in presentation of growth disturbance greater than 24 months had angular deformities in 92% of the cases, compared with 33% in children presenting at less than or at 24 months. Treatment based on type of deformity, age at time of injury, and growth remaining was considered successful in 83%. Patients with angular or linear deformities were more likely to present late, have high energy injuries, be males, and have Salter-Harris types IV and V injuries.

In a retrospective study, Eid et al. [30] reported a series of 151 injuries involving the distal femoral physis. The average age at the time of injury was 12.3 years. Patients were followed for an average of 8.2 years. The complications encountered were not insignificant and the rate of satisfactory outcomes was relatively low (64.9%). The juvenile age group was the most commonly affected. Salter–Harris type II injuries predominated (43.0%), and they did not have a good prognosis as previously suggested. Symptomatic knee ligamentous laxity was found in 12 patients (7.9%). Compartment syndrome had occurred in two patients (1.3%).

The authors concluded that children with a physeal injury of the distal femur should be followed for several years after injury, and preferably until skeletal maturity. The surgeon should always have a high index of suspicion for compartment syndrome. Physeal injuries of the distal femur, and especially Salter and Harris type II, should be reduced anatomically and fixed well. See table 1 for an overview of the extant literature on physeal injuries [31–39].

Length discrepancy, angular deformity, or altered joint mechanics can be caused by disturbed physeal growth resulting from an injury. This may result in long-term disability [22]. There are no precise data about incidence or long-term health outcome of physeal injuries in youth sports.

Apophyseal Injuries and Growth Disturbance

A traction epiphysis is called an apophysis, and is mainly subjected to tensile forces. It is the growth cartilage site where a tendon inserts onto the growing bone [48]. An apophysis is also responsible for peripheral (non-longitudinal) growth of a bone, and is a secondary ossification centre [49]. Acute and chronic injuries of the apophyses usually are not associated with defects of longitudinal bone growth. The anatomy of the apophysis and epiphysis are similar [50], but the growth rate of the apophysis is slower than that of the nearby epiphyseal plate [48, 51]. This could be caused by the increased number of collagen fibres in the apophysis because of the tensile forces exerted on this structure [48]. Overuse apophyseal conditions typically affect skeletally immature patients [48, 52]. Apophyseal injuries are common in sport given that intensive work outs may generate pathological changes in the apophysis [53].

A common pitfall is the radiographic overestimation of chronic apophyseal injuries [54]. Usually, apophyseal injuries are not associated with growth disturbance, even though angular malalignment can be a residual drawback of these injuries, which tend to resolve without growth complication in the short-term. Some studies report stress-related premature partial or complete apophyseal closure [14]. Painful ossicles in the distal patellar tendon may follow an Osgood-Schlatter lesion. These ossicles are rarely symptomatic, but require surgical management. Other sequelae of an Osgood-Schlatter lesion are a permanent bump, or a displaced avulsion fracture of the tibial tubercle [14]. Increased forces imposed by overuse activities may cause fragmentation or separation of the apophysis. These could be considered adaptive changes to physical stress, and commonly are not disabling [14].

Spine Pathology

Young gymnasts and divers are exposed to overuse and acute spinal injuries. Damaging effects such as repetitive microtrauma and/or acute macrotrauma may be revealed by plain radiography. Damage to the pars interarticularis resulting in spondylolysis or spondylolysisthesis, discal pathology, and abnormalities of the vertebral endplates and vertebral ring apophyses of the thoracolumbar spine are examples of spinal injuries in young athletes [55–65]. Table 2 provides a summary of the available work on spine pathology in young athletes and a discussion of key studies follow.

Foster et al. [59] tested 82 high-performance young male fast bowlers in cricket (mean age 16.8 years). Eleven percent of the players sustained a stress fracture to a vertebra(e) (L4 to S1), and 27% sustained a soft tissue injury to the back. Morita et al. [63] investigated 185 adolescents under the age of 19 years with spondylolysis. All but 5 were active in sport (soccer, baseball, volleyball, basketball, athletics, judo). The pars defect was classified into early, progressive and terminal stages. Of the 346 pars defects in 185 patients, 39.6% were early, 29.5% progressive and 30.9% in the terminal stages. Conservative management produced healing

Table 1. Physeal injuries and growth disturbance

Author	Type of injury	Age	Sport	Results
Landin et al. [40]	65 physeal ankle fractures (59 Salter-Harris 111 and IV lesions of the medial malleolus, Tillaux fractures, and triplane fractures)	3–16 years	Not reported	Not reported
Lombardo et al. [41]	34 fractures through the distal femoral epiphyseal plate followed Non-displaced: 8 Type. Displaced, reduced 8, 1 Type I; 3 Type II; 2 Type III; 2 Type IV Displaced, not reduced: 8 type II; 3 type III; 1 type IV	Non-displaced 10 years Displaced, reduced 10 years Displaced, not reduced 11 years	Skating, football, bicycle	Limb-length discrepancy of 2.0 cm or more occurred in 36% and varus or valgus deformity in 33%
Hynes et al. [42]	26 patients 18 Salter-Harris type II and 8 type III fractures	5–15 years	Not reported	21 patients showed a regular "normal" pattern of line and healed with no deformity. 3 patients had medial physeal arrest revealed by abnormal lines. 2 had a minor central physeal arrest without subsequent deformity.
Nenopoulos et al. [43]	83 physeal and epiphyseal injuries of the distal tibia with intra-articular involvement	11–14 years	Not reported	Varus deformity, 10°–15° in relation to the normal opposite leg, 4 patients 1 patient had painful limitation of ankle joint movement; 2 patients had overgrowth of the medial malleolus with no functional impairment
Berson et al. [29]	24 patients with growth disturbance following distal tibial physeal fractures (12 SH2, 2 SH3, 7 SH4, and 3 SH5 distal tibial physeal fractures)	3–15 years	Not reported	Patients with a delay in presentation of growth disturbance greater than 24 months had angular deformities in 92% compared with 33% in children presenting less than or at 24 months
Goldberg et al. [26]	53 cases of fractures of the distal tibial epiphysis	5–16 years	Football, basketball, skiing, gymnastic, skateboarding	

Author	Type of injury	Age	Sport	Results
Ilharreborde et al. [44]	20 patients with Salter-Harris type 2 distal femoral injuries	8–15 years	4 sports-related accidents (ski, soccer, judo)	70% of complications Epiphysiodesis (12), femoral over-lengthening (1) or associated loss of knee motion (5)
Eid et al. [30]	151 injuries involving the distal femoral physis Salter–Harris type I 39, type II 65, type III 19, type IV 22, type V 6	Average age 8.2 years	Not reported	Shortening (38.4%), angular deformity (51.0%), loss of knee joint motion (28.5%), ligamentous laxity (13.9%), thigh atrophy (27.8%)
Stephens et al. [45]	20 patients with fractures of the distal femoral epiphyseal cartilage	10–14 years	Not reported	5 of 15 SHI resulted in shortening which averaged 2.3 cm
Cannata et al. [46]	63 lesions to the distal physis of the forearm bones in 157 patients 14 type 1A, 4 type 1C, 84 type 2A, 13 type 2B, 17 type 2C, and 25 type 2D	5–17 years	Not reported	Shortening (2) open and subsequently infected lesions as well as in 5 uncomplicated lesions of the 157 distal radial physeal injuries (4.4%), and in 3 of the 6 distal ulnar physeal injuries (50%). 38 additional patients had radioulnar length discrepancy that ranged from 2 to 9 mm, and 53 patients had styloid nonunion, but all of them were asymptomatic
Barmada et al. [32]	92 fractures: 8 (8.5%) medial malleolar (SH III and IV) injuries, 19 triplane fractures (21%) 14 Tillaux fractures 45 SH II fractures	Medial malleolar average age 12.6 years Triplane fractures average age 14.0 years Tillaux fractures average age 14.8 years	Football, basketball, soccer, biking	Twenty-five fractures (27.2%) were complicated by PPC (premature physeal closure) SH III and IV (medial malleolar type) fractures resulted in the highest percentage of PPC by fracture type (38%) SHI and II resulted in PPC in 36% of cases, followed by triplane fractures (21%) and Tillaux fractures (0%)
Krueger-Franke et al. [47]	85 patients with epiphyseal fractures of the lower extremity 85 epiphyseal fractures 30 were SalterHarris type I injuries, 25 type II, 8 type III and II were type IV fractures, while II were avulsion fractures	4–17 years	Soccer, skiing	Complications were documented in 9 instances, including 3 leg length discrepancies, 4 axis deviations. one avascular necrosis of the femoral head and one case of osteomyelitis, of which 6 required corrective surgery

Table 2. Spinal injuries in young athletes

Author	Type of injury and patients	Age	Sport	Results
Annear et al. [55]	20 former fast bowlers, spondylolysis, spondylolisthesis and degenerative change	34–68 years	Bowlers (cricket)	Fast bowlers are noted to have an increased incidence of spondylolysis (20%) There was a high incidence of radiological thoracolumbar degenerative facet joint and disc disease in former fast bowlers
Morita et al. [63]	185 adolescents with spondylolysis.	6–18 years	Football, basketball, soccer, volleyball, baseball, athletics, judo	Of the 346 pars defects in 185 patients, 39.6% were early, 29.5% progressive and 30.9% in the terminal stages Conservative management produced healing in 73.0% of the early, 38.5% of the progressive and none of the terminal defects
Foster et al. [59]	82 high-performance young male fast bowlers Spine injuries	15–22 years	Bowlers (cricket)	Eleven percent of the players sustained a stress fracture to a vertebra(e) (L4 to S1), while 27% sustained a soft tissue injury to the back
Dixon et al. [57]	42 male and 74 female elite (artistic) gymnasts Spondylolysis	Males 12–22 years Females 9-19 years	Gymnastic	Prevalence of spondylolysis 9.5% for female and 7.1% for males Spondylolysis affected 8 females with 10 pars defects (incidence 10.8%)
Semon and Spengler [66]	506 consecutive college football players 135 (27%) had low-back pain	Not reported, College-aged players	Football	12 cases of lumbar spondylosis were observed (21%)
Jackson et al. [61]	100 young female gymnasts engaged in high-level competition	6–24 years	Gymnastic	The incidence of pars interarticular defects was 11%; 6% had spondylolisthesis
McCarroll et al. [66]	145 freshman players	Not reported, College aged players	Football	15.2% of the defect was found than exists in the general population Only 2.4% of these players developed the problem in college
Hardcastle et al. [60]	24 fast bowlers, selected for special training in Western Australia	18–24 years	Cricket	Pars interarticularis defects were diagnosed in 54% and intervertebral disc degeneration in 63%

in 73.0% of the defects classified to be at an early stage, in 38.5% of those classified to be at a progressive stage, and in none of the defects classified to be at the terminal stage. Clearly, early diagnosis is important.

Dixon et al. [57] retrospectively studied 42 male and 74 female elite (artistic) gymnasts regarding the prevalence of spondylolysis. Of these patients, 44 females and 21 male gymnasts suffered from low back pain. Ten of these symptomatic patients had radiographically confirmed spondylolysis. Another 22 gymnasts were radiographically normal when investigated for low back pain. The incidence of spondylolysis per gymnast while on a scholarship was 9.5% for females and 7.1% for males.

Semon and Spengler [66] studied the records of 506 consecutive college football players over an 8 year period. Of these athletes, 135 (27%) had low-back pain. Because of persistent low-back symptoms, 58 players had roentgenograms of the lumbosacral spine, and 12 cases of lumbar spondylosis were observed (21%). From the 58 players for whom roentgenograms were available, two groups were compared with respect to time lost from games and practices. One group (n = 8) had low-back pain complaints with lumbar spondylosis. The randomly selected control group (n = 12) had low-back pain with no evidence of spondylolysis on roentgenograms.

At present, few studies are available in the literature about the late sequelae of sport participation. Spondylolysis or spondylolisthesis are associated with certain types of sport which are characterized by extreme hyperextension and rotation of the lumbar spine. For example, gymnastics and ballet, weight-lifting, wrestling, football, swimming and some light athletics [14, 55].

Morita et al. [63] reported elongation of the pars interarticularis as the pars defect progressed: this is likely to be a consequence of the defect in the adolescent rather than a contributing cause.

McCarrol et al. [65] evaluated prospectively the incidence of lumbar spondylolysis and spondylolisthesis in 145 freshman football players who were followed through their careers from 1978 to 1983. Even though a higher percentage (15.2%) of the defects was found than in the general population, only 2.4% of these players developed the problem in college.

Annear et al. [55] examined 20 former fast bowlers to determine the incidence of spondylolysis, spondylolisthesis and degenerative change. Fast bowlers are noted to have an increased incidence of spondylolysis. In this series, there was a high incidence of radiographically evident thoracolumbar degenerative facet joint and disc disease in former fast bowlers.

Hardcastle et al. [60] studied a group of 16- to 18-year-old fast bowlers, identifying a high incidence of back pain, always associated with a radiographical abnormality. Pars interarticularis defects were diagnosed in 54%, and intervertebral disc degeneration in 63%.

A possible relationship has been hypothesized between back pain and the spinal abnormalities observed in young athletes [55, 57, 58, 60, 61, 65, 66]. However, there is no evidence about the long-term effects of spinal trauma in athletes.

Knee Injury and Osteoarthritis

There is no definitive evidence in the literature about the relationship between acute knee injuries during adolescence and osteoarthritis developed in adulthood. Nevertheless, in a long-term follow-up of young athletes with meniscus surgery, more than 50% of subjects presented knee osteoarthritis [67].

Anterior cruciate ligament (ACL) injury is common in young athletes, but little is known about the effect of age as a risk factor for ACL injury because of a lack of age-related exposure studies. Regardless of management, athletes who suffered an ACL injury usually retire from active sports at a higher rate than athletes without this injury.

Long-term follow-up studies showed that 12–20 years after knee injury (meniscus or ACL) more than 50% of those injured will experience knee osteoarthritis compared to 5% in the uninjured population [2, 67]. Hence, it is reasonable to suggest that proper management of knee injuries in childhood or adolescence may reduce future impairments.

Dislocations

Dislocations in adolescents are typically traumatic. Glenohumeral dislocation is uncommon prior to closure of the growth plate. Recurrence is highly likely due to age and the traumatic nature of the injury [68]. Soft tissue injuries are commonly associated with shoulder dislocation, especially affecting the rotator cuff and biceps tendon. An excessive throwing action in sports such as baseball may damage the glenoid labrum. Elbow dislocation is common in gymnastics and football, and can be associated with fractures of the medial epicondyle of the humerus. Also, fractures of the neck of the radius or injury to the median or ulnar nerve may accompany elbow dislocation.

In young athletes, shoulder dislocations are usually posterior or posterolateral. Emergency reduction is required at all ages, and active rehabilitation encouraged. The return to sport activities is reasonable when the child has regained full range of movement, which is likely after 8–12 weeks.

A twisting injury of the knee is a common cause of patellar subluxation or dislocation. The typical mechanism of injury is that the femur is twisted medially with the foot planted on the ground. A direct trauma may also cause dislocation [20]. Patella alta predisposes to patellar instability, and may be accompanied by chronic low-grade knee pain from patellofemoral stress syndrome [18].

Soft Tissue Injuries

Muscle injuries may occur from a direct blow, sudden explosive action or occasionally from a more trivial action. Quadriceps contusions may cause local muscle bleeds associated with injury [11]. Chronic compartment syndrome may also occur, even in young athletes, typically in runners [69]. Tendinopathy of the lower extremity is common in young athletes. Achilles tendinopathy can be caused by excessive eccentric weight bearing, and tibialis anterior tendinopathy may result from direct pressure in skates or ski boots. Ankle sprains are more common in patients suffering from weak and deconditioned peroneal muscles and cavovarus deformity of the foot [17]. As ligaments in youth are considerably more elastic than in adults, these kind of injuries are well tolerated in lax individuals [17, 70].

Strategies for Injury Prevention

The principal concern for the young athlete is injury risk reduction. Risk factors for paediatric musculoskeletal injury in sport are well established [62, 71]. For example, after the adolescent growth spurt, the decrease in flexibility from the relative lengthening of bone may predispose to injury if stretching exercises before the sport activity are not performed. However, recent evidence has shown that in adults stretching before exercise does not reduce the incidence of injury [72, 73]. It is not clear whether this is also the case in children. Nutrition plays an important role in the success of young athletes, and is particularly important in young female athletes [74, 75]. Amenorrhoeic and anorexic youngsters are, because of their reduced bone mineral density, at higher risk of injury [76] and prevention of amenorrhoea, anorexia and the athletic female triad is a crucial part of any sport injury prevention strategy in young female athletes.

It should be kept in mind that players have to be matched for body size, athletic ability and biological maturity with appropriate body protection and supervision [77]. Different sports may cause different musculoskeletal injuries.

Author	Prevention strategies
Frisch et al. [78]	Active prevention programmes focusing specifically on the upper extremity are scarce Initiatives enhancing the awareness of trainers, athletes and therapists about risk factors and systematic prevention measures should be encouraged
Lippi et al. [79]	The current anti-doping policy should be replaced with a more efficient and practical strategy to identify and monitor abnormal and harmful deviations of the biochemistry and haematology
Shanmugam et al. [12]	Most injuries caused in children's sports are minor and self-limiting, suggesting that children and youth sports are safe The training programmes should take into account their physical and psychological immaturity, so that growing athletes can adjust to the changes in their bodies
Moreira et al. [80]	Moderate activity may enhance immune function, whereas prolonged, high-intensity exercise temporarily impairs the immune competence Athletes, when compared with lesser active individuals, experience higher rate of upper respiratory tract infections (URTI) after training and competitions. In non-athletes, increasing physical activity is associated with a decreased risk of URTI
Khanna et al. [81]	The only thing that appears clinically justified in adhesion prevention of flexor tendons of the hand is the need for early post-operative mobilization of digits after tendon injury or repair but the best method of mobilization remains controversial
Gougoulias et al. [82]	Participation in recreational sports is possible in most patients who were active in sports before lower limb osteotomy Intensive participation in sports after osteotomy may adversely affect outcome and lead to failures requiring re-operation Patients may be able to remain active in selected sports activities after a lower limb osteotomy for osteoarthritis More rapid progression of arthritis is, however, a possibility

Health professionals should know about these differences and about the physical and psychological immaturity of the young athlete, which is more influential than chronological age with regard to injury prevention. An overview of injury prevention strategies is provided in table 3 and a discussion of key considerations is provided below.

The duration, intensity, frequency and recovery of training programmes should be carefully evaluated and monitored for each child to avoid injuries of the musculoskeletal system. Incomplete recovery and therefore residual symptoms may create long-term injury problems for the young athlete. Few studies are available which document long-term sequelae of youth athletes. Also there is a lack of evidence about the health-related quality of life of young athletes in comparison with the general population.

Other measures to prevent injuries in young athletes include a proper selection of sporting events by coaches and parents; appropriate equipment and enforcement of rules. Use of safe playing conditions and adequate supervision are obviously important factors in sport injury prevention in the child as well as in the adult athlete.

Thorough documentation of different injuries is also essential for physicians to optimise their management of injuries in the young athlete. Age-appropriate designations for injury types specific to children and youth should be always carried out. Injury rates based on time-at-risk exposure data are also important for prevention, and future research should aim to provide reliable data. Analytical as well as descriptive components should be included in a well-designed prospective cohort study, so that possible risk factors and viable preventive measures might also be evaluated. The multivariate nature of sports injuries should also be taken into account, including as many relevant risk factors as possible [83].

It has been thought that periods of rapid growth are related to an increased risk of injury: consequently, training programmes may be designed to reduce the training loads during these periods to reduce the risk of injury. Studies which test the effectiveness of pre-participation musculoskeletal screening are also recommended. Active prevention measures should be included in therapy and training programmes to reduce the (re)injury rate and to enhance athletic performance.

Content, duration, and frequency of training, and also athlete compliance have been highlighted as important factors in sport injury prevention in the young in a recent systematic review [78]. Home-based programmes have been found to result in better compliance; however, athletic trainers and therapists should also be included in systematic prevention measures [78], and interact regularly with the physician and epidemiologist. Last, dialogue between young athletes and their parents should be considered an important factor in the prevention and management of sport injuries during youth.

Dropping Out of Sport Because of Injury

Where prevention fails and young athletes do become injured, a consequence of injury can be drop out. There are few well-controlled epidemiological studies of the rate of drop out in young athletes as a result of injury [11, 84–86]. In Australia, about 8% of the adolescents annually drop out because of injury [58]. Some young athletes drop out of sports completely, while others stop participation in one sport to continue participation in other sports [87–89]. 'No longer interested in the sport' (highest for both boys and girls), 'no longer fun', 'the coach played favourites/was a poor teacher', and 'wanting to participate in other activities' are the main reasons reported for sport drop out in youngsters [90].

The most common injuries which can cause sport drop out are chronic rotator cuff injury, navicular stress fracture, loose bodies in the ankle joint, medial and lateral meniscus lesions, anterior cruciate ligament rupture, and osteochondritis dissecans of the elbow joint [87, 88].

Conclusions

Although sport carries the inevitable risk of injuries in children, these negative effects are balanced by the many social, psychological and health benefits that a serious commitment to sport brings [91–93]. To maximise the benefit and minimise the risk of injury, it is important that systems are in place which allow identification of young athletes who are at high injury risk, facilitate coach and trainer education to optimise training programmes and reduce injury risk, as well as educate parents and young athletes in injury prevention [94–98]. Developing more extensive and thorough documentation of sports injuries in elite young athletes will also improve injury management and knowledge of the longer-term outcomes of injuries.

References

1 Maffulli N, Baxter-Jones AD, Grieve A: Long term sport involvement and sport injury rate in elite young athletes. Arch Dis Child 2005;90:525–527.

2 Smith AD, Tao SS: Knee injuries in young athletes. Clin Sports Med 1995;14:629–650.

3 Klenerman L: ABC of sports medicine: musculoskeletal injuries in child athletes. BMJ 1994;308:1556–1559.

4 d'Hemecourt P: Overuse injuries in the young athlete. Acta Paediatr 2009;98:1727–1728.

5 Baxter-Jones AD, Helms P, Maffulli N, Baines-Preece JC, Preece M: Growth and development of male gymnasts, swimmers, soccer and tennis players: a longitudinal study. Ann Hum Biol 1995;22:381–394.

6 Caine D, Cochrane B, Caine C, Zemper E: An epidemiologic investigation of injuries affecting young competitive female gymnasts. Am J Sports Med 1989;17:811–820.

7 Caine DJ, Maffulli N: Epidemiology of children's individual sports injuries: an important area of medicine and sport science research. Med Sci Sports Exerc 2005;48:1–7.

8 Caine DJ, Nassar L: Gymnastics injuries. Med Sport Sci 2005;48:18–58.

9 Maffulli N, Helms P: Controversies about intensive training in young athletes. Arch Dis Child 1988;63:1405–1407.

10 Erlandson MC, Sherar LB, Mirwald RL, Maffulli N, Baxter-Jones AD: Growth and maturation of adolescent female gymnasts, swimmers, and tennis players. Med Sci Sports Exerc 2008;40:34–42.

11 Maffulli N: The growing child in sport. Br Med Bull 1992;48:561–568.

12 Shanmugam C, Maffulli N: Sports injuries in children. Br Med Bull 2008;86:33–57.

13 Soligard T, Myklebust G, Steffen K, Holme I, Silvers H, Bizzini M, Junge A, Dvorak J, Bahr R, Andersen TE: Comprehensive warm-up programme to prevent injuries in young female footballers: cluster randomised controlled trial. BMJ 2008;337:a2469.

14 Maffulli N, Longo UG, Gougoulias N, Loppini M, Denaro V: Long-term health outcomes of youth sports injuries. Br J Sports Med 2010;44:21–25.

15 Bright RW, Burstein AH, Elmore SM: Epiphyseal-plate cartilage: a biomechanical and histological analysis of failure modes. J Bone Joint Surg Am 1974;56:688–703.

16 Flachsmann R, Broom ND, Hardy AE, Moltschaniwskyj G: Why is the adolescent joint particularly susceptible to osteochondral shear fracture? Clin Orthop Relat Res 2000;381:212–221.

17 Stanish WD: Lower leg, foot, and ankle injuries in young athletes. Clin Sports Med 1995;14:651–668.

18 Maffulli N, Baxter-Jones AD: Common skeletal injuries in young athletes. Sports Med 1995;19:137–149.

19 Booth FW, Gould EW: Effects of training and disuse on connective tissue. Exerc Sport Sci Rev 1975;3:83–112.

20 Castiglia PT: Sports injuries in children. J Pediatr Health Care 1995;9:32–33.

21 Dalen N, Edsmyr F: Bone mineral content of the femoral neck after irradiation. Acta Radiol Ther Phys Biol 1974;13:97–101.

22 Caine D, DiFiori J, Maffulli N: Physeal injuries in children's and youth sports: reasons for concern? Br J Sports Med 2006;40:749–760.

23 Falk B, Dotan R: Temperature regulation and elite young athletes; in Armstrong N, McManus AM (eds): The Elite Young Athlete. Med Sports Sci. Basel, Karger, 2011, vol 56, pp 126–149.

24 Maffulli N: Epiphyseal injuries of the proximal phalanx of the hallux. Clin J Sport Med 2001;11:121–123.

25 Salter RB, Harris WR: Injuries involving the epiphyseal plate. J Bone Joint Surg 1963;45:587–622.

26 Goldberg VM, Aadalen R: Distal tibial epiphyseal injuries: the role of athletics in 53 cases. Am J Sports Med 1978;6:263–268.

27 Ogden JA: Skeletal Injury in the Child. Philadelphia, Lea & Febiger, 1982.

28 Gregg JR, Das M: Foot and ankle problems in the preadolescent and adolescent athlete. Clin Sports Med 1982;1:131–147.

29 Berson L, Davidson RS, Dormans JP, Drummond DS, Gregg JR: Growth disturbances after distal tibial physeal fractures. Foot Ankle Int 2000;21:54–58.

30 Eid AM, Hafez MA: Traumatic injuries of the distal femoral physis: retrospective study on 151 cases. Injury 2002;33:251–255.

31 Arkader A, Warner WC Jr, Horn BD, Shaw RN, Wells L: Predicting the outcome of physeal fractures of the distal femur. J Pediatr Orthop 2007;27:703–708.

32 Barmada A, Gaynor T, Mubarak SJ: Premature physeal closure following distal tibia physeal fractures: a new radiographic predictor. J Pediatr Orthop 2003;23:733–739.

33 Burkhart SS, Peterson HA: Fractures of the proximal tibial epiphysis. J Bone Joint Surg Am 1979;61:996–1002.

34 Cass JR, Peterson HA: Salter-Harris Type-IV injuries of the distal tibial epiphyseal growth plate, with emphasis on those involving the medial malleolus. J Bone Joint Surg Am 1983;65:1059–1070.

35 Criswell AR, Hand WL, Butler JE: Abduction injuries of the distal femoral epiphysis. Clin Orthop Relat Res 1976;115:189–194.

36 Goldberg VM, Aadalen R: Distal tibial epiphyseal injuries: the role of athletics in 53 cases. Am J Sports Med 1978;6:263–268.

37 Kawamoto K, Kim WC, Tsuchida Y, Tsuji Y, Fujioka M, Horii M, Mikami Y, Tokunaga D, Kubo T: Incidence of physeal injuries in Japanese children. J Pediatr Orthop B 2006;15:126–130.

38 Lalonde KA, Letts M: Traumatic growth arrest of the distal tibia: a clinical and radiographic review. Can J Surg 2005;48:143–147.

39 Nietosvaara Y, Hasler C, Helenius I, Cundy P: Marked initial displacement predicts complications in physeal fractures of the distal radius: an analysis of fracture characteristics, primary treatment and complications in 109 patients. Acta Orthop 2005;76:873–877.

40 Landin LA, Danielsson LG, Jonsson K, Pettersson H: Late results in 65 physeal ankle fractures. Acta Orthop Scand 1986;57:530–534.

41 Lombardo SJ, Harvey JP: Fractures of the distal femoral epiphyses – factors influencing prognosis: a review of thirty-four cases. J Bone Joint Surg Am 1977;59:742–751.

42 Hynes D, O'Brien T: Growth disturbance lines after injury of the distal tibial physis: their significance in prognosis. J Bone Joint Surg Br 1988;70:231–233.

43 Nenopoulos SP, Papavasiliou VA, Papavasiliou AV: Outcome of physeal and epiphyseal injuries of the distal tibia with intra-articular involvement. J Pediatr Orthop 2005;25:518–522.

44 Ilharreborde B, Raquillet C, Morel E, Fitoussi F, Bensahel H, Pennecot GF, Mazda K: Long-term prognosis of Salter-Harris type 2 injuries of the distal femoral physis. J Pediatr Orthop B 2006;15: 433–438.

45 Stephens DC, Louis E, Louis DS: Traumatic separation of the distal femoral epiphyseal cartilage plate. J Bone Joint Surg Am 1974;56:1383–1390.

46 Cannata G, De Maio F, Mancini F, Ippolito E: Physeal fractures of the distal radius and ulna: long-term prognosis. J Orthop Trauma 2003;17:172–179; discussion 179–180.

47 Krueger-Franke M, Siebert CH, Pfoerringer W: Sports-related epiphyseal injuries of the lower extremity: an epidemiologic study. J Sports Med Phys Fitness 1992;32:106–111.

48 Caine D, DiFiori J, Mattulli N: Physeal injuries in children's and youth sports: reasons for concern? Br J Sports Med 2006;40:749–760.

49 Zilkens KW, Defrain W: Apophyseal avulsion fractures in adolescents–a typical sports injury. Aktuelle Traumatol 1985;15:260–263.

50 Hebert KJ, Laor T, Divine JG, Emery KH, Wall EJ: MRI appearance of chronic stress injury of the iliac crest apophysis in adolescent athletes. AJR Am J Roentgenol 2008;190:1487–1491.

51 Ogden JA: Skeletal Injury in the Child. New York, Springer, 2000.

52 Ouellette H, Thomas BJ, Nelson E, Torriani M: MR imaging of rectus femoris origin injuries. Skeletal Radiol 2006; 35:665–672.

53 Moeller JL: Pelvic and hip apophyseal avulsion injuries in young athletes. Curr Sports Med Rep 2003;2:110–115.

54 Sanders TG, Zlatkin MB: Avulsion injuries of the pelvis. Semin Musculoskelet Radiol 2008;12:42–53.

55 Annear PT, Chakera TM, Foster DH, Hardcastle PH: Pars interarticularis stress and disc degeneration in cricket's potent strike force: the fast bowler. Aust NZ J Surg 1992;62:768–773.

56 Burnett AF, Khangure MS, Elliott BC, Foster DH, Marshall RN, Hardcastle PH: Thoracolumbar disc degeneration in young fast bowlers in cricket: a follow-up study. Clin Biomech 1996;11:305–310.

57 Dixon M, Fricker P: Injuries to elite gymnasts over 10 yr. Med Sci Sports Exerc 1993;25:1322–1329.

58 Ferguson RJ, McMaster JH, Stanitski CL: Low back pain in college football linemen. The Journal of sports medicine 1974;2:63–69.

59 Foster D, John D, Elliott B, Ackland T, Fitch K: Back injuries to fast bowlers in cricket: a prospective study. Br J Sports Med 1989;23:150–154.

60 Hardcastle P, Annear P, Foster DH, Chakera TM, McCormick C, Khangure M, Burnett A: Spinal abnormalities in young fast bowlers. J Bone Joint Surg Br 1992;74:421–425.

61 Jackson DW, Wiltse LL, Cirincoine RJ: Spondylolysis in the female gymnast. Clin Orthop Relat Res 1976;117:68–73.

62 Micheli LJ, Glassman R, Klein M: The prevention of sports injuries in children. Clin Sports Med 2000;19:821–834, ix.

63 Morita T, Ikata T, Katoh S, Miyake R· Lumbar spondylolysis in children and adolescents. J Bone Joint Surg Br 1995; 77:620–625.

64 Rossi F, Dragoni S: Lumbar spondylolysis: occurrence in competitive athletes. Updated achievements in a series of 390 cases. J Sports Med Phys Fitness 1990;30:450–452.

65 McCarroll JR, Miller JM, Ritter MA: Lumbar spondylolysis and spondylolisthesis in college football players: a prospective study. Am J Sports Med 1986; 14:404–406.

66 Semon RL, Spengler D: Significance of lumbar spondylolysis in college football players. Spine 1981;6:172–174.

67 Moretz JA 3rd, Harlan SD, Goodrich J, Walters R: Long-term follow up of knee injuries in high school football players. Am J Sports Med 1984;12:298–300.

68 Hovelius L: Anterior dislocation of the shoulder in teen-agers and young adults. Five-year prognosis. J Bone Joint Surg Am 1987;69:393–399.

69 Bernhardt DT, Landry GL: Sports injuries in young athletes. Adv Pediatr 1995;42:465–500.

70 Stanitski CL: Common injuries in preadolescent and adolescent athletes: recommendations for prevention. Sports Med 1989;7:32–41.

71 Purvis JM, Burke RG: Recreational injuries in children: incidence and prevention. J Am Acad Orthop Surg 2001;9:365–374.

72 Pope RP, Herbert RD, Kirwan JD, Graham BMJ: A randomized trial of pre-exercise stretching for prevention of lower-limb injury. Med Sci Sports Exerc 2000;32:271–277.

73 Shrier I: Stretching before exercise: an evidence based approach. Br J Sports Med 2000;34:324–325.

74 McManus AM, Armstrong N: Physiology of elite young female athletes; in Armstrong N, McManus AM (eds): The Elite Young Athlete. Med Sport Sci. Basel, Karger, 2011, pp 23–46.

75 Jeukendrup A, Cronin L: Nutrition and elite young athletes; in Armstrong N, McManus AM (eds): The Elite Young Athlete. Med Sport Sci. Basel, Karger, 2011, pp 47–58.

76 Jones BH, Bovee MW, Harris JM 3rd, Cowan DN: Intrinsic risk factors for exercise-related injuries among male and female army trainees. Am J Sports Med 1993;21:705–710.

77 Baxter-Jones AD: Growth and development of young athletes. should competition levels be age related? Sports Med 1995;20:59–64.

78 Frisch A, Croisier JL, Urhausen A, Seil R, Theisen D: Injuries, risk factors and prevention initiatives in youth sport. Br Med Bull 2009;92:95–121.

79 Lippi G, Franchini M, Guidi GC: Doping in competition or doping in sport? Br Med Bull 2008;86:95–107.

80 Moreira A, Delgado L, Moreira P, Haahtela T: Does exercise increase the risk of upper respiratory tract infections? Br Med Bull 2009;90:111–131.

81 Khanna A, Friel M, Gougoulias N, Longo UG, Maffulli N: Prevention of adhesions in surgery of the flexor tendons of the hand: what is the evidence? Br Med Bull 2009;90:85–109.

82 Gougoulias N, Khanna A, Maffulli N: Sports activities after lower limb osteotomy. Br Med Bull 2009;91:111–121.

83 Bahr R, Holme I: Risk factors for sports injuries: a methodological approach. Br J Sports Med 2003;37:384–392.

84 Gould D, Petlichkoff L: Participation motivation and attrition in young athletes; in Smoll FL, Magill RA, Ash MJ (eds): Children In Sport. Champaign, Human Kinetics,1988, pp 161–178.

85 Jackson DW, Silvino N, Reiman P: Osteochondritis in the female gymnast's elbow. Arthroscopy 1989;5:129–136.

86 Singer KM, Roy SP: Osteochondrosis of the humeral capitellum. Am J Sports Med 1984;12:351–360.

87 Caine D, Knutzen K, Howe W: A three-year epidemiological study of injuries affecting young female gymnasts. Phys Therap Sport 2003;4:10–23.

88 Kolt GS, Kirkby RJ: Epidemiology of injury in elite and subelite female gymnasts: a comparison of retrospective and prospective findings. Br J Sports Med 1999;33:312–318.

89 Lindholm C, Hagenfeldt K, Ringertz BM: Pubertal development in elite juvenile gymnasts: effects of physical training. Acta Obstet Gynecol Scand 1994;73:269–273.

90 Grimmer KA, Jones D, Williams J: Prevalence of adolescent injury from recreational exercise: an Australian perspective. J Adolesc Health 2000;27:266–272.

91 Brady TA, Cahill BR, Bodnar LM: Weight training-related injuries in the high school athlete. Am J Sports Med 1982;10:1–5.

92 Ostrum GA: Sports-related injuries in youth: prevention is the key-and nurses can help! Pediatr Nurs 1993;19:333–342.

93 Sewall L, Micheli LJ: Strength training for children. J Pediatr Orthop 1986;6:143–146.

94 Maffulli N, Longo UG, Gougoulias N, Caine D, Denaro V: Sport injuries: a review of outcomes. Br Med Bull 2010 Aug 14. [Epub ahead of print] PubMed PMID: 20710023.

95 Maffulli N, Longo UG, Spiezia F, Denaro V: Sports injuries in young athletes: long-term outcome and prevention strategies. Phys Sportsmed 2010 Jun;38:29–34. PubMed PMID: 20631461.

96 Longo UG, Franceschetti E, Maffulli N, Denaro V: Hip arthroscopy: state of the art. Br Med Bull 2010 Jul 6. [Epub ahead of print] PubMed PMID: 20605889.

97 Longo UG, Loppini M, Denaro L, Maffulli N, Denaro V: Rating scales for low back pain. Br Med Bull 2010;94:81–144. Epub 2010 Jan 10. PubMed PMID: 20064820.

98 Longo UG, Lamberti A, Maffulli N, Denaro V: Tendon augmentation grafts: a systematic review. Br Med Bull 2010;94:165–188. Epub 2010 Jan 4. PubMed PMID: 20047971.

Prof. Nicola Maffulli
Centre for Sports and Exercise Medicine
Barts and The London School of Medicine and Dentistry
Mile End Hospital, 275 Bancroft Road, London, E1 4DG (UK)
Tel. +44 20 8223 8839, Fax +44 20 8223 8930, E-Mail n.maffulli@qmul.ac.uk

Author Index

Subject Index